Current and Future Developments in Surgery

(*Volume 2*)

(*Oesophago-gastric Surgery*)

Edited by

Sami M. Shimi

Consultant Oesophago-gastric Surgeon, Department of Surgery
Ninewells Hospital and Medical School, University of Dundee
Dundee, Scotland, UK

General:

1. Any dispute or claim arising out of or in connection with this License Agreement or the Work (including non-contractual disputes or claims) will be governed by and construed in accordance with the laws of the U.A.E. as applied in the Emirate of Dubai. Each party agrees that the courts of the Emirate of Dubai shall have exclusive jurisdiction to settle any dispute or claim arising out of or in connection with this License Agreement or the Work (including non-contractual disputes or claims).
2. Your rights under this License Agreement will automatically terminate without notice and without the need for a court order if at any point you breach any terms of this License Agreement. In no event will any delay or failure by Bentham Science Publishers in enforcing your compliance with this License Agreement constitute a waiver of any of its rights.
3. You acknowledge that you have read this License Agreement, and agree to be bound by its terms and conditions. To the extent that any other terms and conditions presented on any website of Bentham Science Publishers conflict with, or are inconsistent with, the terms and conditions set out in this License Agreement, you acknowledge that the terms and conditions set out in this License Agreement shall prevail.

Bentham Science Publishers Ltd.
Executive Suite Y - 2
PO Box 7917, Saif Zone
Sharjah, U.A.E.
Email: subscriptions@benthamscience.org

**BENTHAM
SCIENCE**

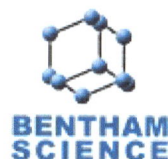

CONTENTS

Foreword

In this increasing age of sub-specialisation in medicine in general and surgery in particular, learning organ specific details for diagnosis and treatment is a challenge to every clinician. This e-book 'Oesophago-gastric Surgery' will therefore come as a welcome addition to the specialist literature on the subject. It has been put together, written and edited by a multi-disciplinary specialist team from Ninewells Hospital in Dundee, Scotland, who have covered the full range of oesophago-gastric conditions and their treatment. The book is meant primarily for surgical trainees, both with a general and specialist upper GI interest, as well as consultants who wish to gain up-to-date knowledge of this area. It goes into great detail in all the areas of benign, pre-malignant and malignant disease. The book is well referenced and provides very clear figures and diagrams to help the reader understand many of the complexities of treatment. While the incidence of squamous cell carcinoma of the oesophagus is falling, and of adenocarcinoma is rising, the management of the pre-malignant condition of Barrett's oesophagus has therefore, become increasingly important. The role of surgery in the management of gastro-oesophageal reflux and other benign conditions has increased significantly over the last 20 years with advances in minimally invasive surgery. This has brought the medical and surgical endoscopists into a much closer relationship than in the past, with recognition that treatment can now be tailored to the underlying condition and the patients' needs. The background pathophysiology on which both diagnosis and management are based on particularly useful and is a credit to the editorial team and the authors involved. Overall, this is a well-written, detailed and up to date e-book, which covers all the relevant areas of oesophago-gastric surgery and will be a very welcome addition to the eBook series.

Simon Paterson-Brown
Consultant General and Upper Gastro-intestinal Surgeon
Royal Infirmary of Edinburgh
Scotland
UK

Preface

The natural evolution of surgical knowledge and technology meant that the traditional general surgeon concept is no longer sustainable. This has necessitated the need for sub-specialization. Along the route, the influence of volume on outcomes was established. The end result seen today is an endorsement of subspecialisation by all the Surgical Colleges, professional societies and health care systems. "Super specialization", is a separate discussion for the coming decade. The traditional textbooks on general surgery can no longer provide the core knowledge for specialist training.

This book addresses the core knowledge needs of higher surgical trainees in oesophago-gastric surgery and provides a reference manual for established consultants in oesophago-gastric surgery and other specialties. It provides a practical and user-friendly reference to all relevant topics. A comprehensive but concise approach was adopted to detail the main relevant topics. Detailed discussion of rarer topics was left for the commonly practiced Internet searches. The chapters in this book are practice based. They were written by experienced clinicians who have gone through the sub-specialisation process with full awareness of the specialist educational curriculum specified by the surgical colleges and professional societies. With this book being one of the "e-book" series, it means that busy practitioners can have instant access to this book on the Internet to refresh knowledge and gain additional insight.

I am grateful to all the contributors who have shared their knowledge enthusiastically. To our readers, we hope that you enjoy reading this book, enjoy the knowledge riches in its pages and for those who are preparing for professional examinations, we wish you success.

Sami M. Shimi
Consultant Oesophago-gastric Surgeon
Department of Surgery
Ninewells Hospital and Medical School
University of Dundee
Dundee, Scotland
UK

DEDICATION

This book is dedicated to my family who encouraged and supported me throughout the various stages of editing this book and authoring some of the chapters.

I also dedicate this book to my surgical colleagues and trainees who enlightened me with their wisdom, surgical craft and educational needs.

Finally, I dedicate this book to all my patients who entrusted me and filled my life with the joy which I derived from treating them.

"A surgeon without knowledge, creativity and skill is like a house without a roof, water or electricity."

List of Contributors

Asa Dahle-Smith   Department of Oncology, Ninewells Hospital and Medical School, Dundee, Scotland, UK

Elizabeth Vaughan   Department of Surgery, Ninewells Hospital and Medical School, Dundee, Scotland, UK

Hugh Dalziel   Department of Gastroenterology and Surgery, Ninewells Hospital and Medical School, Dundee, Scotland, UK

Jamie Young   Department of Surgery, Borders General Hospital, Melrose, Roxburghshire, Scotland, UK

Maria Coats   Department of Surgery, Ninewells Hospital and Medical School, Dundee, Scotland, UK

Prdeep Patil   Department of Surgery, Ninewells Hospital and Medical School, Dundee, Scotland, UK

Petty Russell   Department of Oncology, Ninewells Hospital and Medical School, Dundee, Scotland, UK

Sami M. Shimi   Department of Surgery, Ninewells Hospital and Medical School, Dundee, Scotland, UK

Shaun McLeod   Department of Anaesthesia, Ninewells Hospital and Medical School, Dundee, Scotland, UK

CHAPTER 1

Benign Disorders of the Stomach

Elizabeth Vaughan and **Sami M. Shimi**[*]

Department of Surgery, Ninewells Hospital and Medical School, Dundee, Scotland, UK

Abstract: Dyspepsia describes a constellation of symptoms centred in the upper abdomen. In functional dyspepsia, no discernible organic pathology is found. Diagnosis and management of these patients are challenging but centred on individual symptom management. In organic dyspepsia, patients are found to have a number of disorders to account for their symptoms. These include gastritis and peptic ulceration. Gastritis refers to a group of diseases characterized by inflammation of the gastric mucosa. It can be acute or chronic in nature and may involve part or all the stomach. *H. pylori* infection gives rise to Type B atrophic gastritis where the inflammatory changes are accompanied by atrophy and intestinal metaplasia. There is an increased risk of intestinal type gastric cancer. Other types of gastritis are less common. Peptic ulcer disease and its complications remain a significant cause of morbidity and mortality. It is most commonly caused by *H. pylori* infection or the use of non-steroidal anti-inflammatory drugs. Management involves the use of PPIs together with eradication therapy of *H. pylori*. The management of perforation and gastric outlet obstruction is mainly surgical. The management of upper gastro-intestinal bleeding consists of resuscitation and haemostasis mainly by endoscopic therapy. In-hospital mortality from bleeding peptic ulcers remains high. Acute gastric dilatation and gastric volvulus are surgical emergencies. The management must commence early by resuscitation followed by prompt surgical management. Mortality remains high in vulnerable and compromised patients.

Keywords: Dyspepsia, Endoscopic therapy, Functional dyspepsia, Gastric dilatation, Gastric outlet obstruction, Gastric volvulus, Gastritis, Gastropexy, Gastro-enterostomy, *H. pylori*, Peptic Ulcers, Pyloroplasty, Upper GI bleeding.

DYSPEPSIA

Dyspepsia describes acute, chronic or recurrent symptoms of pain or discomfort centred in the upper abdomen. The term includes both organic and functional dyspepsia with the latter being the most common cause of these symptoms. The currently accepted standard for the diagnosis of functional dyspepsia is the Rome III criteria, developed by a multi-national group of experts in the field [1]. In

[*] **Corresponding author Sami M. Shimi:** Department of Surgery, Ninewells Hospital and Medical School, Dundee DD1 9SY, Scotland, UK; Tel: +44 1382 383550; E-mail: s.m.shimi@dundee.ac.uk

organic dyspepsia, a discernible organic cause for the symptoms is found and treatment of the cause is rewarded by amelioration of the symptoms. The causes of organic dyspepsia include benign and malignant conditions of the gastro-duodenal segments and appendages (Gallbladder, bile ducts, liver and pancreas) of the gastro-intestinal tract. Functional dyspepsia as described by the Rome III criteria, describes pain, discomfort or burning in the epigastrium, early satiety (inability to ingest a normal sized meal), satiety with fullness during or after a meal, or a combination of these symptoms. There is chronicity to the symptoms, which occur at least weekly, and over a period of at least 6 months, in the absence of an organic explanation. Bloating and nausea often coexist with dyspepsia but are nonspecific and are thus not included in its definition. Heartburn is also excluded from the described symptom criteria for dyspepsia since it is thought to arise primarily from the oesophagus and suggests gastro-oesophageal reflux disease (GORD) although it may occur concomitantly. A number of symptoms overlap between functional dyspepsia and gastroparesis. In excess of 25% of patients with functional dyspepsia have evidence of delayed gastric emptying. Conversely, a significant number of patients with gastroparesis meet the criteria for functional dyspepsia. Peptic ulcers and gastritis are each found in around 10% of patients undergoing assessment for dyspepsia. Medications such as aspirin or NSAIDs are another frequent and often overlooked cause of dyspepsia.

Recently, the terminology used to describe functional dyspepsia has also changed. Patients are no longer grouped according to the predominant reported symptom such as ulcer-like, reflux-like, or dysmotility-like functional dyspepsia. Instead, they are described as having one of two syndromes, the epigastric pain syndrome and the postprandial distress syndrome [2]. The epigastric pain syndrome consists of intermittent pain or burning in the epigastrium, occurring at a frequency of once per week at least. The postprandial distress syndrome is marked by bothersome postprandial fullness occurring after normal-sized meals or by early satiety that prevents the person from finishing a regular meal. This occurs at least several times per week.

Functional dyspepsia has been historically attributed to a disturbance of gastric physiology, such as slow gastric emptying, failure of the gastric fundal relaxation in the postprandial period, or gastric hypersensitivity to gastric distension. Duodenal hypersensitivity to acid or distension has also been reported in patients with functional dyspepsia. Gastroenteritis or Infections due to *H. pylori* may also lead to functional dyspepsia. Inflammation of the stomach and/ or duodenum due to any cause can also lead to functional dyspepsia. Functional dyspepsia is a syndrome, which is meal-induced. Food content, which alters the gut-hormone responses or causes allergic intolerance, may play an important role. Functional dyspepsia is associated with psychological stress, especially anxiety, and this may precede the onset of the disorder in some individuals. This suggests a gut driven brain disorder or central pain processing disorder. Some patients with functional dyspepsia may have an organic mechanism for their symptoms. Some of these organic mechanisms are apparent on simple tests but the majority are not.

Diagnosis

No particular symptoms can reliably distinguish between organic and functional dyspepsia. The clinical challenge in assessing patients with dyspepsia remains in discriminating between functional dyspepsia and organic conditions of the stomach or duodenum that may provoke similar symptoms. For patients with alarm symptoms or patients with new onset dyspepsia and over a threshold age of 55 years, prompt endoscopy is recommended. This age limit however is variable between different health-care systems in different countries. Alarm symptoms warranting upper GI endoscopy, in patients with new onset dyspepsia include dysphagia, odynophagia, persistent vomiting, unintentional weight loss of $\geq$ 3kg, GI bleeding, anaemia or the discovery of an epigastric mass.

Upper GI endoscopy performed during a symptomatic period while the patient is off acid-suppressant therapy is important to making a diagnosis of functional dyspepsia. The findings may exclude other potential causes of symptoms. At the time of endoscopy, biopsies of the stomach (and small bowel if celiac disease is suspected) can be obtained to detect *H. pylori* infection and, peptic ulcer disease (PUD) or gastritis. *H. pylori* eradication is indicated in all positive cases. If endoscopy confirms PUD then antibiotic treatment with triple (or quadruple) therapy for one or two weeks is recommended.

In addition, a number of other investigations may be considered in the assessment of patients with dyspeptic symptoms. These include ultrasound of the liver and biliary system; cross-sectional imaging of the abdomen, including the pancreas, using either CT or MRI; small bowel radiography; enteric angiography; and hydrogen breath testing. The presenting symptoms, clinical features, severity, and refractoriness of the symptoms should dictate the choice of test(s).

Management

In the general population, the prevalence of dyspepsia can be as high as 40%, however an organic cause can be found in a minority of patients who seek medical attention. The management represents a considerable financial burden to any health care system. Some of the causes of dyspepsia are amenable to medical treatment including peptic ulcer disease (PUD) and functional dyspepsia. Patients who test positive to *Helicobacter pylori* would benefit from eradication of the infection and prevention the onset of PUD. Patients presenting with new onset dyspepsia, age greater than 55 years, or alarm features require upper gastrointestinal (GI) endoscopy to exclude malignancy in the oesophagus or stomach. In younger individuals without alarm features, upper GI endoscopy for is not cost-effective compared with the *H. pylori* "test and treat" approach [3]. Test and treat and empirical acid-suppression using a proton pump inhibitor (PPI) have similar costs and effects. Screen testing and treatment of *H. pylori* in PPI users and the community may reduce the costs of managing dyspepsia at the population level. Upper GI endoscopy is indicated in young individuals who have failed a 4-8 week trial of PPI therapy (in an area of low prevalence of *H. pylori*) or failed to respond to eradication of *H. pylori* (in an *H. pylori* endemic region) [4].

Patients found to have organic disease are best managed according to algorithms for the specific disorder. Patients labelled, as having functional dyspepsia can be more difficult to manage. Up to 30% of these patients will respond to advice on meal content, reassurance and simple over the counter medication given for a short period and directed at specific symptoms. Others with persistent symptoms may benefit from an *H. pylori* 'test and eradicate' policy. A trial of acid suppression therapy (if it has not been tried previously) is worthwhile in all patients with functional dyspepsia particularly in those who have tested negative for *H. pylori* or in those with positive *H. pylori* testing results in whom eradication therapy has not alleviated their symptoms. Antacids, sucralfate, and bismuth are not efficacious in functional dyspepsia. All patients, who do not respond to empiric PPI therapy, have normal upper GI endoscopy, and who either are negative for *H. pylori* or have cleared infection following treatment yet continue to have dyspeptic symptoms are in a group which continues to challenge primary and secondary care. Prokinetic agents may be considered and can be useful in a small group of patients particularly the post-prandial distress syndrome sub-group. A misdiagnosis should be considered at different stages along the management pathway. In the absence of a different diagnosis, reassurance, distraction techniques and education of the patient with functional dyspepsia are important in the management. In particular, patients should be reassured that there is no on-going malignant process and that functional dyspepsia does not limit survival. Second-line pharmacotherapy should be considered for some patients; however, the benefits may be limited. Antidepressants and psychological treatments may be tried in this challenging group of patients.

In the majority of patients with functional dyspepsia, the natural history is chronic and fluctuating, with periods of time when the patient is may be asymptomatic. These may be followed by episodes of symptom relapse. Population studies suggest that up to 50% of patients will have resolution of their symptoms and 15 to 20% of patients will have persistent symptoms. The remaining patients will have fluctuating symptoms and develop another functional gastro-intestinal disorder.

GASTRITIS

Gastritis refers to a group of diseases characterized by inflammation of the gastric mucosa. It can be acute or chronic in nature. The inflammation may involve the entire stomach (pangastritis) or a region of the stomach (*e.g.* antral gastritis). Since the majority of individuals with gastritis are undiagnosed, data for the incidence and prevalence of gastritis are limited to groups of presenting clinical syndromes.

Chronic Gastritis

This can be infectious or non-infectious. *Helicobacter* pylori infection is the commonest cause of chronic gastritis. Other forms of infectious gastritis include: *Helicobacter heilmannii*–associated gastritis; granulomatous gastritis associated with gastric infections in mycobacteriosis, syphilis, histoplasmosis, mucormycosis, South American blastomycosis, anisakiasis or anisakidosis; chronic gastritis associated with parasitic infections; and viral infections, such as cytomegalovirus and herpes virus infection. Data on the incidence and prevalence of these is limited to certain communities.

Non-infectious gastritis is associated with autoimmune gastritis, reactive or chemical gastropathy (usually related to chronic entero-gastric reflux or NSAIDs intake), uraemic gastropathy, lymphocytic gastritis (including gastritis associated with celiac disease), eosinophilic gastritis, non-infectious granulomatous gastritis, radiation injury to the stomach (mainly therapeutic irradiation), ischaemic gastritis, gastritis secondary to chemotherapy and graft-versus-host disease. In many patients, gastritis has no known cause and when discovered present as chronic, inactive gastritis with various degrees of severity and sequel.

Acute Gastritis

Many patients with chronic gastritis of different origins may present with acute gastritis, with progression to chronic gastritis because of persisting injury. This is usually the case of gastritis associated with entero-gastric reflux, long-term intake NSAIDs, aspirin, excessive alcohol consumption, heavy smoking, uraemia, the use of systemic anticancer chemotherapy, therapeutic radiation, severe stress (trauma, burns, surgery), shock, mechanical trauma, such as gastric intubation associated mucosal damage, ingested acids and alkali in self harm, ischemia, systemic bacterial and viral infections.

Histological Classification

The Sydney system was introduced in 1990 as a basis for the classification of gastritis. The system was updated in 1996 in Houston and the classification is now referred to as the Sydney-Houston classification [5]. The system recommends sampling of the mucosa for evaluation of gastritis by using at least 5 biopsies, including 2 biopsies from the antrum, 2 from the corpus or body, and 1 from the incisura angularis. The system is based on the histological appearance of the gastric mucosa in different parts of the stomach. The system is based on five histological parameters:

1. Chronicity of inflammation is based on mononuclear infiltrates. Lymphocytic and plasmacytic inflammatory reaction indicates chronic gastritis.
2. Activity of inflammation is based on polymorphonuclear infiltrates.
3. The presence of glandular atrophy is based on loss of normal glands.
4. The presence of intestinal metaplasia
5. The presence and extent of colonization of biopsies by *H. pylori* in non-metaplastic epithelium.

As a result, the gastric mucosa can be categorized as *normal*, chronic, active (or both) gastritis, *non-atrophic H. pylori gastritis* and *atrophic gastritis* (*H. pylori* positive or negative). The presence of intestinal metaplasia and it gradation should also be described. Special forms of gastritis have also been described with specific histological features. In addition, the histological parameters are graded as mild, moderate or severe [6]. Patients with a histologically 'normal' stomach only develop ulcers due to ingestion of drugs such as NSAIDs and rarely due to Crohn's disease or Zollinger Ellison syndrome.

Non-atrophic H. pylori Gastritis

In this variety, the gastric antrum and duodenal bulb are mainly affected and 30% of patients develop ulcers. The acid output is not impaired and may be increased as a result of inflammation. There is however an increased risk of diffuse type gastric cancer.

Atrophic Gastritis

This can occur in the absence of *H. pylori* (type A) or be caused by *H. pylori* infection (type B). In both types, the risk of peptic ulceration is low. Gastric secretory function is impaired.

Type A Atrophic Gastritis

This affects mainly the body of the stomach and is autoimmune in aetiology (anti-parietal cells antibodies present). It develops in patients with pernicious anaemia and is associated with achlorhydria, absence of intrinsic factor secretion and vitamin B_{12} malabsorption. Since the antrum is spared, serum gastrin levels are grossly elevated. The chronic hypergastrinaemia, may lead to the development of neuroendocrine tumours. There is also an increased risk of diffuse gastric cancer.

Type B Atrophic Gastritis

This is the result of infection with *H. pylori* and can improve following eradication of *H. pylori*. It is more common than type A variety. The inflammatory changes tend to commence in the pyloric region and spread proximally to the antrum and body of the stomach. The inflammatory changes are accompanied by atrophy and intestinal metaplasia, which are marked in the body of the stomach. There is an increased risk of intestinal type gastric cancer.

H. pylori Associated Chronic Gastritis

Helicobacter pylori infection is usually acquired during childhood. There is an incubation period of 7-10 days preceding mild symptoms, which comprise epigastric pain, flatulence and halitosis, anorexia and occasionally mucous vomiting. The acute phase is often sub-clinical. Achlorhydria is present during the acute phase. The symptoms, if present persist for an average of one week before resolving. But although the symptoms resolve, the infection persists in the majority of cases.

The acute infection often develops into chronic gastritis if the responsible infective agent is not eradicated or treated adequately. Over many years, the gastric mucosa undergoes a sequence of adaptive changes which may lead to glandular atrophy, intestinal metaplasia with goblet cells, increased risk of gastric dysplasia and carcinoma, and mucosa-associated lymphoid tissue lymphoma. The changes can be localised, regional or involve the whole stomach (pan-gastritis).

H. pylori infection is regarded as the main cause of the commonest form of chronic gastritis. It is also widely accepted that *H. pylori* infection is the initiating factor for, and possibly the direct cause of, atrophy and intestinal metaplasia. These alterations in the gastric mucosa can predispose to peptic ulceration in a sub-set of individuals. Given that the infection is usually in the antrum and antrum-corpus transitional zone, this is the site of predilection for gastric ulcers. Different patterns of *H. pylori* gastritis are associated with profound alterations in acid output. In antral-predominant gastritis, acid production from the largely unaffected corpus is enhanced whereas corpus inflammation is associated with hypochlorhydria. These changes have an important bearing on the pathogenesis of peptic ulceration.

Under the microscope, *Helicobacter pylori* infection is associated with the pattern of chronic active gastritis, with the presence of neutrophils and mononuclear cells (lymphocytes and plasma cells) in the mucosa, respectively. The term *active gastritis* is preferred to *acute gastritis* because *H. pylori* gastritis is a long-standing chronic infection with on-going activity. Lymphoid aggregates and lymphoid follicles may be observed within the lamina propria. Rarely lymphocytes may be found in the epithelium. The organisms of *Helicobacter pylori* are found within the gastric mucus layer that overlays the apical side of gastric surface cells. Lower numbers of organisms may be found in the lower portions of the gastric foveolae. In patients on acid suppression therapy, *Helicobacter pylori* organisms may be found within the deeper areas of the mucosa in association with glandular cells.

Helicobacter pylori–associated gastritis can be found with different levels of severity; mild (rare neutrophils seen), moderate (obvious neutrophils within the glandular and foveolar epithelium), and severe (numerous neutrophils with glandular micro abscesses and mucosal erosion or ulceration).

Chronic gastritis associated with *Helicobacter pylori* can manifest as a pangastritis involving the whole area from the cardia to the gastric body and pylorus, or it may predominantly involve the antrum. Patients found to have gastric ulcers generally have antral-predominant gastritis. By contrast, patients with gastric cancer more commonly have pangastritis, or at least multifocal gastritis. The latter generally have significant intestinal metaplasia and gastric oxyntic glandular atrophy coexisting in the rest of the stomach. It is important to look for histological evidence of atrophic gastritis because it is associated with increased risk of gastric cancer. In comparison with the general population, patients with chronic atrophic gastritis may have up to a 16-fold increased risk of developing gastric cancer.

Eradication of *H. pylori* infection is usually followed by resolution of gastritis. This in turn reduces the risk of further peptic ulceration. Whether such intervention can remove the increased risk of progression to gastric cancer is yet to be determined. Although strong claims have been made for a synergistic association between *H. pylori* and NSAIDs in causing chronic gastric and duodenal ulcers, the evidence remains controversial. An association in this respect has not progressed to establishing causality.

Other Forms of Gastritis

There are various specialized forms of gastritis with characteristic histological appearances.

Chronic Reactive (Chemical) Gastritis

This results from damage to the gastric mucosa by exogenous and endogenous irritants. Drugs, *e.g.* NSAIDs, alcohol or bile reflux, are the main causative irritants. Histologically, there is foveolar hyperplasia, severe congestion, oedema and fibrosis of lamina propria with little inflammatory infiltrate. The usual location of drug-induced damage is the antral and prepyloric regions. These lesions are produced by blockade of the cyclooxygenase pathway with reduction of the cytoprotective prostaglandins. Thus, prostaglandin sparing NSAIDs and low dose steroids are less likely to cause erosive gastritis. The alcohol induced mucosal damage also affects the mucosal micro vessels with resulting haemorrhage and thrombosis. Other causes of haemorrhagic erosions include cor pulmonale, severe chest infections, cirrhosis and blood disorders. Bile gastritis results from enterogastric bile reflux. It is a form of chemical gastritis with distinctive pathological change, which consists of sub nuclear vacuolization of the foveolar epithelium.

Autoimmune Gastritis

This form of gastritis presents as a chronic gastritis with oxyntic cell injury, and glandular atrophy essentially restricted to the oxyntic mucosa of the gastric body and fundus [7]. Antiparietal cell and anti-intrinsic factor antibodies cause it. The histologic changes vary in different phases of the disease. In the early phase, there is multifocal infiltration of the lamina propria by mononuclear cells and eosinophils and focal T-cell lymphocyte infiltration of oxyntic glands with glandular destruction. Hyperplasia of focal mucous cells (pseudopyloric metaplasia), and parietal cells hypertrophic changes are also observed. In the florid phase, there is increased lymphocytic accumulation, oxyntic gland atrophy, and focal intestinal metaplasia. The end stage is characterized by diffuse chronic atrophic gastritis associated with multifocal intestinal metaplasia involving the gastric body and fundus. In contrast to the gastric body, the antrum is spared [8]. Recently, a distinct form of autoimmune gastritis was reported in a small group of patients with systemic autoimmune disorders which is characterized by atrophic pangastritis. Although autoimmune gastritis is a relatively rare disease, it is the most frequent cause of pernicious anaemia in temperate climates. In patients with pernicious anaemia, the risk of gastric adenocarcinoma is thought to be at least 2.9 times higher than in the general population. There is also an increased risk of gastric carcinoid tumours. Western countries are seeing a constant increase in autoimmune gastritis coupled with a decline in the incidence of *Helicobacter pylori*-associated gastritis. Autoimmune gastropathy is due to autoantibodies aggression targeting parietal cells through a complex interaction against the parietal cell proton pump, intrinsic factor, and sensitized T cells. Given the specific target of this aggression, autoimmune gastritis is typically focal and restricted to the gastric corpus and fundic mucosa. In advanced cases, the oxyntic epithelia are replaced by atrophic and metaplastic mucosa, creating the phenotypic background in which both gastric neuroendocrine tumours and intestinal-type adenocarcinomas may develop. Despite improvements in understanding the phenotypic changes occurring in this autoimmune variety, no reliable biomarkers are available to identify patients at higher risk of developing a gastric cancer.

Eosinophilic Gastritis

This occurs as part of eosinophilic gastroenteropathy, which usually presents in young people. It is basically an allergic reaction. It usually affects the pyloric region and the adjacent duodenum become diffusely thickened due to oedema of the submucosa and muscle layers. There is an esinophilic infiltrate and occasionally giant cells. The gastric antrum is most severely affected. Histologically, there is extensive esinophilic infiltration, oedema and lymphangiectasia. Serum IgE is elevated and most patients also have peripheral eosinophilia. The clinical features include symptoms of delayed gastric emptying, and gastrointestinal bleeding. The treatment is with sodium cromoglycate and steroids.

Lymphocytic Gastritis

This is a rare form of chronic gastritis, which may be encountered in patients with coeliac disease. It is probably the result of an abnormal immunological reaction to unidentified luminal antigens. Histologically it is characterized by T-lymphocyte infiltration of the gastric epithelium. Endoscopically, nodules, erosions and enlarged mucosal folds are characteristic.

Suppurative (Phlegmonous) Gastritis

This is a rare and often fatal bacterial infection producing severe inflammatory changes in the stomach with systemic sepsis. Haemolytic streptococci are the commonest infecting organisms. The condition often complicates a pre-existing gastric lesion. The condition is more commonly encountered in elderly and compromised patients. The presentation is usually one of severe progressive peritonitis. The only lifesaving treatment is with gastric resection and antibiotics. At surgery, the stomach looks dusky and the serosal surface is covered with a fibrinous exudate. The gastric infection can progress to necrotizing gastritis, which results in gangrene of the stomach. It is caused by a mixed infection with fusiform and spirochaete bacteria.

AIDS Gastritis

In patients with acquired immunodeficiency syndrome (AIDS), inflammatory oedema of the pyloric ring is caused by infection with cryptosporidiosis. Clinically, patients present with symptoms of gastric outlet obstruction and cryptosporidial oocysts can be recovered from stools. AIDS patient can rarely be infected with toxoplasma gondii. The infection causes diffuse thickening of the gastric folds as seen on endoscopy. Biopsies of the mucosa show necrosis and intracellular trophozoites in gastric epithelial, smooth muscle and endothelial cells.

Granulomatous and Crohn's Gastritis

There are infectious and non-infectious causes of granulomatous gastritis. Non-infectious diseases make up the usual causes of gastric granulomas including Crohn's disease, sarcoidosis, and isolated granulomatous gastritis. Sarcoid-like granulomas may be observed in cocaine users, and foreign material is occasionally observed in the granulomas.

Gastritis can be found in Crohn's disease patients. The histological features are similar to those of intestinal Crohn's disease with patchy, acute inflammation with some gastric pit or glandular abscesses, on a background of lymphoid aggregates. Non-caseating epithelioid granulomas may also be present in about a third of cases of Crohn's disease gastritis. Characteristically, there is focal chronic active ulceration with epithelial erosions in the absence of *H. pylori* infection.

Granulomatous gastritis is a form of infectious gastritis. These are rare and include tuberculous gastritis. The tuberculous infection of the stomach is usually secondary to active pulmonary tuberculosis. Multiple ragged ulcers and discrete tubercles are seen at endoscopy. Serosal inflammation is common and a regional lymphadenopathy is usually found. Treatment is with anti-tuberculous chemotherapy.

Emphysematous Gastritis

This is characterized by air-filled cysts in the gastric wall and is usually accompanied by pneumatoides cystoids intestinalis. Gas-filled cysts in the wall of the stomach can also occur in association with chronic obstructive airways disease or emphysema in the presence of pyloric obstruction.

Gastritis Cystica Polyposa

This is a rare, late sequel of gastric surgery. Patients usually present with abdominal pain, nausea, vomiting or GI bleeding. Endoscopically, a hypertrophic nodular gastritis is seen.

Presentation and Clinical Features

Data for the incidence and prevalence of gastritis are unavailable. Dyspeptic symptoms are reported in 10% to 20% of patients taking NSAIDs. Older age is a key risk factor for *H. pylori* and chronic atrophic gastritis. Globally more than 50% of people are infected with *H. pylori* but the incidence is declining.

The vast majority of patients with chronic gastritis are either asymptomatic or have vague ill-defined dyspeptic symptoms or lethargy due to anaemia. The clinical presentation of gastritis is not associated with any specific gastrointestinal signs or symptoms. Acute gastritis is usually symptomatic. The signs and symptoms of acute gastritis include gnawing or burning ache or pain in the epigastric region that may be exacerbated or relieved by eating. Intermittent nausea, vomiting and early satiety are sometimes reported. Some patients present with episodes of haematemesis with or without melaena. Microcytic anaemia, due to iron deficiency, is a common presenting sign and is caused by chronic blood loss from the inflamed stomach and achlorhydria, which impairs iron absorption. Macrocytic and rarely megaloblastic anaemia can also lead to presentation or can be found incidentally.

Diagnosis

Diagnosis of gastritis is rarely suspected from a patient's presentation. However, the persistence of dyspeptic symptoms in young people or new onset dyspepsia in those over 55 years warrants endoscopy when the diagnosis could be made and confirmed by representative biopsies. A panel of serum biomarkers has recently been advocated in the non-invasive diagnosis of atrophic gastritis and a meta-analysis corroborates it high sensitivity and specificity [9].

Risk of Cancer with Gastritis

Mild gastritis is unlikely to cause long-term complications. However, severe gastritis in patients with normal / high acid secretion, will result in antral predominant gastritis that may go on to give rise to a duodenal ulcer. Those with a low acid secretion will develop a pangastritis. If severe this may give rise to a gastric ulcer and if this continues long term will give rise to atrophy and intestinal metaplasia that in the course of time represents a risk for the development of non-cardia gastric cancer. The risk of gastric cancer is associated with corpus predominant atrophy and intestinal metaplasia. A corpus gastritis rather than an antral predominant gastritis is the main predictor for gastric cancer. Chronic atrophic gastritis (CAG) is an essential precursor lesion in the development of intestinal type of gastric cancer.

Medical Management of Gastritis

The management is principally directed to the effects of gastritis (*e.g.* Bleeding, anaemia, vomiting *etc.*), the removal of the underlying cause when possible and specific therapy when indicated. Acid suppression therapy reduces gastric acid output to enable healing of the gastric mucosa. Anaemia should be treated with iron or cyanocobalamin injections depending on the type of anaemia. Avoidance of irritants such as alcohol and NSAIDs should be advised. If *H. pylori*, was found on the basis of appropriate tests, it should be eradicated. If dysplasia id found on biopsy, these patients should have surveillance endoscopy with multiple biopsies.

Surgical Management of Gastritis

Surgery is reserved for management of the complications of gastritis. Alkaline reflux gastritis (entero-gastric reflux) can been seen as a complication following operations on the stomach that alter, remove or bypass the pyloric sphincter mechanism. Symptomatic alkaline reflux has also been found in patients without previous gastric surgery and has been linked with previous cholecystectomy. Reflux gastritis is associated with abdominal pain, weight loss and bilious vomiting and is caused by enterogastric reflux of alkaline intestinal contents, particularly bile.

Unlike many other forms of gastritis that can be managed medically, the only effective treatment for symptomatic bile gastritis after previous gastric surgery is surgical diversion of the duodenal contents away from the stomach or gastric remnant. The Roux-en-Y procedure, Braun entero-enterostomy and isoperistaltic jejunal interposition segment (Henley loop) procedures have been used for this purpose. Although there is a risk of post-operative disabling stasis syndrome following a Roux-en-Y procedure, it's technical simplicity and lower morbidity rate has made it a popular choice for many surgeons when attempting surgical diversion of bile from the stomach.

Roux-en-Y or Braun Gastrojejunostomy

Following a Billroth I or Billroth II gastrectomy, reflux gastritis can be treated by conversion to a Roux-en-Y gastrojejunostomy. The Roux limb diverts the alkaline contents 45-60 cm below the gastric mucosa thereby reducing the potential for reflux. However, if a vagotomy was not performed at the time of the initial operation then a Roux-en-Y operation with the associated diversion of buffering alkali has the potential to cause ulceration. In these cases, life-long treatment with acid suppression therapy is necessary.

Ideally, a retro colic, iso-peristaltic GE should be formed. The procedure can be done laparoscopically with early recovery and rapid discharge from hospital. However, after previous gastric surgery, adhesiolysis can be time consuming (Fig. **1**).

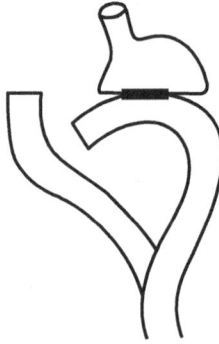

Fig. (1). Roux en Y gastroenterostomy.

Access

- For open surgery, a limited transverse upper abdominal incision is ideal. However, depending on preference, or the presence of a previous scar, a small midline upper abdominal incision can provide adequate access.
- For laparoscopic surgery, an infra-umbilical port should be used for the endoscope/ camera. Two ports on each side of the abdomen should be used for dissection and retraction.

Exploration

- The procedure should commence with a limited abdominal exploration to assess the feasibility of gastroenterostomy, extent of adhesiolysis required and the feasibility of a retrocolic approach.

Dissection

- The pre-existing Billroth anastomosis should be dissected free from other organs and then taken down or stapled to separate the stomach from the duodenum or jejunum.
- In a retrocolic approach, a window is created in the transverse colon mesentery to the left of the middle colic vessels.
- A 5 cm length of the dependent part of the stomach is withdrawn to the infra-colic compartment.
- A loop of proximal jejunum approximately 15 – 20 cm from the ligament of Treitz is identified.

Reconstruction (Braun)

- The jejunum is approximated to the dependent part of the stomach using either sutures or a linear stapling device.
- The two sides of the jejunum on either side of the gastroenterostomy are approximated using either sutures or a linear stapling device.

Reconstruction (Roux-en-Y)

- The jejunum is transected.
- The distal limb of the transected jejunum is approximated to the dependent part of the stomach using either sutures or a linear stapling device.
- The proximal limb of the transected jejunum is approximated end to side to the distal limb of jejunum approximately 50 cm distal to the gastroenterostomy using either sutures or a linear stapling device.
- The abdomen should be closed.

Post-Operative Course

- The patient should be nursed on an appropriate ward with appropriate monitoring of vital parameters.
- The patient should be nursed without oral intake and all fluids and medication should be administered intravenously for at least 24 hours.
- After 24 hours, the volume of fluid intake is stepped up gradually over 48 hours. At the end of this period, small amounts of semi-solid food could be introduced and if tolerated, substituted with more solid food.
- The patient should be ready for discharge home when sufficiently mobile and independent.

Anticipated Complications

- Primary or secondary haemorrhage from the edges of the gastroenterostomy should be managed by endoscopic haemostasis or surgery if necessary.
- Respiratory infection or compromise should necessitate antibiotics and pulmonary toilet by physiotherapy. Depending on the level of respiratory compromise, additional measures may be necessary such as positive airway pressure (CPAP) or ventilation.

De Meester Duodenal Switch Procedure

If the original anastomosis is to be spared then the De Meester duodenal switch procedure is an operation, which can achieve bile diversion (Fig. **2**). The key steps of dissection and reconstruction would change to the following:

Dissection

- The duodenum should be dissected free from other organs and divided 4 cm beyond the pylorus and proximal to the ampulla.
- A loop of proximal jejunum approximately 15 – 20 cm from the ligament of Treitz is identified.
- The loop selected of jejunum (based on a vascular arcade) is divided at its mid-point.

Reconstruction

- The distal end of jejunum (alimentary limb) is brought through a window created in the transverse mesocolon.
- The alimentary limb of jejunum is anastomosed to the proximal duodenum.
- The proximal end of the divided small bowel, now the distal end of the biliopancreatic limb, is anastomosed to the ileum 100 cm from the ileocaecal valve to create a 100 cm common channel. The proximal end of the divided small bowel, now the distal end of the biliopancreatic limb, is anastomosed to the ileum 100 cm from the ileocaecal valve to create a 100 cm common channel.
- A cholecystectomy is required.

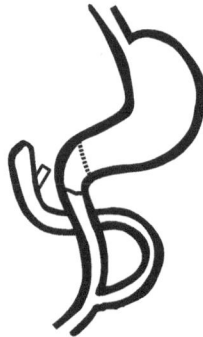

Fig. (2). Duodenal switch procedure.

PEPTIC ULCERATION

Worldwide, peptic ulcer disease (PUD) is a significant cause of morbidity and mortality, with a significant burden in low- and middle-income countries. These ulcers consist of a breach in the mucosa of the stomach and duodenum that extends through the muscularis mucosa and into the submucosa or deeper. Peptic ulcer disease is most commonly caused by *Helicobacter pylori* (*H. pylori*) infection or the indiscriminate use of non-steroidal anti-inflammatory drugs. Peptic ulcers can occur anywhere in the GI tract, but duodenal are most common followed by gastric ulcers. Duodenal ulcers typically arise within 2 cm of the pylorus, are highly associated with *H. pylori* infection (90%), and frequently resolve with appropriate *H. pylori* therapy. Gastric ulcers are less likely to be associated with *H. pylori* infection and are classified into five types based on their location and association with acid secretion (Table **1**).

Table 1. Modified Johnson Classification of peptic ulcers [10].

Type	Location	Common Complications	Acid Secretion	Notes
Oesophageal	Gastroesophageal junction and distal oesophagus	Haemorrhage	High	
Gastric				
I	Gastric body on lesser curvature near the incisura angularis	Perforation	Normal or low	Older patients, Associated with *Helicobacter pylori*
II	Two ulcers; gastric body and duodenal ulcer	Haemorrhage, obstruction, or perforation	High	Younger patients, Association with active or quiescent duodenal ulcers
III	Pre-pyloric	Haemorrhage, perforation	High	Younger patients, Similar to type II gastric ulcers and duodenal ulcers
IV	High on lesser curvature	Haemorrhage	Low	Likely a variant of type I gastric ulcers, Difficult to treat surgically
V	Anywhere	Perforation	Normal	Related to NSAID use
Duodenal	95% occur within 2 cm of pylorus	Haemorrhage, obstruction, or perforation	Normal or high	

The appearance of an ulcer can be either the classic erosive, concave, crater-like ulcer or convex, perhaps resembling a colonic polyp. In general, the erosive concave type tends to be located in the stomach proper while the convex type tends to be found in the pylorus/duodenum. Classification of peptic ulcers is based on the region and number of ulcers in the affected region [10]. In general, ulcers are described as gastric or duodenal. More specific descriptions site the region of the stomach or duodenum where the ulcer is located. This is important clinically since the pathogenesis determines the location of the ulcer. In addition, when checking for ulcer healing, it is helpful to know the precise location of the ulcer.

Epidemiology

In the UK, the incidence rate of uncomplicated peptic ulcer disease is about 0.75 cases per 1000 persons per year. The incidence is 12% higher in males than females. Peptic ulcer disease is more common in patients in their 20s and 30s, whereas gastric cancer tends to arise in the 40s and 50s. Duodenal ulcers are four times as common as gastric ulcers. In the developed world, *H. pylori* incidence has been slowly declining over the past 50 years and NSAID use has increased. This has resulted in a decline in duodenal ulcers and an increase in gastric ulcers (the main site of ulcers caused by NSAIDs). Around 10%–15% of individuals infected with *H. pylori* develop peptic ulcer disease.

Aetiology

Genetic factors play some role in the aetiology of peptic ulceration with increased prevalence of duodenal ulcers in patients with blood group O negative and individuals with hyper-pesinogenaemia. Dietary factors also play a role in the aetiology such as spicy food, alcohol, coffee and caffeinated fizzy drinks. Chemical ulcerogens are one of the main aetiological factors such as non-steroidal anti-inflammatory agents (NSAIDs) and less commonly aspirin and corticosteroids. Infections are also responsible as ulcerogens. The most common infective ulcerogen responsible for peptic ulceration (Gastric and duodenal) is H *pylori*. Other less common infective agents include cytomegalovirus and herpes simplex type I. Peptic ulcers can also arise secondary to severe physiological stress *e.g.* trauma, burns, head injury, sepsis. Other less common causes include malignancy, Crohn's disease, liver cirrhosis and Zollinger-Ellison syndrome [11]. The aetiology of peptic ulcer disease is varied and incompletely understood. Environmental ulcerogens (chemical and infective) are the most common. They tend to act together with other factors to impair the mucosal resistance to injury and the healing of mucosal lesions. However, the main two factors in the aetiology of peptic ulcers are non- steroidal anti-inflammatory drugs (NSAIDs) and *H. pylori*.

Non-steroidal anti-inflammatory drugs cause gastrointestinal injury through both topical and systemic effects. The latter is mediated mainly by blocking prostaglandin synthesis through inhibition of the cyclooxygenase (COX) enzymes, COX-1 and COX-2. However, COX inhibition is not the sole mechanism of NSAID-induced gastrointestinal injury and that other prostaglandin-independent mechanisms are equally important in the pathogenesis of peptic ulceration. After mucosal injury, NSAIDs inhibit both the early events of healing necessary to repair the initial superficial injury as well as the later events of cell proliferation and angiogenesis, leading to delayed ulcer healing.

Topical injury initiates the initial mucosal erosions by disrupting the gastric epithelial cell barrier, but prostaglandin depletion is essential for the development of clinically significant duodenal and gastric ulcers.

Acutely, *H. pylori* infection or colonization may produce a hypochlorhydric environment. This is thought to be a protective mechanism for the organism and occurs due to the increase of urease, which hydrolyses urea and converts it to ammonia and carbon dioxide. *H. pylori*-positive patients have a 10 to 20% lifetime risk of developing peptic ulcer disease. Although gastric colonization with *H. pylori* induces histologic gastritis in all infected individuals, only a minority, develop any apparent clinical signs of this colonization and the rest remain as "carriers" without overt symptoms. *H. pylori* contribute to mucosal injury by multiple mechanisms. Ulcers mostly occur at sites where mucosal inflammation is most severe. Patients infected with CagA+ strains usually have a higher inflammatory response and are significantly more at risk for developing mucosal injury and subsequent peptic ulceration. There is a strong correlation between toxin activity and the pathogenicity of *H. pylori*. The s1/m1 type of VacA, which produces a vacuolating cytotoxin, is the most virulent in Western populations. *H. pylori* infection produce the mucosal injury by the induced hypergastrinaemia through disruption of the gastrin release negative feedback, direct mucosal damage by released toxins and by the inflammatory response to infection.

H. pylori infection and NSAID use, independently and significantly increase the risk of peptic ulcer disease and ulcer bleeding. In addition, there is synergism for the development of peptic ulcer and ulcer bleeding between *H. pylori* infection and NSAID use. Although not all individuals infected with *H. pylori* develop peptic ulceration, peptic-ulcer disease is rare in *H. pylori* negative who do not take NSAIDs.

Pathology

Peptic ulcers occur *in situ*ations where there is a breach in the gastro-duodenal mucosal lining caused by the damaging forces of gastric acid and pepsin, combined with superimposed injury from immunologic or environmental agents. Ulcers may occur with normal or excessive secretion of hydrochloric acid and pepsin, causing an imbalance between gastric luminal factors and degradation in the defensive function of the gastric mucosal barrier. Mucosal defences include mucus, secretion of bicarbonate, mucosal blood flow, cell renewal, prostaglandins and a tight junction between the epithelial cells. Factors that increase acid secretion or break down the mucosal defence barriers include pepsin, bile acids, NSAIDs, *H. pylori*, alcohol and pancreatic enzymes. When acid and pepsin invade a weakened area of the mucosal barrier, histamine is released. Histamine will stimulate the parietal cells to secrete more acid. With the continuation of this vicious cycle, erosion occurs to form an ulcer.

Peptic ulcers may occur in the stomach, duodenum (anterior or posterior aspect of first part of the duodenum), lower oesophagus and in Meckle's diverticulum (containing gastric mucosa). Gastric ulcers occur mostly in the lesser curvature of the stomach and duodenal ulcers occur mainly in the duodenal cap.

Presentation and Clinical Features

Peptic ulceration is characterized by symptoms including epigastric pain, nausea, vomiting, bloating, loss of appetite, haematemesis and melena. The traditional description of abdominal pain upon food intake is suggestive of a gastric ulcer. By contrast, duodenal ulcer pain occurs 2 to 5 hours after eating, on an empty stomach or nocturnally. Food intake, antacids, or anti-secretory therapy, usually relieves the pain. Chronic ulcers may be asymptomatic and are often NSAID-induced, with UGI bleeding or perforation being the first clinical manifestation. A history of gastroesophageal reflux disease and use of NSAIDs or glucocorticoids should raise the suspicion for peptic ulceration. Perforation of the stomach or duodenum into the peritoneal cavity is an uncommon but serious complication.

Diagnosis

Patients under 55 years of age suspected of having peptic ulcer disease without alarm symptoms should undergo non-invasive testing for *H. pylori.* Endoscopy should be considered for patients older than 55 years of age and in those patients presenting with alarm (red flag) symptoms.

Non-invasive tests for *H. pylori* include the urea breath test (UBT), the faecal antigen test (FAT), and HP antibody tests. The UBT and FAT are more wide spread and are the preferred methods for diagnosing an active infection prior to eradication with antibiotics. These tests should be carried out in the absence of PPI administration for 1 to 2 weeks before testing [12].

The UBT is the test of choice for confirming eradication and is most accurate at least 4 weeks following completion of eradication treatment. The FAT is more cumbersome due to the handling and storage of stool samples and is less validated for post-treatment testing. Antibody testing is only useful when the result is negative. A positive antibody result requires confirmation by a UBT or FAT, as the results may remain positive for years after exposure to *H. pylori.* Antibody testing is of no value in testing for eradication. (Table **2**)

In patients having endoscopic evaluation for *H. pylori*, the rapid urease test (RUT) is preferred provided they have not taken PPIs in the past 1 to 2 weeks, or an antibiotic or bismuth in the past 4 weeks, before endoscopy. Histology of retrieved biopsy samples is recommended in patients who have taken one of the previously mentioned medications prior to endoscopy. Culture and polymerase chain reaction are methods capable of identifying antibiotic sensitivities of *H. pylori*. However, these tests are difficult to perform and are not widely available. They are indicated in antibiotics resistant strains, which manifest through failure to eradicate them.

Table 2. Tests for *Helicobacter pylori* [12].

Test	Sensitivity	Specificity	Notes
Non-invasive			
Urease breath test	95%	90%	Determines active infection but must stop PPI 2 wks before; takes 30–60 min and is used to confirm eradication.
Faecal antigen detection	90%	95%	Determines active infection but is positive for up to 12 wks after eradication.
Serology	85%	79%	Cannot be used to confirm eradication because antibodies persist.
Endoscopic			
Biopsy urease test	90%	95%	Decreased sensitivity with on-going PPI, H_2 antagonist, antibiotic, and bismuth treatment or with recent GI bleeding.
Histology	90%	95%	Multiple available stains can be used; increased sensitivity with increased number of biopsies.
Culture	80%	100%	Difficult and expensive; reserved for persistent infections and antibiotic sensitivity testing of resistant strains.

The diagnosis of peptic ulceration is made by direct endoscopic inspection, biopsy and histological confirmation. In patients 55 years or older, or with one or more alarm symptoms, endoscopy with biopsy is recommended to rule out cancer and other serious causes of such alarm symptoms.

Patients with gastric ulcers should be re-endoscoped after 6 weeks to check healing and to exclude a malignant ulcer. Duodenal ulcers can largely be managed expectantly and do not necessarily need a repeat inspection provided symptoms subside. Testing for *H. Pylori* infection should be performed in patients with active PUD or history of PUD. Detecting and treating *H. pylori* infection can reduce the risk of recurrence.

Risk of Cancer from Peptic Ulceration

Patients with a history of gastric ulceration are more likely to develop gastric cancer and patients with a history of duodenal ulceration are at a decreased risk for gastric cancer. Although the explanation is not clear, it reflects the incidence of chronic *H. pylori* gastritis in different parts of the stomach and the effects of this on gastric acid secretion. *H. pylori* infection is at least the triggering factor for, atrophy and intestinal metaplasia. These alterations in the gastric mucosa predispose to peptic ulceration, which are maximal in the antrum-corpus transitional zone. This is the site of predilection for gastric ulcers. By contrast, in antral-predominant gastritis, acid production from the largely unaffected corpus is enhanced and this contributes to duodenal ulceration particularly in the presence of *H. pylori*.

Medical Management

The purpose of treating *H. pylori*–infected patients with antibiotics is to eliminate the organism, resulting in greater rates of ulcer healing, lower recurrence rates, healing of gastritis and reduced risk of gastric cancer.

Eradication of *H. pylori* with antibiotics together with an anti-secretory agent is more effective than anti-secretory therapy alone. Eradication treatment options include triple therapy containing one anti-secretory agent and two antibiotics, or quadruple therapy of one anti-secretory agent, two antibiotics, and bismuth salt.

Amoxicillin and clarithromycin are the preferred antibiotics as part of triple therapy (metronidazole is substituted for amoxicillin in patients with a penicillin allergy). In quadruple therapy Metronidazole and tetracycline are used. Triple therapy is less complex, better tolerated and is usually chosen as first-line treatment. Either treatment options should be continued ideally for 10 to 14 days. Shorter 7- and 10-day treatment regimens are reasonably efficacious, but 14 days is more effective. *H. pylori* eradication rates with first-line triple therapy vary from 70% to 95%. Eradication rates are 4% to 5% higher when the treatment duration is increased from 7 days to 10 days or 14 days. If a second course of therapy is needed because of treatment failure, a different regimen should be utilized. If a patient has a history of macrolide antibiotic use, quadruple therapy should be used in the first instance. For selecting a PPI, there is no appreciable difference within the class of anti-secretory agents. Currently, there are no data to support substitution of ampicillin for amoxicillin, doxycycline for tetracycline, or azithromycin or erythromycin for clarithromycin. Clarithromycin resistance has increased in certain geographic regions and should be considered when choosing antimicrobial therapy. Bismuth-based quadruple therapy results in eradication rates of 57% to 95%, which is highly dependent on patient adherence. If a patient continues to carry *H. pylori* after two different courses of eradication therapy, compliance with treatment and drug resistance must be considered. If the latter is suspected, an antral gastric biopsy should be obtained and cultured immediately in enriched media on antibiotic sensitivity plates and stored at exacting temperature and humidity. This is usually done in reference laboratories that need to be alerted prior to collecting the biopsy.

Anti-secretory Agents

Proton Pump Inhibitors (PPIs)

These agents decrease gastric acid secretions by inhibiting the H^+/K^+-adenosine triphosphatase pump in the gastric parietal cells, leading to a significant reduction of gastric acid secretion. PPIs through a secondary mechanism reduce pepsin by increasing the gastric pH. This in turn promotes decreased mucosal damage and promotes an environment for ulcer healing. A gastric acid pH level greater than 4 encourage peptic ulcer healing and this should be the aim of treatment. Different PPIs achieve different acid suppression extent providing a choice. In terms of acid suppression, PPIs are generally more effective than H_2 receptor antagonists (H2RAs). PPIs are well tolerated with the most common adverse effects include GI upset, somnolence, headache, dizziness, and nausea. Patients, who do not tolerate one brand of PPI, can usually tolerate a different brand although this is not universal [11].

Hydrogen Receptor Antagonists (H2RAs)

These agents selectively inhibit the H2 receptors of parietal cells, leading to reduce acid secretion. This reduces further damage and allows for ulcer healing. All H2RAs at the appropriate dose have similar efficacy in reducing acid secretion and promoting ulcer healing. H2RAs are also well tolerated, but they are used less commonly than PPIs. The most common adverse effects being somnolence, headache, dizziness, and GI upset. Cimetidine has been reported to have an increased risk of causing gynecomastia, impotence, neutropenia, agranulocytosis, and increased serum creatinine, although the frequency of these side effects is rare. Ranitidine and cimetidine are the two main H2RAs in common use.

Antibiotics

Amoxicillin, clarithromycin, metronidazole, and tetracycline all have antimicrobial activity against *H. pylori*, which is a gram-negative bacterium.

Amoxicillin is a beta-lactam antibiotic that inhibits bacterial cell wall synthesis, resulting in bactericidal activity against susceptible organisms such as *H. pylori*. Since amoxicillin has the basic molecular structure of penicillin, it should be avoided in patients with penicillin allergies.

*Clarithromycin*is a macrolide antibiotic that binds to the 50S ribosomal subunit of susceptible organisms, inhibiting RNA-dependent protein synthesis and resulting in bacteriostatic activity. Serious reported adverse effects include QT interval prolongation on ECG, ventricular arrhythmias, and hepatotoxicity. Susceptible patients prescribed clarithromycin should be screened by electrocardiography (ECG).

*Metronidazole*is a nitroimidazole antibiotic, which disrupts the helical DNA structure, and causes strand breakage, leading to inhibition of protein synthesis and subsequent cell death in susceptible organisms. It is also considered bactericidal. Serious, but rare, reported adverse effects include confusion, seizures, hepatitis, pancreatitis, and neuropathy. Patients prescribed metronidazole should avoid alcohol for the duration of treatment due to the potential for disulfiram-like reactions.

*Tetracyclines*exhibit bacteriostatic activity by binding to the 30S ribosomal subunit of susceptible organisms, thereby inhibiting bacterial protein synthesis and leading to microbial cell death. They are considered bactericidal. The most common adverse effects are diarrhoea, nausea, tooth discoloration and photosensitivity. Tetracyclines are contraindicated in pregnant women and children under 8 years old mainly due to tooth discoloration.

Mucosal Protective Agents

Bismuth has multiple ulcer-healing mechanisms. These include antibacterial activity against *H. pylori,* inhibition of pepsin activity, and the increase of prostaglandin, mucus, and bicarbonate production. Bismuth does not inhibit acid production by itself. The most common reported adverse effects are blackened tongue and stools during treatment, which tend to disappear after cessation of use. Bismuth is contraindicated in patients with an aspirin allergy, history of coagulopathy, active influenza, history of GI bleed, or chicken pox infection due to the risk of developing Reye's syndrome.

Misoprostol is a synthetic prostaglandin E1 analogue that replaces prostaglandins, which are inhibited by NSAIDs. Misoprostol inhibits acid secretion to a small extent and provides mucosal protection. For the treatment of NSAID-induced ulcers, it is less effective than PPIs in ulcer healing. It is however effective in reducing the risk for NSAID-induced ulcers when administered concurrently with the NSAID. The most common reported adverse effects are nausea, diarrhoea, flatulence, and headache. Misoprostol should be administered with meals and at bedtime to reduce the incidence of diarrhoea. The main contraindication is pregnancy.

Sucralfate is an aluminium salt from sucrose octasulfate which is not absorbed by the gut. It binds to the gastric mucosa, forming a protective layer that prevents gastric damage from bile salts, pepsin, and gastric acid. This allows healing of the gastric mucosa or the ulcerated tissue. The most commonly reported adverse effect is constipation. Sucralfate should be taken on an empty stomach to avoid binding with dietary proteins and phosphate which would reduce its availability.

Complications of Peptic Ulcer Disease and Their Management

The common complications of PUD include bleeding, perforation and gastric outlet obstruction. Peptic ulcer haemorrhage is the most common complication with up to 15% of patients experiencing some degree of bleeding. Ulcers caused by NSAIDs are at an increased risk of bleeding than those caused by *H. pylori*. Posterior duodenal ulcers can erode the gastro-duodenal artery. Lesser curve gastric ulcers can erode the left gastric artery. The majority of ulcers stop bleeding spontaneously but for those that don't bleeding can be treated endoscopically by injection of the ulcer with adrenaline or sclerosants, laser photocoagulation and coagulation with bipolar diathermy. Endoscopic therapy stops the bleeding in more than 90% of patients but bleeding recurs after endoscopic therapy in 10-25%. If bleeding is massive or refractory to radiological embolization surgery is required. Surgical intervention should also be considered when stigmata of re-bleeding are found on endoscopy or when a large vessel is seen in the ulcer base.

Surgical Control of Bleeding Peptic Ulcer

The vast majority of patients with a bleeding peptic ulcer will have had a diagnostic endoscopy with endoscopic attempts at haemostasis. The majority of those patients who have failed endoscopic haemostasis will have had at least one attempt at embolization of the bleeding vessel. Those presenting for surgery will be patients with profuse haemorrhage from the outset, those with endoscopic stigmata of recurrent bleeds and those who have failed endoscopic and embolic haemostasis. In all these circumstances, it is important to ensure that these patients are adequately resuscitated with normalization of their coagulation parameters as far as possible. The controversy regarding the recommended operation for peptic ulcer bleeding is largely unsettled. Minimal and definitive approaches have traditionally been described. The minimal approach involves ulcer haemostasis only whereas the addition of acid reduction procedures (vagotomy, antrectomy) is classified as a definitive approach. Unless the ulcer is large (more than 3 cm in diameter) or malignant, a minimalist approach is recommended. The availability and safety of PPIs have obviated the need for acid reduction surgical procedures, which carry a considerable burden of morbidity. The goal of the procedure is to achieve rapid luminal control of haemorrhage and suture closure of the ulcer bed. In a minority of situations, additional control of the feeding named vessel is advocated.

Access

- For open surgery, a transverse upper abdominal incision provides sufficient access. However, depending on preference, a midline upper abdominal incision can provide more rapid access particularly in a deteriorating patient. Access should be simultaneous with a diagnostic endoscopy to ascertain the source of bleeding if an endoscopy was not previously done.
- Laparoscopic surgery, in general can take longer and is not strictly speaking used in the control of haemorrhage in a rapidly deteriorating patient.

Exploration

- The falciform ligament should be divided to allow upward retraction of the liver for adequate access.
- A mechanical retractor should be used to achieve adequate surgical exposure.
- The procedure should commence by identifying the position of the pyloric ring with the aid of the pre-pyloric vein of Mayo and manual palpation.

Dissection

- Two, stay sutures should be placed on the duodenum (or stomach) at the site of duodenotomy (or gastrotomy).
- A generous longitudinal duodenotomy (or gastrotomy) should then be made.
- The duodenotomy (or gastrotomy) could be extended across the pylorus if the source of bleeding is still unclear.
- Direct finger pressure on the bleeding site will control the haemorrhage and allow the anaesthetist to resuscitate and stabilise the patient.
- Careful lavage of blood and clots with gentle suction will help dislodge clots overlying the bleeding vessel.
- If the bleeding site is not obvious, kocherisation of the duodenum may help.
- Non-absorbable 0 or No. 1 sutures on a medium, round bodied or taper-cut semi-circular needle are used to control the vessel(s) in the base of the ulcer.
- The sutures should be placed with cognisance of the positions of the pancreatic or common bile duct. The pyloroduodenotomy is then closed.
- Large, deep ulcers may require a partial gastrectomy or wedge resection. Under-running of the bleeding ulcer may be appropriate for small Dieulafoy lesion.
- Suture ligation of named vessels (*e.g.* Gastroduodenal artery) may be necessary.

Reconstruction

- The duodenotomy (gastrotomy) is closed.
- A naso-gastric tube should be left *in situ* with the end near the duodenotomy (or gastrotomy).
- The abdomen should be closed.

Post-operative Course

- The patient should be nursed in a high dependency unit with monitoring of vital parameters and adequate analgesia.
- The patient should remain without oral intake for 48 hours. This will allow the duodenotomy (or gastrotomy) to heal.
- The naso-gastric tube should be aspirated regularly and the aspirate inspected.
- Serum amylase and liver enzymes should be checked early.
- The patients should be on a continuous infusion of PPIs.
- All blood parameters should be normalized. Although serum urea may be found elevated due to absorption of blood products from the small bowel, serum creatinine provides a better indication of renal function.
- The naso-gastric tube should be removed as soon as the patient has reached haemodynamic stability.
- *H. pylori* should be eradicated.

Anticipated Complications

- Primary or secondary haemorrhage should necessitate either re-operation if the haemorrhage is profuse or angiographic imaging to determine the source and attempt radiological embolization if less profuse.
- Respiratory infection or compromise should necessitate antibiotics and pulmonary toilet by physiotherapy. Depending on the level of respiratory compromise, additional measures may be necessary such as positive airway pressure (CPAP) or ventilation.
- Leakage from the duodenotomy or gastrotomy should necessitate antibiotics and antifungal agents, cessation of oral intake, drainage and considerations for sealing the leak. This could be done conservatively with a monitoring policy until the site is healed. Alternatively, a self-expanding covered stent could be placed across the leak to provide a scaffold for healing.
- Pancreatitis could occur as a result of pancreatic injury during the ligation. Supportive measures should be instituted for all affected body systems until resolution of the inflammation. Repeated cross sectional imaging is necessary to monitor recovery or untoward further deterioration in the pancreas.
- Abscess formation can occur due to a surgical site infection and manifest in septic deterioration. The site and size of the abscess could be delineated by cross

sectional imaging. Drainage of the septic collection either surgically or radiologically should lead to noticeable improvement.

- Multi-system organ failure can occur as a result of sepsis or large blood transfusions. Broad-spectrum antibiotics should be commenced and the source of sepsis should be identified by cross sectional imaging and managed. All affected body systems should be supported until discernible improvements are achieved.

- Metabolic and nutritional consequences of gastric surgery can be encountered particularly if resection has been undertaken or septic complications intervene. Consideration of enteral or parenteral feeding is essential in these circumstances.

Surgical Repair of Perforated Peptic Ulcer

The incidence of perforation from PUD in the general population (not taking NSAIDs) is about one per 10,000. Perforation leads to peritonitis and patients present with intense abdominal pain. Anterior peptic ulcers perforate more commonly than posterior ulcers, causing generalized chemical peritonitis. If the perforation is diagnosed promptly and treated expediently, the mortality rate is 6% to 14%, with poorer outcomes in patients with advanced age or major illness. In elderly and frail patients, surgical treatment is not possible. In these patients, treatment with antibiotics combined with nasogastric aspiration can lead to spontaneous healing of the perforation in up to 20 of these challenging patients.

The surgical procedure most recommended for gastro- duodenal peptic ulcer perforation is peritoneal lavage and closure of the perforation with omental patch.

Access

- For open surgery, a transverse upper abdominal incision is ideal. However, depending on preference, a midline upper abdominal incision can provide adequate access.

- For laparoscopic surgery, an infra-umbilical port should be used for the endoscope/ camera. A midline sub-xiphisternal port should be used for a liver retractor. Two ports on each side of the abdomen should be used for dissection and retraction.

Exploration

- The procedure should commence with abdominal exploration to determine the extent of peritonitis, the size and position of the perforated ulcer.
- A mechanical retractor should be used to achieve adequate surgical exposure.
- Peritoneal fluid is sent for bacteriology analysis.
- Suction and irrigation peritoneal lavage is performed to reduce contamination

and clarify the site of the perforated ulcer.

Dissection

- An omental patch should be selected and dissected on a vascular pedicle.

Reconstruction

- Representative biopsies of the edge of the ulcer should be obtained.
- Direct closure of the ulcer with several interrupted absorbable sutures.
- The omental patch is laid over the site of closed perforation and sutured in place using several absorbable sutures.
- A naso-gastric tube should be left *in situ* with the end near the site of perforation.
- Peritoneal toilet should be carried out using warm saline solution.
- Abdominal (peritoneal) drains may be left *in situ* depending on the extent of peritonitis.
- The abdomen should be closed.

Post-operative Course

- The patient should be nursed in a high dependency unit with monitoring of vital parameters and adequate analgesia.
- The patient should remain without oral intake for 48 hours. This will allow the ulcer closure to heal.
- The naso-gastric tube should be aspirated regularly and the aspirate inspected.
- The patients should be on a continuous infusion of PPIs.
- Broad-spectrum antibiotics should be prescribed. *H. pylori* status should be checked and appropriate therapy commenced.
- All blood parameters should be normalized. Although serum urea may be found elevated due to absorption of blood products from the small bowel, serum creatinine provides a better indication of renal function.

Anticipated Complications

- Respiratory infection or compromise should necessitate antibiotics and pulmonary toilet by physiotherapy. Depending on the level of respiratory compromise, additional measures may be necessary such as positive airway pressure (CPAP) or ventilation.
- Leakage from the ulcer site should necessitate antibiotics and antifungal agents, cessation of oral intake, drainage and considerations for surgical re-exploration. In very ill patients, this could be done conservatively with a monitoring policy until the leaking site is healed. Alternatively, a self-expanding covered stent could be placed across the leaking site to provide a scaffold for healing.

- Abscess formation can occur due to the preceding peritonitis and manifest in septic deterioration. The site and size of the abscess could be delineated by cross sectional imaging. Drainage of the septic collection either surgically or radiologically should lead to noticeable improvement.
- Multi-system organ failure can occur as a result of sepsis. Broad-spectrum antibiotics should be commenced and the source of sepsis should be identified by cross sectional imaging and managed. All affected body systems should be supported until discernible improvements are achieved.

GASTRIC OUTLET OBSTRUCTION

Gastric outlet obstruction (GOO), also known as pyloric stenosis, is defined as a clinical and pathophysiological consequence of any disease process that produces a mechanical impediment to gastric emptying. It implies complete or incomplete obstruction of the distal stomach, pylorus or proximal duodenum. The most common pathophysiology is intrinsic or extrinsic obstruction of the duodenum or pyloric channel, but the mechanism of obstruction depends on the underlying aetiology.

Epidemiology

Until the late 1970s, benign peptic ulcer disease was responsible for the majority of GOO cases. Better management of peptic ulcer disease (PUD) through pharmacological therapy and the decreasing incidence of *H. pylori* have both contributed to lower the incidence of obstruction caused by PUD. The incidence of GOO has been reported to be between 5% and 12%. In recent decades up to 80 per cent of GOO cases are attributed to malignancy.

Aetiology

Gastric Outlet Obstruction may arise as a result of a heterogeneous group of diseases, which can be benign or malignant. Throughout the world, the most common benign aetiology is PUD but this accounts for 5% of GOO cases. Other benign causes include pyloric stenosis, gastric polyps, pancreatic pseudocysts, ingestion of caustics, congenital duodenal webs, gallstone obstruction of the second part of duodenum (Bouveret syndrome), and bezoars. Other benign causes include inflammatory conditions such as NSAID induced strictures, pancreatitis, cholecystitis, benign tumours including adenomas, lipomas and stromal tumours and post-surgical scarring in patients who had previous surgery. In children, pyloric stenosis is the most important cause of GOO. Pyloric stenosis occurs in 1 per 750 births, is more common in boys than in girls and is more common in first-born children. Pyloric stenosis usually arises as a result of gradual hypertrophy of the pyloric ring circular smooth muscle.

In PUD, ulcers within the pyloric channel and first portion of the duodenum are usually responsible for obstruction of the stomach outlet. Obstruction can occur in the acute setting secondary to acute inflammation and oedema around a mucosal injury or, more commonly, in a chronic setting secondary to gradual scarring and fibrosis.

Malignant causes of GOO account for 60% of cases and include primary cancers from the stomach, pancreas, bile duct or colon. Pancreatic cancer is the commonest malignancy causing GOO and occurs in 10-20% of patients with pancreatic cancer. Other local tumours, which may obstruct the stomach outlet, include ampullary cancer, cholangiocarcinomas, duodenal and gastric cancer. Other distant tumours may also metastasise to the stomach and cause obstruction.

Pathophysiology

The usual pathophysiology of GOO requires Intrinsic or extrinsic obstruction of the pyloric channel or proximal duodenum. The mechanism of obstruction and clinical manifestation depends on the underlying cause. Persistent obstruction leads to gastric hypertrophy and dilatation with subsequent gastritis and reduced acid secretion. The stomach eventually loses its contractility. Undigested food accumulates, regurgitated or vomited and may represent a constant risk for aspiration pneumonia.

Presentation and Clinical Features

The onset of symptoms varies, depending upon the aetiology of the obstruction. Patients present with intermittent symptoms that progress until obstruction is complete. Persistent nausea and non-bilious vomiting are the cardinal symptom of GOO. Although commonly not reported by patients, the presence of recognizable food more than 8-12 hours after eating is indicative of gastric retention. In the early stages it may be intermittent and usually occurs within one hour of ingestion of a meal. Weight loss and malnutrition are usually reported and indicative of chronicity. In the acute or chronic phase of obstruction, continuous vomiting may lead to dehydration and electrolyte abnormalities. Patients also tend to complain of bloating, epigastric fullness and pain. On examination, some patients are found to have a succession splash and / or an epigastric mass. Patients with GOO resulting from incomplete obstruction, typically present with symptoms of gastric retention, including early satiety and bloating. Dehydration and metabolic insufficiency tend to result if GOO goes untreated for a significant period.

Diagnosis

Clinical examination may reveal a dilated stomach demonstrated as a tympanic fullness or mass in the upper abdomen. The patient may have a succession splash reflective of retained gastric material.

Laboratory studies may document anaemia and liver function tests may be elevated as part of the malignant spectrum. Dehydration and electrolyte abnormalities can be evaluated by routine laboratory tests on serum samples. Increases in blood urea nitrogen (BUN) and creatinine are usually late features of dehydration. *H. pylori* tests may be positive and help to raise the clinical suspicion of PUD aetiology.

Repeat vomiting over a long period causes loss of hydrochloric acid and produces an increase of bicarbonates in the plasma to compensate for the lost chloride and sodium (metabolic alkalosis). Alkalosis shifts the intracellular potassium to the extracellular compartment, and the serum positive potassium is increased factitiously. The result is a hypokalaemic hypochloraemic metabolic alkalosis. With continued vomiting, the renal excretion of potassium increases in order to preserve sodium. The adrenocortical response to hypovolaemia intensifies the exchange of potassium for sodium at the distal renal tubules, with subsequent aggravation of the hypokalaemia.

Plain abdominal radiography may show an enlarged gastric bubble. A calcified pancreas or a large gallstone may be evident in the duodenum. Contrast studies including gastrografin or barium studies may be helpful in elucidating the aetiology. CT with oral contrast can have the added benefit of detailing the pyloric or gastric wall thickness, lymph nodes or pancreatic lesion not visualized on routine imaging.

Upper GI endoscopy is essential to visualize the gastric lumen with the added advantage of providing representative tissue biopsies from an obstructing lesion. In cases of GOO, the stomach is usually full of undigested food debris. In order to increase the diagnostic yield, patients with GOO should have gastric lavage and food abstinence prior to endoscopy.

Medical Management

Patients with persistent or severe symptoms of GOO warrant hospital admission. These patients can be malnourished, dehydrated and with significant electrolyte abnormalities. Urgent cautious administration of intravenous fluids is used for intravenous volume resuscitation and to correct electrolyte disturbances. The metabolic alkalosis of GOO responds to the administration of sodium chloride. Potassium deficits should be corrected after rehydration and after replacement of chloride. Parenteral feeding is indicated in malnourished patients and patients assessed at risk of malnutrition. Gastric lavage *via* NG tube is essential to reduce the risk of aspiration and reduce gastric distension. It is also important prior to diagnostic endoscopy. GOO due to benign ulcer disease may be treated medically if results of imaging studies or endoscopy determine that acute inflammation and oedema are the principal causes of the outlet obstruction. Intravenous proton pump inhibitor will help to relieve pain in patients with oedema and spasm. Nitrogen Urea breath test should be done to detect *H. Pylori*. If positive, the infection should be treated. Approximately 50% of patients with GOO attributed to PUD will respond to this regimen. Refractory cases, with fibrotic scarring, will require definitive treatment with endoscopic balloon dilatation or surgical management.

Endoscopic Therapy

Endoscopic therapy has reduced the number of patients with GOO needing to undergo larger and more invasive surgical procedures. This is particularly important in patients with advanced malignancy who develop GOO as one of the manifestations. It is also useful for benign disease and is recommended as a first-line therapy. Pneumatic balloon dilatation gives the best results with single short benign strictures. The use of self-expandable metal stents to treat malignant gastric outlet obstructions in appropriate patients has been an effective alternative to surgical bypass with lower morbidity and mortality rates, shorter hospitalization, and a lower overall cost of the treatment. This is particularly so for palliative therapy. Endoscopic snare polypectomy can also alleviate intermittent obstruction by a polyp. Endoscopic drainage of a large pancreatic pseudocyst is indicated in cases of obstruction.

Pneumatic Balloon Dilatation

This can increase the diameter of the stenotic pylorus from 6 to 16 mm. Success rates are increased if eradication of an underlying *H. pylori* infection was commenced before the dilatation procedure. Those patients who require more than two dilatations are at higher risk of re-stenosis and the need for surgical intervention should be considered early. Patients should fast for at least four hours before the procedure and in severe GOO nasogastric tube lavage is recommended before endoscopy. A liquid diet 24 hours prior to the fasting period also facilitates optimal views.

A through the scope (TTS) balloon is ideal for negotiating the strictured pylorus. Alternatively, over the wire (OTW) balloons could be used over a previously inserted guide wire. Incremental dilatations with increasing diameter are preferable and safer than a single dilatation particularly for severe strictures.

Immediately after the procedure the patient should be monitored for signs and symptoms of perforation and bleeding for 4-6 hours. In patients with a suspected perforation a water-soluble contrast study should be carried out immediately. Bleeding, perforation and self-limiting pain are uncommon complications of endoscopic balloon dilatation.

Endoscopic Stenting

In patients with limited life expectancy, self-expanding metallic stents provide an excellent palliative measure for several reasons. It can be carried out with minimal hospital stay, is relatively cost-effective compared to surgery, has high clinical success rates, relatively safe in the short and long term and allows rapid resumption of oral intake compared with surgical gastro-jejunostomy.

The procedure is done under sedation or general anaesthesia. The facility for endoscopy and fluoroscopy should be available. An upper GI endoscopy is performed to confirm the nature and site of obstruction. A biliary catheter and a floppy guide-wire are used to negotiate the stricture and contrast is injected under fluoroscopic control to assess the length and extent of the stricture. The endoscope is withdrawn leaving the biliary catheter across the stricture. The stent delivery assembly is passed over the guide-wire, and deployed under fluoroscopy.

A range of stents can be used but most centres prefer uncovered or partially covered stents as they are less likely to migrate. Technical success of deployment in most series is well above 90% with early resumption of oral intake. However, stent migration is reported in up to 15% of cases and stent blockage is reported in 20% of cases. Stent blockage is due to tumour in growth in most cases. Partially covered stents tend to migrate less and stent patency duration is usually close to patients' survival duration.

Surgical Management

The primary treatment for infants with pyloric stenosis is with a surgical pyloromyotomy. Adult patients with benign causes of GOO who did not respond to medical or endoscopic management should be evaluated for surgery. The management of GOO secondary to malignancy is more controversial. Resectable tumours should be considered for curative surgical treatment pathways. Patients with unresectable tumours should be considered on an individual basis. In these cases, in which life expectancy may be limited to a few months, palliation *via* endoscopically placed stents should be considered. When this is not possible, gastrojejunostomy is the surgical treatment of choice. This may be followed with oncological treatment. Patients with advanced malignancy and less than 4 weeks expected survival should be offered supportive care.

Open surgery has traditionally been used for surgical management of GOO. However, expertise in laparoscopic surgery has increased substantially. It represents a valid form of therapy with low morbidity, short hospital stays and early discharge from hospital. Laparoscopic procedures for both benign and malignant causes of GOO are in current practice in tertiary referral centres.

Prior to surgery, dehydration, electrolyte abnormalities and malnutrition should be corrected expeditiously. Nasogastric lavage should be carried out to reduce gastric distension with undigested food material. Insertion of a feeding jejunostomy tube at the time of surgery should be considered. This provides access for temporary post-operative feeding in already malnourished patients. In addition, in chronically dilated partial obstructions, the stomach may be slow to recover a normal rate of emptying.

Surgical Procedures

Numerous surgical procedures have traditionally been described to manage GOO. There are no published data that prove which procedure achieves the best results and the choice of surgical procedure depends on the patient's particular circumstances and intraoperative findings. However, with the decline in incidence of peptic ulcer disease (and its complications) and the proven safety and efficacy of PPIs, the use of these surgical procedures have declined considerably.

For peptic strictures the pylorus is usually too scarred or oedematous to consider a pyloroplasty. Under these circumstances the Jaboulay procedure can be considered. Other types of surgical procedures described for peptic strictures include antrectomy and gastrojejunostomy. Laparoscopic gastrojejunostomy with or without truncal vagotomy benefits the patient with decreased hospital stay, less operative pain and shorter recovery period. Gastrojejunostomy (Billroth II reconstruction) can be considered in patients with preserved anatomy like peptic GOO, however if the duodenum is considered unsafe for an anastomosis, a Roux-en-Y loop may be indicated.

Pyloroplasty

Pyloroplasty is a surgical procedure that was developed since the nineteenth century and has been widely used to treat patients with gastric outlet obstruction or delayed gastric emptying. The surgical procedure aims to divide the pyloric sphincter or render it inoperative. This facilitates gastric emptying. The pyloroplasty ensures drainage of the gastric antrum and partially eliminates the antral phase of gastric digestion and retention. Two types of pyloroplasty are commonly used: The Heineke-Mikulicz pyloroplasty and the Finney pyloroplasty. Pyloroplasty should be avoided in the presence of a marked inflammatory reaction or severe scarring and deformity on the duodenal side of the pylorus. Under these circumstances the Jaboulay procedure should be considered. Alternatively, a gastroenterostomy located within 3 cm of the pylorus on the greater curvature could be formed. The Jaboulay reconstruction should be considered when a long incision is made in the anterior wall of the duodenum as part of another surgical procedure such as control of bleeding.

Heineke-Mikulicz Pyloroplasty

The standard procedure, devised by Heinike and Mikulicz involves making a 6 cm longitudinal linear incision through the deep muscle of the pylorus, extending from the stomach into the duodenum (Fig. 3). The incision is then closed with sutures running transversely to leave a large open orifice at the pylorus and to render the pyloric valve incompetent.

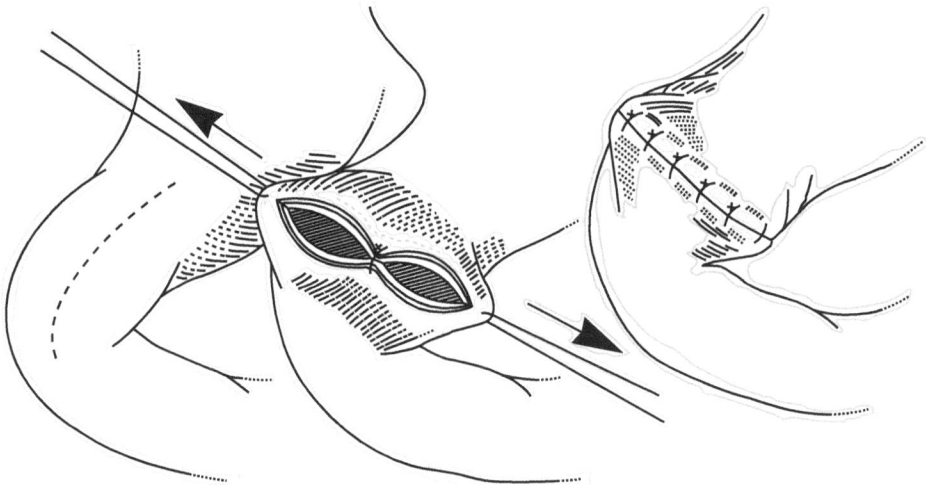

Fig. (3). Heineke-Mikulicz pyloroplasty.

Finney's Pyloroplasty

This is essentially a gastro-duodenostomy with division of the pylorus. Currently, it is rarely performed, however it is still a possible option when scarring of the pylorus is severe. However, in these circumstances most surgeons would opt for a gastroenterostomy.

The incision of the pyloric area is extended onto the antrum and first part of the duodenum. The duodenum should be fully Kocherized and partially detached from the gastro-hepatic ligament to facilitate the descending duodenum being laid alongside the greater curvature of the distal antrum. The greater curve of the prepyloric antrum is attached to the adjacent duodenum with interrupted seromuscular sutures. A u-shaped incision is then made into the stomach through the antrum, pylorus and first part of the duodenum (Fig. **4**). The posterior mucosal septum between the stomach and duodenum is then sutured with a continuous full-thickness suture. Closure of the remaining anterior defect can then be performed with a single row of seromuscular sutures.

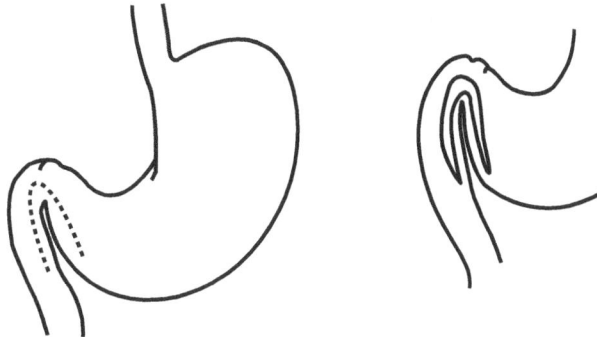

Fig. (4). Finney pyloroplasty.

Jaboulay Pyloroplasty

This procedure is essentially a side-to-side gastro-duodenostomy between the anterior surfaces of the stomach and duodenum. Strictly speaking, it is not a true pyloroplasty since the pylorus is not divided (Fig. **5**).

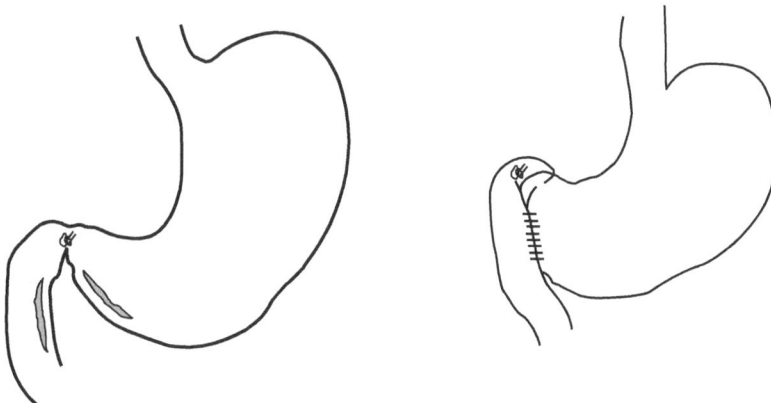

Fig. (5). Jaboulay pyloroplasty.

Antrectomy

Antrectomy (distal gastrectomy) is a procedure in which the distal gastrin-secreting portion of the stomach (antrum) is surgically removed. These procedures were traditionally described for the treatment of peptic ulcers and its complications. With the decline in incidence of peptic ulcers and the proven efficacy and safety of anti-secretory agents, the use of antrectomy has declined considerably. Today, there is no indication for antrectomy in uncomplicated peptic ulcer disease. Antrectomy is indicated in the treatment of gastric ulcers that are (a) refractory to medical therapy; (b) large ulcers complicated by perforation, bleeding, or obstruction; or (c) recurrent after adequate treatment of *H. pylori.*

Gastrectomies are classified by the type of reconstruction used to re-establish gastrointestinal (GI) continuity. A Billroth I procedure is a gastro-duodenostomy, which can be fashioned end-to-end or end-to-side. A Billroth II or gastrojejunostomy reconstruction is usually fashioned end-to-side. Alternatively, a Roux-en-Y gastrojejunostomy can be performed.

Access

- For open surgery, a transverse upper abdominal incision is ideal. However, depending on preference, a midline upper abdominal incision can provide adequate access.
- For laparoscopic surgery, an infra-umbilical port should be used for the endoscope/ camera. A midline sub-xiphisternal port should be used for a liver retractor. Two ports on each side of the abdomen should be used for dissection and retraction.

Exploration

- The procedure should commence with abdominal exploration to determine the site and size of the ulcer.
- A mechanical retractor should be used to achieve adequate surgical exposure.

Dissection

- The greater omentum should be detached from the distal stomach.
- The right gastroepiploic artery and vein are ligated and divided.
- The lesser omentum is then incised in its avascular plane.
- The right gastric artery and vein as well as the pancreatico-duodenal vein and artery are ligated and divided.
- The duodenum is Kocherised and mobilised in order to reduce tension on the anastomosis.

Resection

- The clamped duodenum and stomach are transected at the predetermined resection line.

- The stomach is then closed in two layers starting at the level of the lesser curvature leaving an opening of sufficient calibre for the gastroduodenal or gastrojejunal anastomosis.

Reconstruction

In *Billroth I reconstruction*, the stomach remnant after antrectomy is anastomosed directly to the duodenum either end to end or end to side. The rationale of this reconstruction is the restoration of normal gastrointestinal anatomy with duodenal transit of food. However, Prior duodenal surgery precludes a Billroth I reconstruction, as does a "woody," inflamed, or ulcerated duodenum, which makes a secure anastomosis unlikely.

In *Billroth II (Polya) reconstruction*, a side-to-side anastomosis of the greater curvature of the remnant stomach is made to the proximal jejunum (gastrojejunostomy). The jejunal loop can be brought either behind the transverse colon (retrocolic) or in front of it (antecolic). The jejunum orientation in the anastomosis is usually pro-peristaltic but it can be anti-peristaltic. This reconstruction is less physiological but avoids anastomosis to the duodenum, which is scarred.

In *Roux-en-Y gastrojejunostomy* reconstruction, the proximal end of the jejunum (15 cm from the ligament of Treitz) is transected (usually with a mechanical stapler). The distal limb is brought through the transverse mesocolon (retrocolic) to the supra-colic compartment and anastomosed side to side to the greater curvature of the gastric remnant (gastroenterostomy). The proximal jejunal limb (alimentary limb) is anastomosed to the distal jejunum 50 cm from the gastroenterostomy.

Anticipated Complications

Regardless of the reconstruction technique used, the common complications after antrectomy include anastomotic leaks, gastric outlet obstruction, recurrent ulcer disease, duodenal stump blow out, dumping syndrome, reflux gastritis, afferent or efferent loop syndromes and Roux stasis syndrome. A number of metabolic sequel have also been described after antrectomy. Explosive diarrhoea can also be disabling in a number of patients. Although a number of remedies have been suggested, patients should be warned about the propensity of the complications before surgery.

UPPER GI BLEEDING (NON-VARICEAL)

Gastrointestinal bleeding is among the most common causes of emergency admissions to hospital. It is associated with high diagnosis and treatment costs and has a hospital mortality of around 10%. The main reason for death remains poorly tolerated shock, with destabilisation of underlying cardiopulmonary, liver or renal disease. Patients who have an upper GI bleed while already in hospital for a different morbidity have a higher rate of mortality. Although several reasons have been hypothesised for this, the exact cause is not clear. Non-variceal bleeding of the upper gastrointestinal tract is common and usually stops spontaneously in a large proportion of these patients. However, recurrent bleeding is the most important cause of mortality and morbidity [13]. The source of bleeding is not demonstrated in approximately 4-9% of cases presenting with massive upper gastrointestinal haemorrhage. Bleeding can arise from a variety of lesions in the upper gastrointestinal tract (Table **3**).

Table 3. Common sources of bleeding in the upper gastro-intestinal tract.

Source of Bleeding	Frequency
Duodenal ulcers	20 - 30%
Gastric or duodenal erosions	20 - 30%
Varices	15 - 20%
Gastric ulcers	10 – 20%
Mallory Weiss Tear	5 – 10%
Erosive oesophagitis	5 – 10%
Angiomas	5 – 10%
Arterio-venous malformations	< 5%
Gastro-intestinal stromal tumours	< 5%

Bleeding is more likely, and potentially more severe, in patients with chronic liver disease, those with hereditary coagulation disorders, or in patients taking certain pharmaceutical agents. Drugs associated with GI bleeding include anticoagulants (*e.g*, heparin, warfarin, rivaroxaban), those affecting platelet function (*e.g*, aspirin and certain other NSAIDs, clopidogrel, dipyridamole, SSRIs), and those reducing mucosal defences (*e.g*, NSAIDs).

Evaluation and Management of the Bleeding Patient

The initial assessment of the patient presenting with an upper GI haemorrhage should include assessment of **a**irway patency, **b**reathing and oxygenation, **c**irculatory parameters (pulse, blood pressure and urinary output), **d**isability including comorbidities, and **e**xamination of stigmata of liver disease or undue abdominal tenderness. History of the presentation should focus on the quantity and quality of vomited blood, alcohol intake, drug usage and comorbidities. The patient should be resuscitated promptly and proportionately in accord with the initial assessment. Blood should be transfused if the haemoglobin level drops below 70 g/L. Additional blood products (platelets, fresh frozen plasma or prothrombin complex) should be transfused according to local guidelines. Although controversial, most centres recommend intravenous PPI therapy but stress that their use should not delay endoscopy [14].

Re-bleeding is associated with a 10-fold increase in hospital mortality. At presentation with acute upper gastrointestinal haemorrhage, it is crucial to risk stratify patients. Those at high risk of continuing bleeding or re-bleeding need intensive monitoring and early endoscopic intervention, whereas low-risk patients can be discharged home safely. Several risk stratification systems have been reported. The scoring systems represent a simplified summary of the results of multi-variant analysis and include clinical and/ or endoscopic variables each categorised and scored with 0–6 points, to indicate the risk of intervention requirement.

The Blatchford score [15] is ideal to risk-stratify patients on initial presentation (Table **4**). The Rockall score can also be used but requires endoscopic findings before it is completed [16]. Patients with a Blatchford score of 0 are considered at low-risk and are suitable for discharge and outpatient management. After endoscopy and completion of Rockall score (Table **5**), patients with a low score (<3) could be discharged home while patients with higher scores should be monitored for risk of rebleeding.

Table 4. Blatchford score [15].

Admission Risk Marker	Score Component Value
Blood urea (mmol/L)	
≥6.5 <8.0	2
≥8.0 <10.0	3
≥10.0 <25.0	4
≥25	6
Haemoglobin (g/L) for men	
≥12.0 <13.0	1
≥10.0 <12.0	3
<10.0	6
Haemoglobin (g/L) for women	
≥10.0 <12.0	1

(Table 4) contd.....

Admission Risk Marker	Score Component Value
<10.0	6
Systolic blood pressure (mm Hg)	
100–109	1
90–99	2
<90	3
Other markers	
Pulse ≥100 (per min)	1
Presentation with melaena	1
Presentation with syncope	2
Hepatic disease	2
Cardiac failure	2

Table 5. Rockall risk assessment system [16].

	Score			
Variable	*0*	*1*	*2*	*3*
Age (years)	<60	60–79	≥80	
Shock	"No shock": pulse <100 + systolic BP≥100 mm Hg	"Tachycardia": pulse ≥100 + systolic BP ≥100 mm Hg	"Hypotension": systolic BP <100 mm Hg	
Comorbidity	No major comorbidity		Cardiac failure, ischaemic heart disease, any major comorbidity	Renal failure, liver failure, disseminated malignancy
Diagnosis	Mallory Weiss tear, no lesion identified and no SRH/blood	All other diagnoses	Malignancy of upper GI tract	
Major SRH	None or dark spot only		Blood in upper GI tract, adherent clot, visible or spurting vessel	

Major SRH, major stigmata of recent haemorrhage (active bleeding or visible vessel); GI, gastrointestinal; BP, blood pressure.

Endoscopy provides important prognostic information. Those with low-risk lesions such as a non-bleeding Mallory–Weiss tear, an ulcer with a clean-base or with a pigmented spot in the base can be identified for early discharge. Alternatively, those with blood in the upper gastrointestinal tract, active spurting haemorrhage and a 'non-bleeding visible vessel' can be identified for urgent endoscopy with a planned intervention to reduce the chance of further bleeding.

Active ulcer bleeding infers an 80–90% risk of continuing haemorrhage or re-bleeding. A visible vessel (representing adherent blood clot or a pseudo-aneurysm over the arterial defect) is associated with a 50% risk of re-bleeding during the same hospital admission.

In order to stop and prevent further bleeding, a range of endoscopic techniques may be used. These include injection, thermo-ablative and mechanical therapies. Dual therapy is also possible and useful, for example, adrenaline injection around the bleeding point followed by coagulation therapy or clip application to the visible vessel. Topical haemostatic powders can also be used in upper GI bleeding in selected cases, for example, in those where active bleeding is present and dual therapy is not possible or has failed. Topical therapies include Hemospray, Endoclot and Blood Stopper.

If the initial endoscopic treatment was considered to be suboptimal or the risk of rebleeding is estimated high or potentially life-threatening a repeat endoscopy should be recommended as this reduces rebleeding rate. In those patients where endoscopic therapy has failed to control the bleeding, the remaining options include interventional radiology for angiographic embolisation or surgery. The same options can also be considered for patients who rebleed after dual endoscopic therapy.

After endoscopy, patients at high risk of rebleeding should continue with intravenous high dose PPI therapy. All other patients can switch to oral PPI therapy depending on the endoscopic findings. *H. pylori* positive patients should be prescribed triple or quadruple regimen eradication therapy in accord with local guidelines.

Bleeding Lesions in the Stomach

The commonest causes of massive upper GI bleeding are gastro-duodenal ulcers and erosions and varices. These will be discussed thoroughly elsewhere. However, there are a number of other important lesions in the stomach, which can cause significant upper GI bleeding (Table **3**).

Mallory-Weiss Tears

These occur as a laceration in the mucus membrane at the oesophago-gastric junction and are due to prolonged retching, vomiting or coughing. Alcohol abuse is the usual cause, but other causes of nausea and vomiting (*e.g.* chemotherapy, digoxin toxicity, renal failure, advanced malignancy) may be responsible. They can occur as an iatrogenic adverse event during upper gastrointestinal endoscopic procedures or naso-gastric intubation. Irrespective of the aetiology, MWTs are most frequently found in the lesser curvature of the stomach and the right lateral wall (2- to 4-o'clock position) of the oesophagus. They are a common cause of non-variceal gastrointestinal bleeding. In most cases, the bleeding usually stops spontaneously and active endoscopic or surgical intervention is seldom required. The tear usually heals in a few days without treatment.

Gastric Antral Vascular Ectasia (Watermelon Stomach or GAVE)

This is a rare disorder characterised by upper GI bleeding, chronic iron-deficiency anaemia and endoscopic findings of large dilated veins located at the crests of the mucosal folds running longitudinally along the antrum of the stomach, creating a striped appearance suggestive of a watermelon. The second most common form is a 'honeycomb stomach' characterized by diffuse red spots and the coalescence of many angiodyplastic lesions in the antrum. A third endoscopic form presents as a mushroom shaped lesion formed by a tuft of ectatic blood vessels. It has been reported that patients with cirrhosis are more inclined to have a punctate type appearance and those without cirrhosis present more commonly with the striped macroscopic appearance [17].

Gastric antral vascular ectasia (GAVE) accounts for 4% of non-variceal upper GI bleeding. The condition occurs mainly in older women and is of unknown aetiology. Vascular ectasia can also be found in other areas of the GI tract including the gastric cardia, duodenum, jejunum and rectum. Biopsies confirm diagnosis in 85% of cases.

The aetiology of GAVE is not yet fully understood. GAVE is however most commonly associated with autoimmune disorders. It is also associated with a number of conditions including chronic kidney failure and collagen vascular diseases. The causal connection between cirrhosis and GAVE has not been established. Female sex and old age are also risk factors. Although GAVE has not previously been reported in association with gastric cancer, it is often associated with atrophic gastritis and pernicious anaemia, which are known risk factors for gastric malignancy. Various drugs including corticosteroids, octreotide, hormone therapy and tranexamic acid have been used to stop recurrent bleeds from GAVE but success has been variable and not consistently significant to consider medical therapy as a valid therapeutic option.

Endoscopic therapy is the mainstay of treatment for GAVE and has shown a safety and efficacy profile similar to that of surgery. However, repeated sessions are often necessary. Endoscopic coagulation with an argon plasma coagulator, bipolar probe, or heater probe obliterates the vascular ectasia and reduces the bleeding. Endoscopic band ligation has decreased recurrent bleed rates compared with endoscopic coagulation. Endoscopic laser therapy can also be used however post procedure complications are not infrequent and two weeks after almost all laser sessions a gastric ulcer is frequently observed. Gastric perforation is another reported complication and pyloric stenosis and gastric polyps may occur with repeated laser sessions.

Although endoscopic treatment is an effective treatment for GAVE, surgical antrectomy is a reliable curative treatment. Antrectomy is by far the most commonly used surgical procedure to treat GAVE but other surgical treatments include total and subtotal gastrectomy with Billroth II anastomosis, antrectomy with or without vagotomy and partial gastrectomy with Roux-en-Y reconstruction. Surgery however is associated with significant morbidity and mortality. In general, the surgical approach should be reserved for those who do not respond to endoscopic therapy or those with widespread lesions.

Dieulafoy Lesion (DL)

This is an abnormally large tortuous arteriole that runs within the gastric submucosa and penetrates the wall, occasionally eroding through a minute mucosal defect and causing massive bleeding. It occurs mainly in the proximal stomach within 6 cm of the gastroesophageal junction but can present in any part of the GI tract. Gastric haemorrhage is relatively uncommon and it is thought to cause less than 2% of all gastrointestinal bleeds in adults. However, bleeding from DL can be life threatening as it is often massive and recurrent.

Dieulafoy lesions are thought to be congenital vascular malformations and are most frequently found in the stomach but there have been cases of DLs presenting in the duodenum, colon, jejunum and oesophagus. DLs are twice as common in men than in women and mostly present in the fifth decade of life. There is a suggestion that these lesions may be part of the spectrum of congenital vascular malformations and cases of DL have been reported in new-born infants.

Patients present with an acute GI haemorrhage in the form of melena, haematemesis, hematochezia or iron deficiency anaemia. As there is no surrounding mucosal inflammation on endoscopy, this lesion may be easily missed. Unlike peptic ulceration DLs tends to be clinically silent unless actively bleeding. The lack of clinical suspicion and silent nature of the lesions prior to severe bleeding make the Dieulafoy lesion potentially fatal. A high proportion of patients present with haemodynamic instability and the reported mortality rate can be as high as 80%.

Endoscopic diagnosis can be challenging for several reasons. There is no surrounding mucosal inflammation, the bleeding is often recurrent and intermittent and may not be active at the time of endoscopy. With massive bleeding, the stomach can quickly fill up with blood and obscure views. As the lesion is subtle it may be easily overlooked.

Angiography and contrast enhanced CT in experienced hands are two useful modalities for detecting DLs missed at endoscopy. In the case of angiography, this procedure also offers treatment in the form of embolization. However, the lesion can only be detected if it is actively bleeding [18].

A normal artery of the GI tract usually narrows progressively as it courses along the wall of the end organ distally. In DLs the artery maintains its calibre without narrowing. The abnormally large diameter of the artery can range from 1- 3 mm and importantly there is no evidence of inflammation at the edge of the mucosal defect. The mechanism of final rupture is uncertain but may be due to necrosis of the vessel wall induced by chronic gastritis.

Endoscopic therapy is however the definitive treatment for DL and the reported success rate is in excess of 75% of detected lesions. Endoscopic haemostasis can be achieved with heater probe coagulation, sclerotherapy, mechanical banding or clipping [19]. Angiography can be used to embolise the vessel. However, a vessel supplied with multiple collaterals requires extensive embolization, which can result in ischaemic necrosis of the area supplied by the vessel.

Advances in endoscopic procedures have minimized the need for surgical resection. Surgery in the form of under running of the vessel or wedge gastrectomy is rarely performed for this lesion. Cases managed by laparoscopic trans-gastric resection have been reported. However, the procedure relies on accurate localization of the bleeding lesion, which can be challenging in laparoscopic cases. Currently surgical management accounts for approximately 5% of cases that are refractory to endoscopic or angiographic methods.

Hereditary Haemorrhagic Telangiectasia (HHT) (Rendu-Osler-Weber Syndrome)

This is an autosomal dominant disorder, which is characterized by the presence of multiple arteriovenous malformations (AVMs). There is a lack of intervening capillaries, which results in direct connections between arteries and veins. In most affected individuals the features are age-dependent and the diagnosis is not usually suspected until adolescence or in later adult life. Small AVMs (or telangiectasia) subcutaneous or on mucous membranes often rupture and bleed after insignificant trauma. The most common clinical manifestation is spontaneous and recurrent nosebleeds (epistaxis) beginning on average at a young age (around 12 years). Approximately 25% of affected individuals present with GI bleed, which commonly begins later in adult life (age 50 years). GI bleeding is usually treated with resuscitation, iron replacement therapy and in virtually all cases, endoscopic ablation. Surgical resection of bleeding sites is rarely required.

Gastric Haemangioma

This is a rare tumour, which is usually found in the gastric antrum. It was first described by Lammers in 1893. It accounts for approximately 1.7% of all gastric benign tumours and for 5% of cases of haemorrhage of unknown aetiology. Cavernous haemangiomas are congenital, benign development abnormalities. These tumours are composed of large dilated blood vessels which contain large blood-filled spaces that are caused by dilation and thickening of the walls of the intervening capillary loops. The thin walled blood vessels are prone to rupture in gastric cavernous haemangiomas (GCH) with rapid blood loss. Most GI haemangiomas are of the cavernous type and upper gastrointestinal bleeding is the commonest presenting symptom. Emergency endoscopy is used for both diagnosis and treatment. The lesions may be found incidentally on CT or MRI carried out for other reasons. The lesion appears either as enhancing linear blood vessels or caputmedusae. However, GCH may be misdiagnosed as a stromal tumour. Surgical resection is the definitive treatment, and recurrence following complete resection is virtually unknown.

Portal Hypertensive Gastropathy (PHG)

By definition, PHG requires the presence of portal hypertension. The gastric appearances found on endoscopy correspond with macroscopic changes of the stomach associated with mucosal and submucosal venous dilation with ectatic capillaries. PGH occurs in up to 65% of patients with portal hypertension from hepatic cirrhosis but it can also occur in the setting of non-cirrhotic portal hypertension. In patients with portal hypertension, PHG is often associated with the presence of oesophageal and/or gastric varices. In the setting of cirrhosis, GAVE syndrome can be difficult to differentiate from PHG. This distinction is important therapeutically in that PHG generally responds to a reduction in portal pressures whereas those with GAVE syndrome and coexisting portal hypertension generally do not respond to such therapy.

Approximately 65–90% of patients with hepatic cirrhosis and portal hypertension have mild PHG whereas 10–25% of patients have severe PHG. The likelihood of developing PHG is thought to be dependent on the cause of portal hypertension and the severity of liver disease. In general, patients who develop PHG have more severe liver disease, and PHG can be a marker of more severe liver disease in patients with cirrhosis. However, PHG can occur in patients who do not have cirrhosis. PHG may also be a predictor of variceal haemorrhage. Bleeding from PHG is uncommon (acute bleeding in 2.5% and chronic blood loss in 10.8%) and bleeding related mortality is lower for PHG than for variceal bleeding (12.5%v 39.1%).

In patients, with PHG there is an increased susceptibility to gastric damage. More specifically, an increased susceptibility to NSAIDs drug induced damage. The role of prostaglandins in the development of PHG is uncertain. However, a reduction in prostaglandins by inhibitors causes increased gastric damage. It makes sense to avoid PG inhibitors in these patients.

The total gastric blood flow is increased in PHG. However, there may be a change in the distribution of gastric blood flow. Other defects in the gastric mucosal defences have been described, such as a decreased gastric mucus layer. *Helicobacter pylori* is not involved in the pathogenesis of this pathological entity.

The diagnosis of PHG is made by endoscopy. Four elementary lesions are described: mosaic-like pattern, red point lesions, cherry red spots, and black-brown spots. In mild PHG the gastric mucosa often looks reddened and oedematous with a snakeskin or mosaic pattern. The term scarlatina has also been used to describe the early changes of PHG. Severe PHG is defined by cherry red spots, which are typically very friable and can actively bleed during endoscopy. In PHG, changes in the gastric mucosa and potential bleeding are usually localised to the fundus or gastric body.

Management of PHG is focused on reduction in portal pressure, through the use of systemic pharmaceutical agents. The most important pharmacotherapy for PHG involves the use of β blockers. To reduce portal pressures, particularly for patients with chronic GI bleeding due to PHG, non-selective beta-blockers are first line treatment. Although there are obvious drawbacks to beta-blocker therapy in the acute setting, studies have shown resolution of acute PHG bleeding within 3 days, highlighting their important role for the management of acute as well as chronic PGH bleeding.

Traditionally, surgical porto-caval shunts have been used as means of controlling PHG and associated bleeding. Laterally, interventional radiological procedures have taken a more prominent role in creating transjugular intrahepatic porto-systemic shunting (TIPS). Both mild and severe forms of portal gastropathy improve TIPS with associated reduction in bleeding. TIPS can also be used for the emergency treatment of bleeding in appropriate settings. For those patients with refractory bleeding who are not appropriate candidates for porto-systemic shunting, endoscopic thermal coagulation therapy may be efficacious at least in the short term. Oesophagectomy and total gastrectomy have also been described on patients with uncontrollable PHG and variceal bleeding with considerable mortality. Liver transplantation ultimately reverses portal hypertension and therefore effectively treats PHG.

ACUTE GASTRIC DILATATION

Acute gastric dilation (AGD) leading to ischemia of the stomach can be under-diagnosed and lead to a potentially fatal event. Duplay first described the condition in 1833. It can result from a multitude of conditions including eating disorders, medications, trauma and trauma resuscitation but is most frequently reported as a postoperative complication. Induced aerophagia or rapid consumption of a large volume of fluids without the ability to vent the stomach results in AGD. Although several theories of pathogenesis have been postulated, the pathophysiology is still not fully understood. Without proper and timely diagnosis and treatment, gastric perforation, haemorrhage, and other serious complications can occur. A major, albeit rare, complication of acute gastric dilatation is gastric necrosis. Early recognition, diagnosis and treatment of this complication are essential to minimize morbidity and mortality [20].

Presentation and Clinical Features

Symptoms of acute gastric dilation can initially be vague but typically progress to abdominal distension and tenderness. Pain is often mild in contrast to the massively distended abdomen. More than 90% of patients present with emesis but if the gastroesophageal junction is occluded by a distended / distorted fundus then the patient may be unable to vomit. In severe cases, the patient can present with aspiration pneumonia, peritonitis from gastric rupture or may present with ascites, alkalosis and shock. Submucosal tears can present with haematemesis. Physical examination may reveal a tympanic epigastric region and left upper quadrant with a succession splash emanating from the distended stomach. The dilated stomach may be seen on radiographic images to occupy the whole abdomen. Patients may manifest with evidence of hypovolaemia due to fluid sequestration in the stomach and hypokalemic alkalosis is found on serum biochemistry.

Complications

Necrosis and gastric perforation are complications of delayed diagnosis [21]. Other complications include gastric mucosal tears, upper gastrointestinal bleeding and peritonitis. Cardiogenic shock, hypovolaemia, respiratory failure and pulmonary aspiration are also recognised complications of AGD.

Pathophysiology

The pathophysiology of acute gastric dilatation is not clear. However, the pathophysiology of the sequel is more apparent. The stomach becomes atonic and this has been attributed to reflex inhibition of the myenteric neurones supplying the gastric musculature or to failure of the gastric pacemaker. Vascular insufficiency in the setting of gastric dilation and increased intra-gastric pressure is the critical factor. It is rare to have ischemic events in the stomach due to its copious collateral circulation. Pressure in the stomach lumen beyond 14 mm Hg exceeds gastric venous pressure. This results in cessation of blood flow in the gastric mucosal venous arterio-venous plexuses and mucosal ischaemia. Remarkably, cases of gastric ischaemia have been reported when the arterial blood supply to the stomach has been intact. The chronicity of gastric dilatation is also a factor as some patients with eating disorders have had recorded gastric volumes of up to 15L when as little as 3L of fluid can distend a normal stomach to pressures above 14 mm. Gastric rupture can occur with an intra-gastric pressure of 120 to 150 mm Hg, which can occur with only 4 L of fluid in a normal stomach. External compression such as cardiopulmonary resuscitation is also a rare contributory factor to high pressures and secondary rupture.

Aetiology

Acute gastric dilatation is a recognised complication of abdominal surgery particularly splenectomy and pelvic surgery. Other aetiologies include: anorexia nervosa and bulimia, psychogenic polyphagia, gastric volvulus, medications, diabetes mellitus, acute pancreatitis and electrolyte disturbances. AGD has been reported in trauma patients and although the pathophysiology is multifactorial, several authors have stressed the central role of aerophagia in agitated and confused patients. AGD can be seen with spinal disorders and post after surgery as a result of superior mesenteric artery syndrome (SMAS). In this syndrome, AGD follows vascular compression of the duodenum between superior mesenteric artery, aorta and vertebral column. SMAS may also be precipitated by a binge-eating episode leading to AGD.

Medical Management

Imaging is the key diagnostic modality. Plain radiographs or CT scans will reveal a massively dilated stomach. CT is a more accurate method of identifying associated causes of acute gastric dilation and angiographically enhanced CT can assess gastric wall perfusion. Laboratory investigations should include determination of haemoglobin, electrolytes and urea. An arterial blood gas can assess for alkalosis. Intravenous Fluid resuscitation and correction of electrolytes abnormalities is essential in these acutely compromised patients. Antibiotics may be necessary to cover peritonitis and aspiration pneumonia.

Treatment is focused on early diagnosis, decompression of the stomach, fluid resuscitation and correction of electrolyte abnormalities. Nasogastric tube decompression of the stomach is vital in the emergency management of AGD. Early placement of an NG tube is essential in the management of trauma patients unless there is a clear contraindication. Delayed perforation or bleeding is still possible, even after decompression. Urgent endoscopy in the stable patient may be of use for decompression—particularly if the CT scan suggests gastric or oesophageal aetiology which could be rectified. In addition, endoscopy can assess gastric mucosal perfusion. Most reports on acute gastric dilation note that the majority of ischemic changes occur along the greater curve of the stomach. The lesser curvature and pyloric regions of the stomach tend to be spared. In some patients, rapid gastric decompression can result in profound cardiovascular compromise, multi-organ failure and eventually death. Acute cardiac decompensation can result from the sudden return of lactic acid from the relatively ischaemic stomach. Staged decompression has been suggested as an alternative to prevent these sequels. Delayed gastric haemorrhage after decompression has also been reported.

Surgical Treatment

Emergency surgical treatment is mandated in the presence of instability or evidence of obstruction, necrosis or perforation. When these signs are detected, surgical mortality is in the region of 50 to 60%. Early recognition is essential because treatment delay is associated with a mortality rate in excess of 80%. By contrast, in the absence of surgical treatment, gastric ischaemia has a 100% mortality rate.

The extent of gastric ischemia can dictate the surgical approach. The presence of frank necrosis, and current or impending gastric wall perforation can determine the extent of resection. Adequate resection of the necrotic portion of the stomach is essential. Total gastrectomy has been advocated in cases when surgical resection is necessary. This avoids an anastomosis to an under perfused stomach remnant. A feeding jejunostomy should be placed at the same procedure. Other interventions include partial resection or local debridement and even non-operative therapy. However, with these modalities there is a risk of poor healing of gastric remnant as well as delayed ischaemia. In some patients (diabetics, Prader-Willie Syndrome patients), acute gastric dilatation can be recurrent. A percutaneous endoscopic gastrostomy can be used to regularly vent the stomach in these patients.

GASTRIV VOLVULUS

Gastric volvulus is a rare condition and its incidence is not well defined. It represents rotation of the stomach more than 180 degrees creating a closed loop obstruction as one of the sequel. Berti first described gastric volvulus in 1866.

This condition can be primary or secondary, with secondary volvulus due to para-oesophageal herniation being the commoner variety. Secondary gastric volvulus in adults is commonly due to para-oesophageal herniation and the peak incidence occurs in the fifth decade of life. Approximately 20% of gastric volvulus cases occur in infants under 1 year of age and are often secondary to congenital diaphragmatic defects with subsequent herniation.

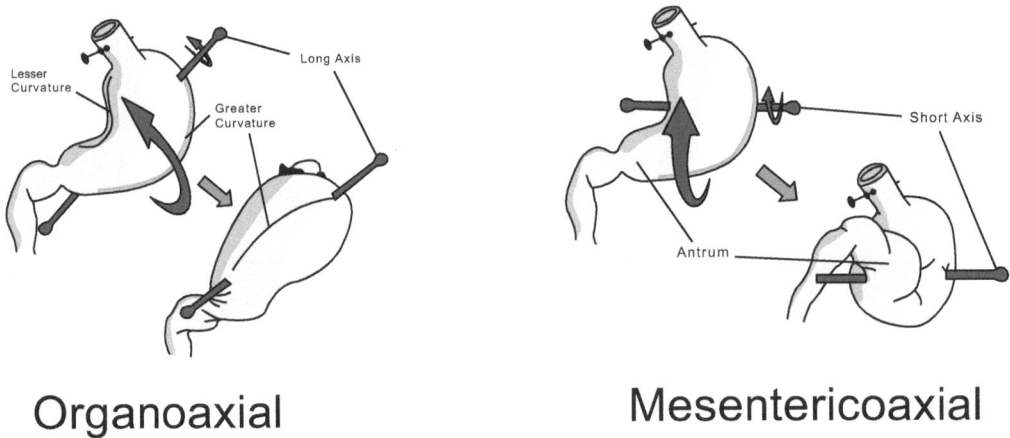

Fig. (6). Anatomic types of gastric volvulus.

There are three anatomic types: organo-axial, mesenteric-axial, and a combination of both (Fig. **6**). Organo-axial volvulus is caused by rotation along the longitudinal cardiopyloric axis. This is the commonest type, accounting for two-thirds of cases. It is usually associated with diaphragmatic defects, most commonly a para-oesophageal hernia. Organo-axial volvulus is far more common than mesenteric-axial volvulus and a combination of both. Mesenteric-axial volvulus occurs when torsion occurs around the transverse axis of the stomach and tends to be associated with gastric ischaemia. Distinction between types is not crucial as the classification is more descriptive than prognostic. Mortality from acute gastric volvulus can be as high as 50%.

Presentation and Clinical Features

The acute presentation of gastric volvulus is dramatic and often obvious, and it is this type that is usually quoted in the literature. Acute volvulus is more common with the organo-axial variety presents with severe pain and ineffectual retching. Distension, tenderness and signs of shock, rapidly follow. The subacute or chronic type, however, is frequently not recognized early in its presentation because it is accompanied by vague and non-specific symptomatology suggestive of other abdominal processes. This condition may present as an acute abdominal emergency or a chronic cause of upper abdominal discomfort. Borchardt's Triad is seen in as many as 70% of cases and is diagnostic of acute gastric volvulus. It includes acute, severe epigastric pain, severe retching and a nasogastric tube cannot be passed to relieve gastric dilatation. Haematemesis may occur due to mucosal sloughing as a result of ischaemia. Patients with chronic gastric volvulus may present with unspecific symptoms, which may go unnoticed. These include dysphagia, gastro-oesophageal reflux, vomiting and altered bowel habit.

Epidemiology

Gastric volvulus is rare. The peak age group of incidence is in the fifth decade and is commonly seen in association with para-oesophageal hernias. Cases in children, which account for between 10 and 20% of all reported cases, are often related to a congenital diaphragmatic defect. Males and females are equally affected and no association with race has been reported.

Diagnosis

Diagnosis of a gastric volvulus is difficult. Features may also be absent in cases of intermittent obstruction. Radiographic findings include herniation of the stomach above the diaphragm, with differential air fluid levels. Barium swallow has a very high sensitivity and specificity for diagnosing a gastric volvulus. It is usually diagnostic and can define the anatomical type of the volvulus. CT scan can help confirm the rotation of the herniated stomach and the transition points. It can also give information about the position and anatomy necessary to hasten surgical intervention [22]. Endoscopic diagnosis can reveal a tortuous appearance of the stomach and difficulty or inability to reach the pylorus

Aetiology and Pathophysiology

Gastric volvulus is usually associated with an underlying pathology such as a diaphragmatic hernia or a para-oesophageal hernia. The stomach is usually fixed to the abdominal cavity by 4 ligaments: gastrocolic, gastrohepatic, gastrophrenic and gastrosplenic. Type 1 Gastric volvulus may result in the absence, elongation or disruption of these gastric ligaments. It can also occur as a result of neoplasia or adhesions. A Type 2 gastric volvulus may result secondary to disorders of gastric anatomy or gastric function. It may also happen in the presence of abnormalities of adjacent organs.

Complications

If undetected gastric volvulus can lead to ulceration, perforation, haemorrhage or ischaemia and full-thickness necrosis. Impaired venous return can lead to poor cardiac output, which leads to hypovolaemic shock, myocardial ischaemia, cardiac arrhythmia, electrolyte imbalance and other detrimental effects.

Management of Gastric Volvulus

Upon diagnosis of the condition the patient should be kept prone and a serious attempt is made to pass a nasogastric to facilitate decompression. Endoscopic reduction may be considered in patients who are unfit for surgery but surgical repair is the mainstay of treatment. Acute volvulus is associated with a high risk of vascular compromise and death and warrants emergency surgery. Chronic gastric volvulus may be treated on a non-emergency basis. There are also some reports of successful conservative management of chronic gastric volvulus. These patients had a high recurrence rate but very few serious complications [23].

The principle aims of surgery for gastric volvulus include de-rotation of the volvulus, reduction of the hiatal hernia contents, repair of the hiatal defect and gastric fixation. Several procedures have been described for the surgical management of gastric volvulus including simple gastropexy, gastropexy with division of the gastrocolic omentum (Tanner's operation), partial gastrectomy, fundo-antral gastro-gastrostomy (Opolzer's operation) and gastrojejunostomy. All these procedures can be carried out with or without repair of the diaphragmatic hernia. There is no consensus on optimal gastropexy method.

Open surgical reduction with or without gastropexy is the most frequently performed procedure. In experienced hands, laparoscopic approaches, *e.g.* laparoscopic gastropexy with para-oesophageal hernia repair, provide a safer, less invasive management strategy with fewer complications. Fixing the stomach to the anterior abdominal wall can also be done by gastrostomy. Gastrojejunostomy can be used to restrict mobility. Endoscopic de-rotation and insertion of a percutaneous endoscopic gastrostomy tube tends to be reserved for elderly patients or those with chronic gastric volvulus.

Gastropexy

Gastropexy is a surgical operation in which the pyloric antrum is sutured to the anterior abdominal wall. The volvulus is reduced and the stomach returned to its normal anatomical position in the abdomen. The stomach is then attached to the anterior abdominal wall and to the diaphragm.

CONSENT FOR PUBLICATION

Not applicable.

ACKNOWLEDGEMENT

Declare none.

CONFLICT OF INTEREST

The authors declare no conflict of interest, financial or otherwise.

REFERENCES

[1]   Tack J, Talley NJ, Camilleri M, *et al.* Functional gastroduodenal disorders. Gastroenterology 2006; 130(5): 1466-79.
[http://dx.doi.org/10.1053/j.gastro.2005.11.059] [PMID: 16678560]

[2]   Talley NJ, Walker MM, Holtmann G. Functional dyspepsia. Curr Opin Gastroenterol 2016; 32(6): 467-73.
[http://dx.doi.org/10.1097/MOG.0000000000000306] [PMID: 27540688]

[3]   Agréus L, Talley NJ, Jones M. Value of the "Test & Treat" strategy for uninvestigated dyspepsia at low prevalence rates of *Helicobacter pylori* in the Population. Helicobacter 2016; 21(3): 186-91.
[http://dx.doi.org/10.1111/hel.12267] [PMID: 26347458]

[4]   Harmon RC, Peura DA. Evaluation and management of dyspepsia. Therap Adv Gastroenterol 2010; 3(2): 87-98.
[http://dx.doi.org/10.1177/1756283X09356590] [PMID: 21180593]

[5]   Dixon MF, Genta RM, Yardley JH, Correa P. Classification and grading of gastritis. The updated Sydney System. International Workshop on the Histopathology of Gastritis, Houston 1994. Am J Surg Pathol 1996; 20(10): 1161-81.
[http://dx.doi.org/10.1097/00000478-199610000-00001] [PMID: 8827022]

[6]   Sepulveda AR, Patil M. Practical approach to the pathologic diagnosis of gastritis. Arch Pathol Lab Med 2008; 132(10): 1586-93.
[PMID: 18834216]

[7]   Coati I, Fassan M, Farinati F, Graham DY, Genta RM, Rugge M. Autoimmune gastritis: Pathologist's viewpoint. World J Gastroenterol 2015; 21(42): 12179-89.
[http://dx.doi.org/10.3748/wjg.v21.i42.12179] [PMID: 26576102]

[8]   Neumann WL, Coss E, Rugge M, Genta RM. Autoimmune atrophic gastritis--pathogenesis, pathology and management. Nat Rev Gastroenterol Hepatol 2013; 10(9): 529-41.
[http://dx.doi.org/10.1038/nrgastro.2013.101] [PMID: 23774773]

[9]   Syrjänen K. A panel of serum biomarkers (gastropanel®) in non-invasive diagnosis of atrophic gastritis. systematic review and meta-analysis. Anticancer Res 2016; 36(10): 5133-44.
[http://dx.doi.org/10.21873/anticanres.11083] [PMID: 27798873]

[10]   Johnson HD, Love AH, Rogers NC, Wyatt AP. Gastric ulcers, blood groups, and acid secretion. Gut 1964; 5: 402-11.
[http://dx.doi.org/10.1136/gut.5.5.402] [PMID: 14218257]

[11]   Peters GL, Rosselli JL, Kerr JL. Overview of peptic ulcer disease. US Pharm 2010; 35(12): 29-43.

[12]   Dore MP, Pes GM, Bassotti G, Usai-Satta P. Dyspepsia: When and how to test for *Helicobacter pylori* infection. Gastroenterol Res Pract 2016; 2016: 8463614.
[http://dx.doi.org/10.1155/2016/8463614] [PMID: 27239194]

[13]   Rockall TA, Logan RF, Devlin HB, Northfield TC. Incidence of and mortality from acute upper gastrointestinal haemorrhage in the United Kingdom. Steering Committee and members of the National Audit of Acute Upper Gastrointestinal Haemorrhage. BMJ 1995; 311(6999): 222-6.

[http://dx.doi.org/10.1136/bmj.311.6999.222] [PMID: 7627034]

[14]   Jafar W, Jafar AJN, Sharma A. Upper gastrointestinal haemorrhage: an update. Frontline Gastroenterol
        2016; 7(1): 32-40.
        [http://dx.doi.org/10.1136/flgastro-2014-100492] [PMID: 28839832]

[15]   Blatchford O, Murray WR, Blatchford M. A risk score to predict need for treatment for upper-
        gastrointestinal haemorrhage. Lancet 2000; 356(9238): 1318-21.
        [http://dx.doi.org/10.1016/S0140-6736(00)02816-6] [PMID: 11073021]

[16]   Rockall TA, Logan RF, Devlin HB, Northfield TC. Risk assessment after acute upper gastrointestinal
        haemorrhage. Gut 1996; 38(3): 316-21.
        [http://dx.doi.org/10.1136/gut.38.3.316] [PMID: 8675081]

[17]   Kar P, Mitra S, Resnick JM, Torbey CF. Gastric antral vascular ectasia: case report and review of the
        literature. Clin Med Res 2013; 11(2): 80-5.
        [http://dx.doi.org/10.3121/cmr.2012.1036] [PMID: 23262190]

[18]   Batouli A, Kazemi A, Hartman MS, Heller MT, Midian R, Lupetin AR. Dieulafoy lesion: CT
        diagnosis of this lesser-known cause of gastrointestinal bleeding. Clin Radiol 2015; 70(6): 661-6.
        [http://dx.doi.org/10.1016/j.crad.2015.02.005] [PMID: 25782338]

[19]   Jeon HK, Kim GH. Endoscopic Management of Dieulafoy's Lesion. Clin Endosc 2015; 48(2): 112-20.
        [http://dx.doi.org/10.5946/ce.2015.48.2.112] [PMID: 25844338]

[20]   Lewis S, Holbrook A, Hersch P. An unusual case of massive gastric distension with catastrophic
        sequelae. Acta Anaesthesiol Scand 2005; 49(1): 95-7.
        [http://dx.doi.org/10.1111/j.1399-6576.2004.00552.x] [PMID: 15675990]

[21]   Powell JL, Payne J, Meyer CL, Moncla PR. Gastric necrosis associated with acute gastric dilatation
        and small bowel obstruction. Gynecol Oncol 2003; 90(1): 200-3.
        [http://dx.doi.org/10.1016/S0090-8258(03)00204-X] [PMID: 12821365]

[22]   Millet I, Orliac C, Alili C, Guillon F, Taourel P. Computed tomography findings of acute gastric
        volvulus. Eur Radiol 2014; 24(12): 3115-22.
        [http://dx.doi.org/10.1007/s00330-014-3319-2] [PMID: 25278244]

[23]   Hsu YC, Perng CL, Chen CK, Tsai JJ, Lin HJ. Conservative management of chronic gastric volvulus:
        44 cases over 5 years. World J Gastroenterol 2010; 16(33): 4200-5.
        [http://dx.doi.org/10.3748/wjg.v16.i33.4200] [PMID: 20806439]

CHAPTER 2

Oesophago-gastric Motility Disorders

Maria Coats[*]

Department of Surgery, Ninewells Hospital and Medical School, Dundee, Scotland, UK

Abstract: Oesophageal motility disorders are notoriously difficult to diagnose and manage. They often manifest as dysphagia, regurgitation or chest pain. Oesophageal manometry is the primary investigation. High-resolution manometry refines the discrimination between different disorders and improves the diagnostic yield. Oesophageal motility disorders can be either primary or secondary to a number of systemic diseases such as diabetes. The main primary disorders include achalasia, diffuse spasm, nutcracker oesophagus and sphincter abnormalities. Pharmaceutical treatment is largely unsuccessful. Endoscopic treatments using pneumatic dilatation or botox injections provide short-term relief of dysphagia. Surgery should be considered for young and fit individuals.

Gastroparesis is a chronic motility disorder of the stomach, which encompasses delayed gastric emptying in the absence of a fixed mechanical obstruction of the pylorus or duodenum. Symptoms include early satiety, nausea, bloating, vomiting, abdominal pain and weight loss. Diagnostic evaluation requires an initial endoscopy to rule out mechanical causes, followed by a gastric-emptying scintigraphy for diagnosis. Gastroparesis can be primary or secondary. Management includes dietary modification, pharmacological agents, endoscopic botox injections to pylorus, gastroenterostomy and gastric electrical stimulation. Most patients continue to be symptomatic despite all management modalities.

Keywords: Achalasia, Cardiomyotomy, Diffuse oesophageal spasm, Gastric electrical stimulation, Gastroparesis, Hypertensive sphincter, Manometry, Motility, Nutcracker oesophagus, Primary motility abnormalities, Secondary motility abnormalities.

OESOPHAGEAL MOTILITY DISORDERS

Oesophageal motility disorders are notoriously difficult to diagnose and manage. They often manifest as dysphagia, regurgitation or chest pain and a careful clinical assessment is critical in order to make an accurate diagnosis and subsequently select patients for the appropriate treatment. Oesophageal motility

---
[*] **Corresponding author Maria Coats:** Department of Surgery, Ninewells Hospital and Medical School, Dundee DD1 9SY, Scotland, UK; Tel: +44 1382 660111; E-mail: mariacoats@nhs.net

disorders may occur due to a complete failure of peristalsis or due to a global weakness of peristalsis resulting in abnormal contractions and functional oesophago-gastric junction outflow obstruction (Fig. **1**).

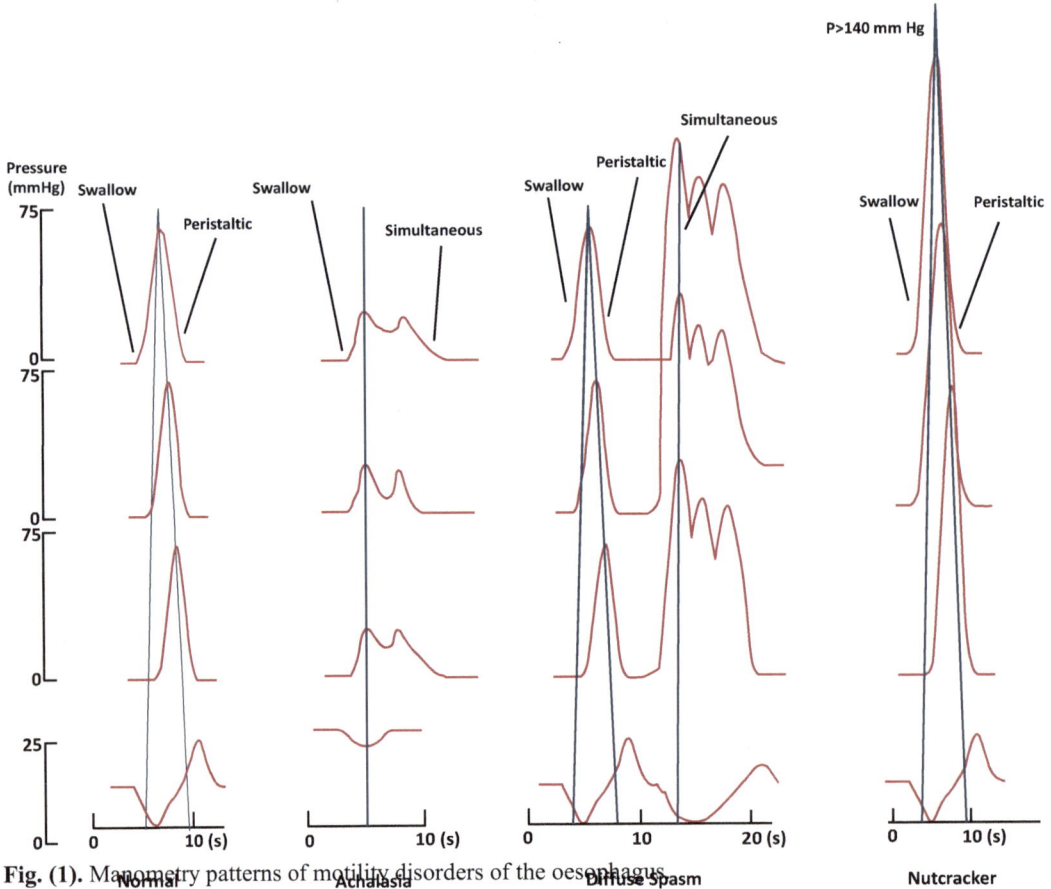

Fig. (1). Manometry patterns of motility disorders of the oesophagus

Oesophageal motility disorders may be classified as primary or secondary. The former is categorised according to the manometric patterns that are observed and for some disorders on the radiological appearances. Primary disorders originate directly from the oesophagus and include achalasia, diffuse oesophageal spasm, nutcracker oesophagus, hypertensive lower oesophageal sphincter (LOS) and non-specific oesophageal motility disorders. Secondary disorders occur as a result of wider systemic disease such as systemic sclerosis, diabetes mellitus, excess alcohol consumption, psychiatric disorders and presby-oesophagus. The oesophageal motility disorder is one of their manifestations. Although this may appear to be a discrete classification, there is much controversy in this area and primary motility disorders have frequently been described as a progression from one type to another.

Presentation

The vast majority of patients with oesophageal neuro-muscular dysfunction present with either dysphagia (with subsequent weight loss) or non-cardiac chest pain. Dysphagia is usually for both solids and liquids can be intermittent and is exacerbated by low temperature liquids. Some patients with dysphagia find that food transit through the oesophagus can be facilitated by sipping fluid after each solid bolus or by repeated swallows and various postural manoeuvres such as expiration against a closed glottis (Valsalva) *etc*.

Oesophageal anterior chest pain is often described as a tightening or gripping pain, which closely simulates angina pectoris. Thus it may radiate to the back, jaw, arm and ear and may even be relieved by sublingual nitrates. This type of pain is commonly found in patients with oesophageal motility disorders or reflux oesophagitis. It may occur in association with meals when it persists for about an hour after meals, but is also experienced in the fasting state and is frequently precipitated by emotion and exercise.

Some patients complain of regurgitation of gastric or oesophageal fluid into the throat accompanied by a sour taste in the mouth. It is often postural and occurs predominantly in the supine position especially at night, with the regurgitated material often staining the pillow. Postural regurgitation is usually precipitated by meals and activities associated with a rise in the intra-abdominal pressure *i.e.* bending and straining. Regurgitation may also occur as an overflow phenomenon due to the accumulation of food in the non-propulsive oesophagus. This spillback into the pharynx and mouth at night may lead to aspiration pneumonitis. In oesophageal motility disorders both overflow and postural regurgitation may occur, although the former is more commonly encountered in these conditions.

INVESTIGATIONS OF OESOPHAGEAL MOTILITY DISORDERS

All symptomatic patients should have the mandatory endoscopy to inspect the mucosa of the oesophagus and stomach, exclude any mucosal inflammation or obstructing lesion and delineate the anatomy of the upper gastro-intestinal tract. It would be inappropriate for any patient to have other tests before endoscopy unless this is not available or practical for the individual patient. Patients with chest pain should also have had cardiac assessment including electrocardiography and cardiac enzyme studies depending on the presentation. Further assessments will then focus specifically on motility disorders of the oesophagus. Indeed, the endoscopy may have found evidence of a dilated, impacted or tortious oesophagus, which are indicative.

Oesophageal Manometry

This technique measures the mechanical function of the oesophageal musculature and its sphincters by recording intra-luminal pressure profiles caused by the contractions. It is indicated in the investigation of patients with non-obstructive dysphagia, non-cardiac chest pain and oro-pharyngeal dysphagia.

Conventional Water-Perfused Catheter Manometry

Intra-luminal pressure recording is carried out using a system of water-perfused catheters or solid-state strain-gauge transducers built into catheters. For sphincter pressure measurements there is a potential for the position of the sphincter to alter in relation to the pressure sensor on the catheter especially in prolonged measurements. In these situations, the Dent sleeve can be used. This is a thin, 6 cm long, open ended, silastic sleeve, which surrounds the pressure sensor ports of a water-perfused catheter. The sleeve operates by traversing the sphincter and records the averaged circumferential and axial pressure forces acting on the sleeve. An alternative is the sphinctometer. This device is usually sited distally in a multi-channel micro-transducer catheter and consists of a side-mounted transducer surrounded by a silicone, oil filled silastic tube of 6 cm length and of the same diameter as the catheter. The water-perfused catheter is connected to a low compliance hydraulic pump, which in turn is connected to a system of strain gauges and a system of readout, most commonly a computer (Fig. **2**).

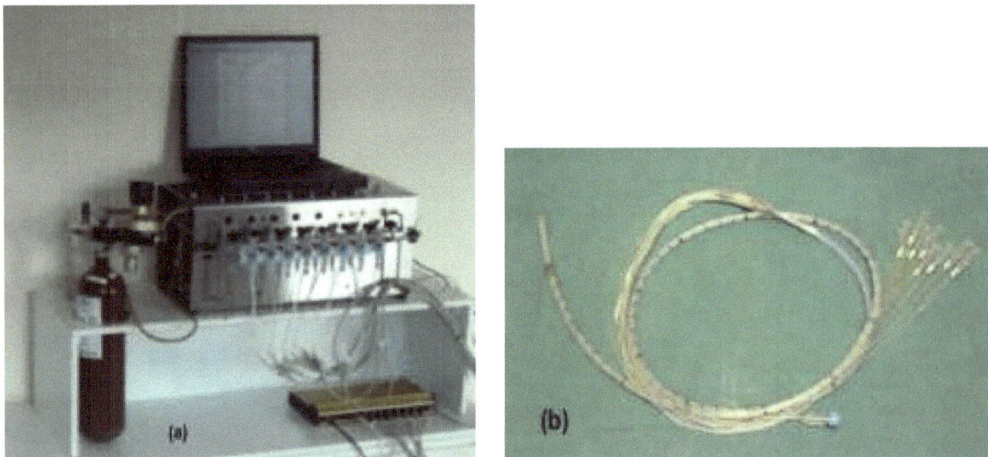

Fig. (2). (a) Stationary manometry is performed using a low compliance gas driven hydraulic pump infusing water through a multi-channel catheter connected to a system of strain-guages which feed the back pressure signal into a digital converter and displayed on the computer screen. **(b)** A multi-channel silicone catheter.

The solid-state strain-gauge micro-transducers can be connected directly to the readout system. The study commences by determination of the position of the lower oesophageal sphincter/ high-pressure zone. This is done by inserting the catheter into the stomach and withdrawing it either rapidly (rapid pull-through), or slowly (station pull-through) taking pressure recordings at each of the stations from both the sphincter and oesophageal body. The rapid pull-through technique provides information on the position and length of the sphincter. The manometry catheter can then be positioned with one pressure sensor in the middle of the sphincteric area and three pressure sensors separated by 5 cm intervals on the catheter lying within the oesophageal body. In stationary manometry pressure recordings are taken from the sensors in response to a number of water swallows separated by 30 seconds. This method provides sufficient information on the position, length and pressure of the lower oesophageal sphincter in addition to pressure, peristalsis and propagation of contractions within the oesophageal body (Fig. **3**).

The information obtained from manometric studies is analysed according to set criteria (Table **1**) to diagnose oesophageal motility disorders.

Table 1. Oesophageal manometry indices and criteria

Index	*Normal*	*Abnormal*
HPZ (sphincter) pressure	10 – 26 mm Hg	< 10.0 mmHg, > 26.0 mmHg
HPZ relaxation	Relaxes when reached by primary wave	No relaxation with swallowing
Oesophageal body contractions	Primary peristaltic waves generated by Wet/dry swallows.	> 10% aperistaltic waves, retrograde, or segmental contractions.
Amplitude	30-140 mmHg	< 30 mmHg, > 140 mm Hg
Duration	2 – 10 seconds	> 15 seconds
Wave form	Mostly single or double peaked wave forms	abnormal and multi-peak wave forms
Additional contractions	Secondary peristaltic waves	Repetitive (tertiary, non-propulsive) contractions.

This method is indicated for the accurate placement of pH electrodes prior to 24-hour ambulatory pH monitoring, in patients suspected of having gastro-oesophageal reflux disease. This method can also be diagnostic in patients with classical motility disorders of the oesophagus.

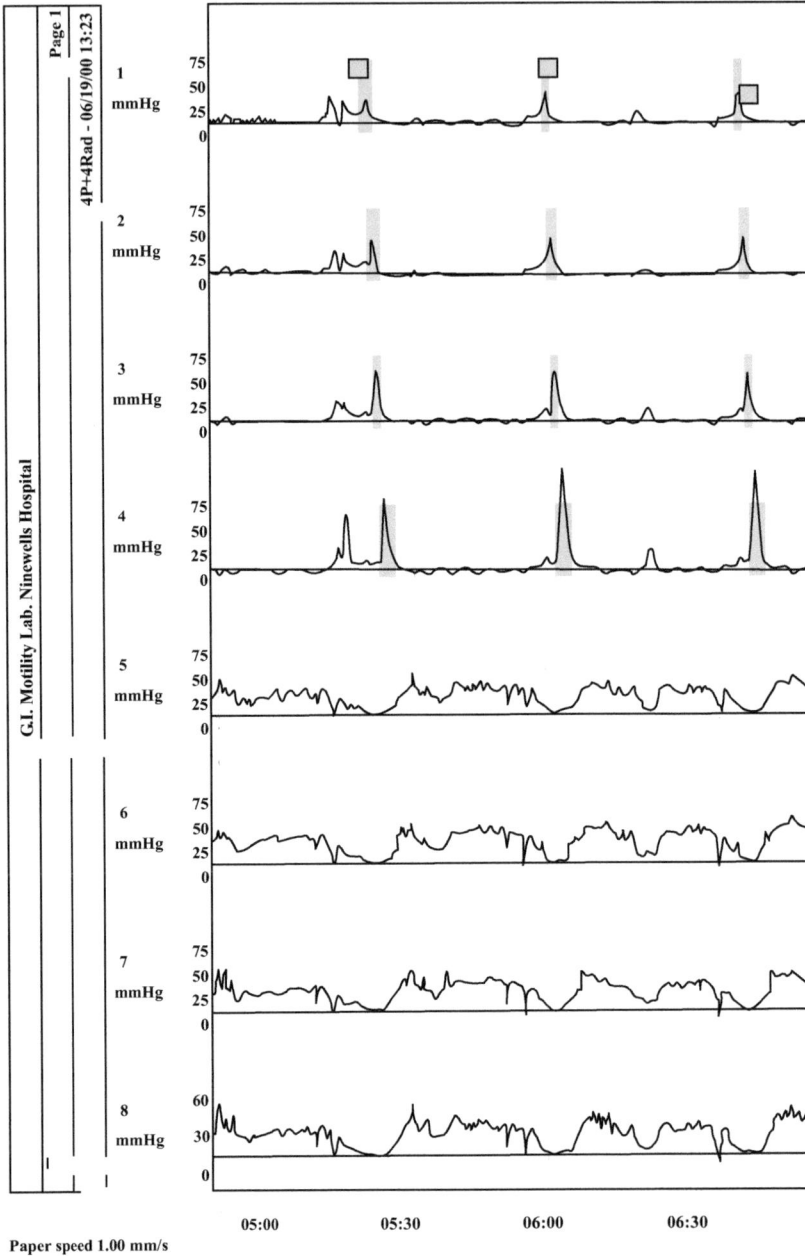

Fig. (3). Stationary manometry recording using an 8 channel catheter with 4 radial channels at the same distance from the tip of the catheter (lower 4) positioned within the lower oesophageal sphincter determined by a station pull-through technique and 4 channels separated by 5 cm intervals along the catheter placed in the body of the oesophagus. The contraction of the oesophagus and lower oesophageal sphincter in response to three wet swallows is demonstrated.

Solid-State Catheter Manometry

In patients where the stationary manometry reveals a motility disorder of the oesophagus and in those patients suspected of having an oesophageal motility disorder, prolonged ambulatory manometry is preferred. This method employs solid-state pressure transducer catheters attached to a portable recording system with event markers triggered by the patient when symptoms occur (Fig. **4**).

They are particularly useful for patients with non-cardiac chest pain who may have transient motility disturbances in the oesophagus and for patients with non-specific motility disorders. Because of the diverse aetiology of these disorders, a combined recording of manometry and pH metry is usually indicated. Analysis of both manometry and pH metry may reveal the disorder causing their symptoms. The investigation may however demonstrate the absence of pathology causing the symptoms.

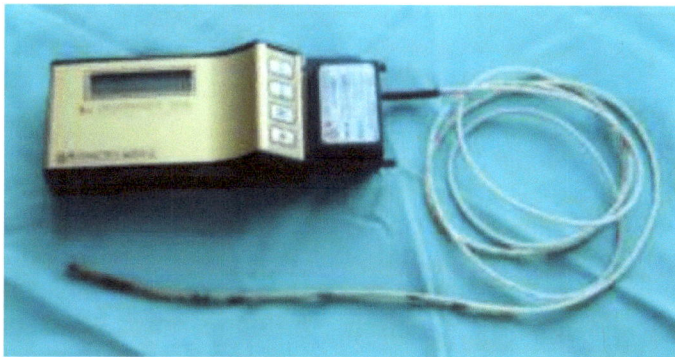

Fig. (4). A portable recording device connected to a catheter on which 3 pressure transducers measure pressure and a pH electrode measures the hydrogen ion concentration.

More recently, vector manometry of the lower oesophageal sphincter has been obtained using a water-perfused catheter with 8 radial channels. Although, this technique has provided illustrative 3-dimensional representation of the lower oesophageal sphincter, the technique suffers from poor reproducibility.

Currently, abnormal motor activity is defined in terms of a few basic patterns seen in oesophageal manometry: incomplete sphincter relaxation, oesophageal spasm, hypertensive contractions, and loss of tone and motility. Only achalasia and severe diffuse oesophageal spasm are specific disorders with manometric abnormalities that are absent in healthy subjects (Table **2**). Other oesophageal motility disorders are poorly defined, inconsistent and often include "abnormalities" that can be found in asymptomatic individuals. Diagnoses based on conventional manometry alone can be subjective and often uncertain.

Table 2. Manometric criteria for oesophageal motility disorders

Motility Disorder	*Manometric Criteria*
Achalasia	Simultaneous contractions (aperistalsis) High LOS pressure Incomplete LOS relaxation
Diffuse oesophageal spasm	Simultaneous contractions (> 10% of swallows) Intermittent normal peristalsis
Nutcracker oesophagus	High amplitude (>140 mm Hg) peristaltic contractions
Hypertensive LOS	High resting LOS pressure (>45 mm Hg) Normal LOS relaxation Normal peristalsis
Non-specific motility disorders	Non-propagated contractions Retrograde contractions Low amplitude (< 30 mm Hg) contractions Prolonged duration (> 6 sec) contractions Multi-peaked and disordered contractions Aperistalsis in oesophageal body with normal LOS Abnormal LOS function

High Resolution Manometry (HRM)

In this test a catheter is used with a sufficient number of pressure sensors within the oesophagus such that intraluminal pressure can be monitored as a continuum much as time is viewed as a continuum in line tracings of conventional manometry. Basically, this means having pressure sensors spaced around 1 cm apart. At that spacing, pressure values between sensors can be estimated by interpolation without significant loss of contractile information. When coupled with sophisticated algorithms to display the manometric data as pressure topography plots, HRM permits the visualization of oesophageal contractility with isobaric conditions among sensors indicated by iso-caloric regions on the high-resolution oesophageal pressure topography (HROPT) plots (Fig. **5**). Pressure activity can be assessed for several swallows through the oesophagus. Time, catheter position and average pressure are then reconstructed into pseudo-3D "topographic plots" that demonstrated the functional anatomy of the oesophagus (Fig. **5**). The advent of high-resolution manometry came with the development of micro-manometric water-perfused assemblies with 21–32 channels and more recently, novel solid-state transducers that allowed construction of catheters with up to 36 pressure sensors. At the same time, advances in computer technology allowed the large volume of data acquired by HRM to be presented in real time as conventional "line plots", and as "spatiotemporal plots" that display the direction and force of oesophageal pressure activity. An electronic "e-sleeve" can be applied during data analysis to provide stable measurements of LOS function similar to that acquired by a conventional sleeve sensor. HRM can precisely quantify the contractility of the oesophagus and its sphincters. However, translating this information into the diagnosis of an oesophageal motility disorder to account for symptoms is a daunting task.

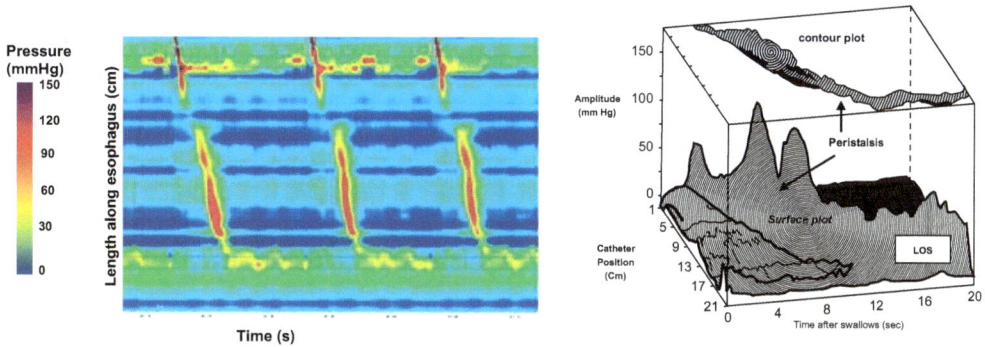

Fig. (5). Topographic display of normal oesophageal pressure data reconstructed from separate measurements at multiple levels during a station pull-through. (left): Iso-coloric (iso—baric) pressure topography plot. (right): Pseudo-3-D surface plot with superimposed contour plot.

The introduction of HRM was accompanied by the introduction of several new parameters that are instrumental in describing the details of oesophageal motor function. The Chicago group first reported normal values for these parameters. On the basis of these normal values the Chicago Classification, first described in 2007, was designed to aid clinical interpretation of HRM and pressure topography [1]. It has since been modified twice by the International High Resolution Manometry Working Group to integrate it with the clinical evaluation of patients enabling further sub classification of types of achalasia and primary motility disorders. It uses an algorithmic approach to diagnose patients symptoms based upon the integrated relaxation pressure (IRP) and distal contractile integral (DCI), which are parameters, obtained through pressure topography studies [2].

Although high-resolution manometry has refined our interpretation of oesophageal muscular disorders, it is an expensive test due to the cost of equipment, maintenance, training and relatively long learning curve to acquire expertise in interpreting the results. The diagnostic yield of HRM is higher than that of pull–through manometry and at least comparable to that of sleeve sensor manometry. Presently the most important advantage of solid-state HRM is that it makes oesophageal manometry easier to perform since it obviates the need for precise positioning of the manometric catheter across the LOS. Oesophageal manometry can be performed by a technician with limited knowledge of oesophageal function. In addition, topographic plotting of signals is a visually attractive way of presenting data. Due to the discriminating ability of HRM over conventional manometry, it is gaining gradual acceptance within the clinical community.

Contrast Radiology

The standard contrast investigation is the barium swallow which is particularly useful in the following categories of patients:

1. Patients with dysphagia unable to have endoscopy.
2. Patients with previous surgery to the oesophagus or oesophago-gastric junction.
3. Symptomatic patients with normal endoscopic findings.

Barium meal is an essential investigation in the evaluation of patients with dysphagia and normal endoscopy. The barium meal examination provides a record of the anatomy. In motility disorders, barium meal examination excludes a mechanical obstruction and may show characteristic features of a motility disorder such as achalasia. A barium-marshmallow swallow or bread and barium swallow is also useful in delineating peristaltic progress in the oesophagus.

Fluoroscopy/Video-Radiology

The use of cine-fluoroscopy/video recording is largely restricted to the investigation of patients with cricopharyngeal dysfunction and oesophageal motility disorders. The three phases of swallowing can be identified with remarkable accuracy and any deviations from the normal pattern are illustrated, evaluated and compared after treatment. Fluoroscopy plays but a minor role in the evaluation of oesophageal motility disorders. Its value is limited to the exclusion of mechanical obstruction in the oesophagus and oesophago-gastric junction.

CT Scanning

In the investigation of patients with motility disorders, Ct scanning is restricted to exclusion of peri-oesophageal lesions, which may interfere with the normal passage of food down the muscular oesophagus. Oral contrast enhanced CT adds little to the diagnosis of motility disorders but may be important in exclusion of other disease processes.

Radio Isotope Studies

These are used to evaluate oesophageal transit of liquid and solid boluses in individuals with motility disorders. When a labelled liquid bolus is used, the patient is placed in the supine position and swallows on demand the labelled liquid previously held in the mouth. Normal individuals clear 90% of the liquid from the oesophagus into the stomach in 4 to 15 seconds. A more physiological modification employs the use of a standardised solid bolus, which is swallowed by the patient in the erect position. The bolus consists of 10 mls, poached egg white labelled with ^{99m}Tc pertechnetate. External scinti-scanning is started as the patient swallows the chewed bolus. The normal transit time for this test is 10 seconds. Special software can generate time versus radioactivity curves, which outline transit in the upper, middle and lower thirds separately in addition to the total oesophageal transit. Using row summation, a condensed image can also be generated. This outlines graphically the spatial arrangement of the labelled egg white bolus (vertical axis) with respect to time on the horizontal axis. Prolonged transit times are encountered in oesophageal motility disorders with an oscillatory pattern encountered in achalasia. The condensed image shows a striking sinuous outline resulting from the up and down oscillations of the bolus in patients with achalasia and diffuse oesophageal spasm.

Endoscopy

Endoscopy is the primary investigation for all patients presenting with oesophageal symptoms. However, it has no specificity or positive diagnostic yield in oesophageal motility disorders. Endoscopy provides a means of excluding other pathology to account for the symptoms. In addition, endoscopy evaluates the oesophageal lumen (and oesophago-gastric junction) for additional findings, which may be consistent with a motility disorder. These include a dilated oesophagus, food debris in the oesophagus, tertiary contractions, *etc.*

PRIMARY OESOPHAGEAL MOTILITY DISORDERS

There is contention over the precise aetiology of primary oesophageal motility disorders and defining them based on manometric studies alone creates challenges for clinicians when managing these patients. It is far better to consider each clinical disorder as a syndrome.

Primary oesophageal motility disorders can be very distressing for patients. Their nutritional state is affected and symptoms are problematic to control. When coupled with the social implications of disordered food intake, it can lead to psychological problems. Patient selection for surgical intervention has to be judged carefully and should not be undertaken lightly as it depends on making the right diagnosis and exclusion of others. It also depends on weighing up the benefits and risks for the intended intervention.

Achalasia

Achalasia (Greek for 'does not relax') is the commonest primary oesophageal motility disorder with an incidence of 0.3 to 1.6 per 100,000 per year and a prevalence of 8 to 10 per 100,000 populations. It affects people at any age but usually presents between 25 and 60 years with a mean age at presentation of 50 years. Achalasia is uncommon in childhood (<16 years) with an incidence reported of 0.18 per 100,000 per year and when diagnosed in this age group is often associated with alacrima and Addison's disease, known as Triple A or Allgrove syndrome.

Sir Thomas Willis first reported achalasia in 1674. He was a British physician who called it a spasm with failure of the Lower Oesophageal Sphincter (LOS) to relax. Willis was the first to describe the successful dilatation of this sphincter using a cork-tipped whalebone. The precise aetiology and pathogenesis of Achalasia remains unknown but is thought to occur as a result of one or more neuromuscular defects. It is characterised by the selective degeneration of nitric oxide producing neurons in the oesophageal wall and preservation of cholinergic neurons. Some studies have reported degenerative changes in neurons of the dorsal motor nuclei of the vagus nerve and Wallerian degeneration in vagal fibres but the most widely accepted mechanism is the reduction of the inhibitory neurons described above. Histological examination of the myenteric plexus (Auerbach's plexus) shows ganglion cells surrounded by lymphocytes and to a lesser extent eosinophils suggesting an inflammatory process. In a normal oesophagus, these neurons produce an inhibitory cholinergic effect that enables relaxation of the LOS. In achalasia, degeneration of these neurons leads to an increased tone of the LOS and a failure in this relaxation mechanism.

Clinical Features

Typically, patients with achalasia present with a slow-onset and progressive history of dysphagia with a mean duration of symptoms of 4.5 years. Dysphagia is often worse with solids than liquids and they may describe having to 'force' food down using certain techniques such as eating upright, using the Valsalva maneuver or breath holding. Symptoms are often exacerbated with emotional stress and cold liquids. Significant weight loss (>20 Kg) is usually seen in advanced disease but 50-60% of patients will describe mild weight loss. This symptom should always raise the suspicion of an underlying malignancy. 75% of patients describe regurgitation of undigested food and may experience excessive drooling on the pillow overnight. Chest pain is a poor prognostic indicator of response to balloon dilatation or surgical treatment if it occurs in younger patients and can affect up to 40% of people. Halitosis occurs due to undigested food sitting in the oesophagus and up to a third of patients complain of heartburn, which fails to respond to acid suppression therapy, as a result of the bacterial fermentation of this food in the lower oesophagus. In advanced achalasia a 'mega-oesophagus' can occur with dilatation of more than 6 cm seen on chest radiographs. This leads to respiratory complications such as recurrent aspiration pneumonia, lung abscesses, pulmonary fibrosis, bronchiectasis and an increased risk of tuberculosis. In very severe situations the gullet becomes tortuous and causes odynophagia or complete dysphagia and patients may develop fever, sweating, breathlessness and expectoration of muco-purulent sputum. Anaemia is usually seen as a result of malnutrition and may be accompanied with vitamin deficiencies [3].

Investigations

The clinical presentation of achalasia is an essential component in making an accurate diagnosis but radiological investigations are useful to confirm and further classify the disease. A *plain chest radiograph* may show a widened mediastinum often with or without an air fluid level suggesting oesophageal dilatation and incomplete clearance of fluid and residue from the gullet. The gastric bubble under the left hemi diaphragm is also usually absent. A *barium contrast swallow* is the best single diagnostic test for achalasia demonstrating aperistalsis or simultaneous contractions resulting in a poor clearance on contrast (>1 min). The classical contrast X-Ray appearances describe a 'bird beak' tapering to the LOS with a smooth narrowing (Fig. **6a**). The subtle sign of an irregular shadow at the top of the barium level in the oesophagus is indicative of retained food residue in the gullet. In advanced disease the oesophagus is chronically dilated and tortuous and a so-called 'sigmoid oesophagus' may be seen (Fig. **6b**).

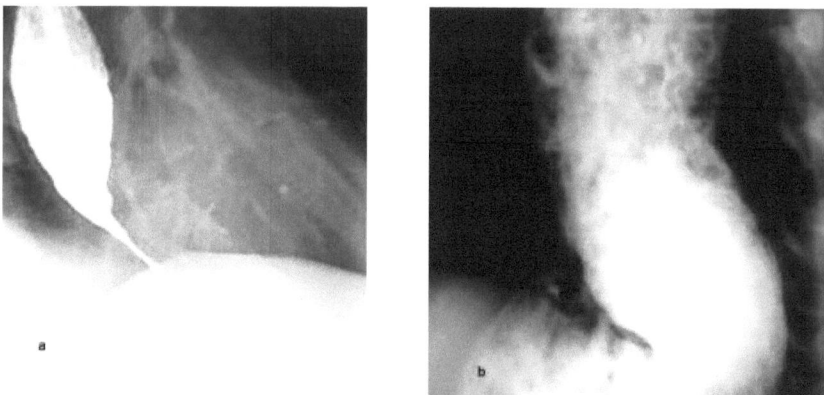

Fig. (6). Barium contrast X-Ray showing the classical appearances of (**a**) Bird-beak and (**b**) Sigmoid oesophagus with food debris.

Upper Gastro-Intestinal Endoscopy

This should be performed to exclude an anatomical anomaly or a stricture secondary to malignancy or peptic ulceration. Appearances of the oesophagus in achalasia range from normal to a mildly dilated oesophagus or a tortuous sigmoid oesophagus. The mucosal lining may be ulcerated and friable in the dilated oesophagus as a result of an inflammatory response to food stasis, oesophagitis or candida infection. Although mucosal biopsies are not essential they may show an infiltrate of eosinophils. The gastro-oesophageal junction is puckered and shows a rosette appearance on retro flexion of the endoscope in the stomach and is negotiable with minimal pressure with the endoscope despite giving the appearance of incomplete relaxation. *Endoscopic ultrasound* should be performed if there is a high index of suspicion from the patient's symptoms of malignancy or if the OGJ is difficult to traverse suggesting a diagnosis of pseudo achalasia.

Manometry Studies

These are the gold standard investigation for confirming the diagnosis of achalasia. The findings of aperistalsis and incomplete relaxation of the LOS are classical for achalasia. Manometry may be conventional (CM) or high resolution (HRM) and although techniques vary they generally involve the passage of a small tube, lined with pressure sensors at 1 cm (HRM) or 3 to 5 cm (CM) intervals, through the nose, across the OGJ into the stomach. Patients fast overnight prior to testing and omit all medications that may affect oesophageal motility for 48 hours prior to the test. They are instructed to drink sips of water and the contractility response of the oesophagus is recorded. A comparison is made between the results of CM and HRM below (Table **3**).

Conventional manometry involves the utility of a 'stationary pull-through' method pulling the manometry catheter in small increments (1 cm) to identify the LOS at the pressure inversion point and this may be uncomfortable for the patient where as high resolution manometry doesn't require this laborious process and enables data acquisition from a single series of swallows with a stationary catheter. As a result, HRM is a shorter, more comfortable and convenient test. However, the main advantage of high-resolution manometry over conventional manometry is the topographical information that can be extrapolated and interpreted from the pressure sensors in order to generate a 'Clouse plot' of colour-coded recordings of low (blue and green) and high (red and yellow) pressures. This has revolutionised the interpretation of data and enabled achalasia to be further classified into three types: I, II and III on the basis of peristalsis, oesophageal contractility and response to water swallows (Fig. **7**).

Table 3. A comparison of the abnormalities detected on conventional manometry and high resolution manometry.

Manometry Features	Conventional Manometry	High Resolution Manometry
LOS	***Impaired LOS relaxation*** - Fall in resting LOS pressure to >8 mmHg (mean) above gastric pressure following a swallow - Complete relaxation to gastric baseline in < 6 secs. ***Basal Pressure*** - >45 mmHg	***Impaired OGJ relaxation*** - Mean 4sec IPR ≥10 mmHg over swallows
Peristalsis	***Aperistalsis in distal 2/3 of Oesophagus*** - No recognisable contractions - Simultaneous contraction with amplitude <40 mmHg	***Aperistalsis*** - Absent (Type I) - Pan-oesophageal pressurization (Type II)
Other	***Vigorous achalasia*** - Preserved peristalsis with amplitude of contractions >40 mmHg	***Spastic achalasia*** *(Type III)*

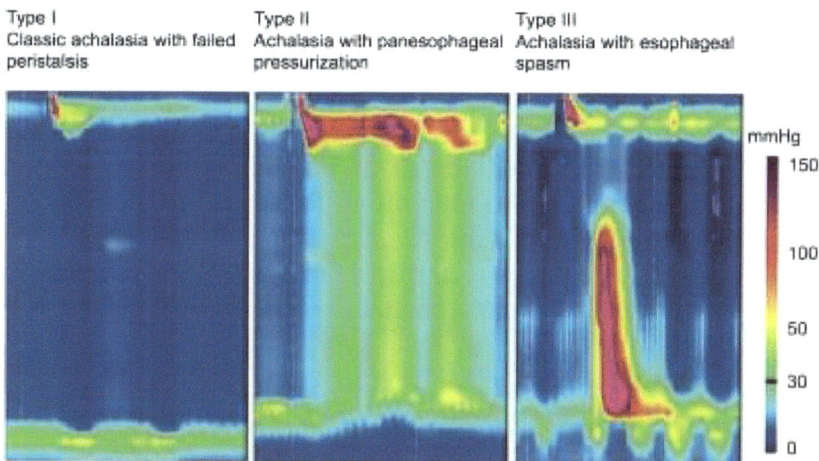

Type I
Classic achalasia with failed peristalsis

Type II
Achalasia with panesophageal pressurization

Type III
Achalasia with esophageal spasm

Fig. (7). High Resolution Manometry (HRM) charts showing different 3 different types of achalasia.

Type I achalasia HRM shows 100% failed peristalsis with minimal contractility of the oesophageal body and minimal oesophageal pressurizations. Type II achalasia HRM shows no normal peristalsis and intermittent periods of groups of high oesophageal pressures (>30 mmHg in ≥10 wet swallows). Type III achalasia HRM shows spastic contractions of the distal oesophagus with preserved segments of distal peristalsis or premature contractions in ≥20 wet swallows. These sub classifications are useful to determine the outcomes of achalasia treatment options [4] (Table **4**).

Table 4. Outcomes of treatment options for Achalasia sub-types I, II and III.

Achalasia Sub-Type	Response to Pneumatic Dilatation	Response to Heller's Myotomy
Type I	96%	85%
Type II	56%	95%
Type III	26%	70%

Management

Treatment options for primary achalasia may be pharmacological, endoscopic or surgical. The mainstay of treatment is to provide symptomatic relief by improving the passage of liquids and food through the oesophagus as the underlying cause of achalasia cannot be reversed [3, 5].

Pharmacological Therapy

This is usually the first-line management for the large number of disease processes in medicine but in achalasia it is the least effective treatment and reserved for patients that have failed botulinum toxin therapy or are unable to undergo definitive surgical treatment. The two most commonly used drugs are long-acting nitrates (*e.g.* Isosorbide dinitrate) and calcium channel blockers (*e.g.* nifedipine). They transiently reduce LOS pressure through smooth muscle relaxation facilitating oesophageal emptying. The benefits are often short lived and side effects of these medications such as headache, hypotension and peripheral oedema are frequently observed leading to poor patient compliance. Results are very variable and calcium channel blockers are reported to effectively reduce LOS pressure by 13-49% and create symptomatic relief in 0-75% of cases. Nifedipine (sublingual) takes its maximum effect 20-45 minutes after ingestion and lasts for a duration of 30-120 minutes. In comparison, Isosorbide dinitrate takes maximal effect in 3-27 minutes but only lasts for up to 90 mins. It is shown to reduce LOS pressure in 30-65% of patients and with studies reporting symptomatic relief in 53-87% of cases. Other drugs shown to reduce LOS pressure that have been used in the management of achalasia with variable results include sildenafil, anti-cholinergics (*e.g.* atropine, dicyclomine), β-adrenergic agonists (*e.g.* terbutaline) and theophylline.

Endoscopic Treatments

These include botulinum toxin (botox) injections and pneumatic dilatation. Botox is a presynaptic inhibitor of acetylcholine receptors and therefore when injected into the distal oesophagus it causes a short-term paralysis of the LOS by blocking the release of acetylcholine from cholinergic neurons. The effect of botox is transient lasting approximately 3-6 months and has a 100% failure rate as its effect diminishes with time [6]. Botox is reported to relax the LOS by up to 50% and provide an immediate response for 89% of patients in the first month. This response falls to 66% by 6 months after a single injection but with repeated injections improves to 77%. In the short-term botox injections are relatively risk free with only a few side effects such as mild chest pain post procedure for a few hours (25%) and heartburn (5%). It is often a favourable treatment choice for the elderly and in those with multiple cardio-respiratory co-morbidities who cannot undergo pneumatic dilation or a surgical intervention. The long-term effects of repeated botox injections are not widely known.

Endoscopic pneumatic dilatation (PD) of the LOS is a more definitive therapy and superior to botox injections. However, patients should be fit enough for surgical intervention in the event of an iatrogenic perforation during the procedure. PD uses non-radiopaque polyethylene balloons of a graded size (30-40 mm) that are dilated with air to pressures of 8-15 psi for up to 60 seconds in order to disrupt the LOS circular fibres. Standard endoscopic balloons reach diameters of 20 mm and are too small for the treatment of achalasia. PD is done under conscious sedation or general anaesthesia. The balloon is positioned to straddle the oesophago-gastric junction (OGJ) - this is a vital step to ensure effectiveness. Fluoroscopy is used to confirm the balloon waist has been adequately obliterated during the procedure and this is an important indicator of outcome and response to treatment. Post procedure, it is recommended that all patients undergo a contrast swallow test to exclude a perforation. PD carries a risk of perforation in up to 16% of cases and the risk is progressively higher with larger balloon diameters. For small perforations, conservative management with antibiotics, stent insertion and parenteral nutrition may suffice. However, in larger perforations with extensive mediastinal contamination, open surgical repair *via* a thoracotomy is usually indicated. Up to 35% of patients develop reflux symptoms post PD and if associated with dysphagia may lead to peptic stricturing that can confuse the patients' symptoms. Proton pump inhibitor therapy is indicated in this patient group. Serial dilatations with progressively larger balloons produce a good response over several months. No more than two dilatations are recommended during each sitting in order to minimise the risk of perforation. Good symptomatic relief has been reported in 75, 86 and 90% with 30, 35 and 40 mm balloon sizes respectively. Reports have suggested that females, age >45 years, type II achalasia on HRM, narrow oesophagus pre-dilatation or LOS pressure post-dilatation of <10 mmHg have the most favourable outcome. Although initial response is often good typically a third of patients will get recurrent symptoms by 3-6 years although some studies have reported a benefit of up to 25 years.

Surgery

The most common surgical intervention for achalasia is a Heller's Cardiomyotomy procedure, which was first reported in 1913 by a young German surgeon, Ernest Heller at the age of 34. He described a double myotomy dividing the external fibres of the OGJ anteriorly and posteriorly in a longitudinal fashion in order to weaken the LOS. This was initially performed through an open laparotomy incision but is now more commonly performed as a minimally invasive procedure by laparoscopy using 4-5 access ports [7]. The modern technique is an anterior myotomy which extends over 6 - 8 cm from the lower oesophagus to the stomach across the OGJ. The anterior vagus nerve is dissected from the line of the myotomy and preserved. The post-operative hospital length of stay is 1-2 days after the laparoscopic procedure. The selection of patients for surgical intervention is important. The surgical procedure is usually indicated for young patients and all those who are fit to have surgery. In addition, those who have failed botox therapy and PD should be considered for surgery. However, due to peri-oesophageal scarring from PD or injections, surgery is more difficult. Children or young adults with achalasia can face a lifetime of repeated treatments with PD or botox with their associated risks and for this patient group definitive surgery should be considered earlier than in the older patient population. Patients who have a hiatus hernia, tortuous oesophagus or lower oesophageal diverticulum are at higher risk of developing complications from non-surgical intervention and these patients also do better with a surgical cardiomyotomy procedure. However, it is worth remembering that surgery and anaesthesia carry minimal risks and the decision to proceed for surgery should always be a fully informed patient's choice. Long-term outcomes are mainly dependent on the manometric type of achalasia [8].

Heller's Myotomy Technical Steps

- A Heller's myotomy is performed under general anaesthesia. The patient is initially positioned supine with the abdomen fully exposed. Subsequently (after establishing pneumoperitoneum), the patient is placed in a steep Trendelenberg position.
- Pneumoperitoneum is typically created using a Verres needle in the sub-umbilical or left upper quadrant position just below the costal margin. In the vast majority of patients, a normal port can be inserted in the sub-umbilical position. For patients with previous surgery, a 'visi-port' or optical entry trocar can be used to gain access to the abdominal cavity through an incision about 10-12 mm distant from the site of previous surgery. Three further ports are placed under direct vision (Fig. **8**). The lateral right upper quadrant port is used to place an expandable liver retractor through a 5 mm incision just below the xiphoid

process and secured externally by a retractor post and flexible arm. The lateral port in the left upper quadrant is used for tissue retraction and the remaining superior ports are the primary working ports for the surgeon.

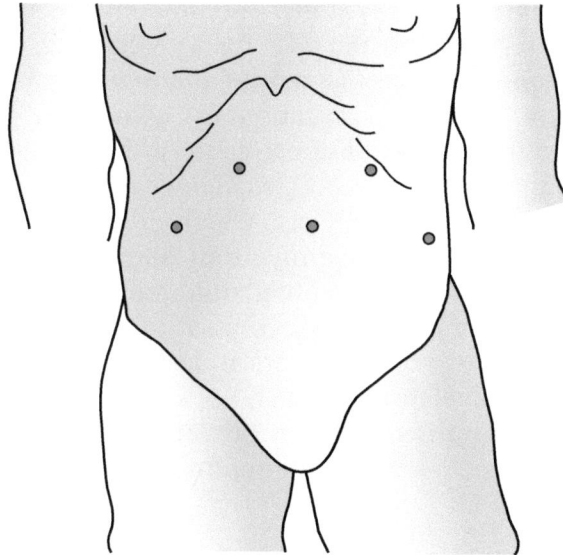

Fig. (8). Laparoscopic port placement for a Heller's Myotomy.

- Once the OGJ is adequately exposed the gastrohepatic ligament (Pars flaccida) and oesophago-phrenic ligaments are divided to expose the oesophageal hiatus with the right and left crus. Some surgeons suffice by dissecting the anterior surface of the oesophagus keeping the posterior hemi-oesophagus attached. Others complete a circumferential dissection of the lower oesophagus in preparation for a fundoplication.
- The anterior vagus nerve should be clearly identified, dissected from the oesophagus and preserved throughout. The fat overlying the oesophago-gastric junction is dissected from left to right until the anterior surface of the OGJ is fully exposed.
- The stomach is retracted caudally using the gastro-oesophageal fat pad to bring the OGJ into view and generate tension on the tissues to perform the myotomy. Simultaneous upper endoscopy may be carried out to identify the high-pressure zone within the oesophagus where the myotomy is made. The mediastinal oesophagus may need to be mobilised to perform a long myotomy and if required, a tension-free fundoplication.
- If a circumferential dissection of the lower oesophagus has been done, a Jakes catheter or similar atraumatic device is placed around the OGJ to facilitate

lateral and medial retraction.

- Once adequately exposed, the longitudinal and then the circular muscle fibres of the lower oesophagus are divided along the antro-lateral surface using mechanical splitting, sharp scissors division, mono-polar hook diathermy or an ultrasonic energy device. The myotomy should commence 5 - 6 cm above the OGJ and extend inferiorly below the OGJ for 2 - 3 cm (Fig. **9**).

- Care should be taken to reduce the risk of thermal injury to the oesophageal mucosa and prevent delayed perforation by controlling any bleeding with pressure and time rather than additional cautery. Minimal bleeding is usually encountered from the lower oesophagus. However, the gastric sub-mucosal plexus is populated with larger vessels, which are prone to bleed.

- Controversy exists as to whether the myotomy should be extended until all the oesophageal fibres have been divided or should routinely extend onto the cardia of the stomach. This part of the dissection is often the most difficult as the distinction between the dissection layers is less well defined and the risk of perforation of the gastric mucosa is higher.

- A gastric perforation, identified intra-operatively, can be primarily sutured with an absorbable monofilament suture with minimal long-term repercussions.

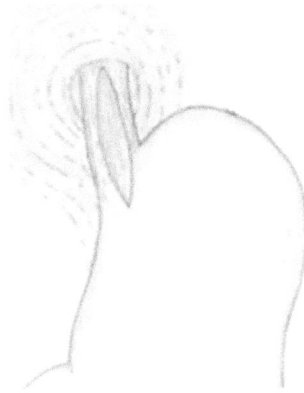

Fig. (9). Heller's cardiomyotomy.

- Post cardiomyotomy some surgeons would routinely perform a fundoplication as the risk of postoperative reflux symptoms without an anti-reflux procedure is 28-31% and with a fundoplication this falls to 9-14%. If an intra-operative gastric perforation occurs then a fundoplication should be performed to buttress the sutured repair. Post myotomy, pH monitoring of the lower oesophagus is reported to be abnormal in 9% and 47% of patients with and without a fundoplication respectively. The most common types of anti-reflux procedures performed post myotomy are an anterior (Toupet) or a posterior (Dor) fundoplication with symptomatic relief in up to 90% of patients. However, some surgeons believe that extensive mediastinal dissection of the lower oesophagus is unnecessary and preservation of phreno-oesophageal membrane reduces the risk of gastro-oesophageal reflux disease.

- In the immediate post-operative period after an uncomplicated operation, patients should be commenced on liquids over night with a soft diet the following day at which point they should be fit for discharge.

- If fundoplication was not done, patients should be commenced on proton pump inhibitors for life. Postoperative nausea should be treated aggressively with anti-emetics to reduce the risk of perforation.

At 10 years after cardiomyotomy, symptomatic relief is sustained in up to 85% of patients and by 20 years 65% still feel the benefit. Therefore, the long-term outcomes of cardiomyotomy are very good with superior results to PD or botox therapy and are recommended as definitive treatments. A poorer outcome is usually attributed to an inadequate myotomy or in patients who complain of significant reflux symptoms.

A subtotal oesophagectomy with cervical anastomosis may be required for patients with end-stage achalasia who have a tortuous mega oesophagus or a sigmoid oesophagus. However it should only be reserved for patients who fail PD or myotomy procedures and are fit enough to undergo major surgery under general anaesthesia [9]. A laparoscopic Heller's myotomy is associated with a 0.1% peri-operative morbidity risk usually due to missed perforations and their sequel whilst an oesophagectomy carries up to a 5% risk of mortality and a 10% risk post-operative complications including anastomotic leak, recurrent laryngeal nerve injury, delayed bleeding or chylothorax. Therefore, this surgery should not be undertaken lightly and careful patient selection is essential.

Recent Advances and Emerging Therapies

A new hybrid technique has been developed in Japan termed POEM (per oral oesophageal myotomy), which is based upon the principals of natural orifice transluminal endoscopic surgery (NOTES) and was first performed in 2008 [10]. A forward viewing endoscope is used and hydro-dissection of the sub-mucosal layer in the mid oesophagus is performed with an injection of saline and indigo carmine. Then a small (2 cm) incision is made at this site and a sub-mucosal tunnelling method is employed to create a space extending 2-3 cm inferiorly onto the stomach. Haemostasis is controlled with cautery and the circular fibres of the lower oesophagus are then divided 2-3 cm from the mucosal entry site and progressing distally. The initial mucosal incision may be anterior (11 to 2 O'clock) or posterior (5 O'clock) depending on operator preference although a posterior approach is thought to provide better relief of dysphagia and an anterior approach for reflux symptoms. At the end of the procedure, the sub-mucosal dissection plane is sprayed with a prophylactic antibiotic solution and the mucosal entry site closed with haemostatic clips. The whole procedure takes approximately 2-3 hours. Post operatively the patient is restricted to water for 48 hours and requires routine intravenous antibiotics for 3 days with oral therapy to continue for a further 4 days. The long-term outcomes of this procedure are largely unknown at this stage but reports so far suggest more than a 90% satisfactory response rate. The surgical community have not fully adopted this procedure yet.

Diffuse Oesophageal Spasm

Diffuse Oesophageal Spasm is an uncommon primary motility disorder of unknown aetiology. It was first described in 1889 by Osgood in a series of 6 patients presenting with chest pain and dysphagia. It is characterised by spontaneous non-propulsive contractions of the oesophagus. The LOS pressures are elevated and high amplitude, prolonged contractions are seen on manometry after swallowing, which are interspersed with normal peristaltic waves.

The diagnosis is often difficult from the history as patients may present with chest pain radiating to the back and jaw and often undergo cardiac investigations such as coronary angiography in the first instance. However, they also complain of dysphagia, odynophagia and regurgitation. These symptoms may be preceded by the ingestion of gassy beverages or following hot and cold drinks but they can also occur spontaneously with no stimulus. Studies have suggested reflux is also seen in 38-51% of patients and although weight loss is not a classical feature it has been reported in up to 30% of cases.

The pathogenesis of this disorder is undetermined and may be related to the inhibitory neurons in the distal oesophagus. Animal models have shown that the inhibition of nitric oxide causes spontaneous contractions of the oesophagus and when nitric oxide is replaced normal peristaltic function is restored. This suggests that nitric oxide may play a role in the mechanism of the disease. Other physiological studies have suggested that the oesophageal mucosa is sensitive to cholinergic and olfactory stimuli and the use of inhaled anti-cholinergic agents can improve symptoms. Interestingly, the psychological profile of these patients frequently show emotional disturbances and stressful events can trigger their symptoms.

The gold standard investigation of choice is oesophageal manometry, which demonstrates simultaneous contractions in the distal oesophagus in more than 10% of wet swallows with contraction amplitude of greater than 30 mmHg. The advancement of high-resolution oesophageal pressure topography has enabled better diagnostic accuracy of diffuse oesophageal spasm disorder. These pressure topography studies measure distal latency, which is the time interval between the relaxation of the upper oesophageal sphincter and the point where the velocity slows which delineates the tubular oesophagus from the oesophageal ampulla. If the distal latency is less than 0.4 seconds in 20% of wet swallows and a normal LOS pressure is measured, then a diagnosis of diffuse oesophageal spasm can be confidently made. The manometry findings in this motility disorder may overlap with that of achalasia and some reports have suggested that diffuse oesophageal spasm may progress to achalasia over time [11].

As with achalasia, it is important to perform routine upper endoscopy to exclude an anatomical anomaly or oesophago-gastric lesion that may cause obstruction. High frequency endoscopic ultrasound may show a thickened oesophageal muscle layer suggestive of hypertrophy but this is a non-specific finding. Barium swallow studies will be abnormal in 60% of patients and a 'corkscrew' or 'rosary bead' oesophagus, although a classical feature of the disease, is seen in less than 5% of cases (Fig. **10**).

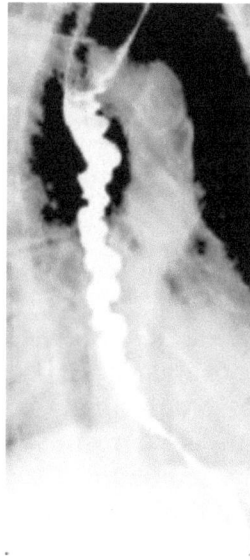

Fig. (10). A 'corkscrew' oesophagus seen on barium contrast swallow in Diffuse Oesophageal Spasm.

Oesophageal scintigraphy is a radio nucleotide transit study that may show incomplete oesophageal clearance and provocation tests with cholinergic compounds (*e.g.* edrophonium chloride 10 mg IV) may show hypersensitivity of the oesophageal musculature but these have generally not proved to be helpful in distinguishing between diffuse oesophageal spasm and achalasia. Acid reflux may be seen in association with this disorder and therefore 24-hour pH monitoring may help demonstrate this.

Once investigations have excluded a cardiac origin for the chest pain treatment can be focused on palliating symptoms. However, with an unclear aetiology, response to treatments may be variable and often unsatisfactory. A trial of proton pump inhibitor therapy may be offered for 8-12 weeks to treat any co-existing reflux disease in the first instance. In the absence of an adequate response to this, long-acting nitrates may be used intermittently to provide short-term symptomatic relief. Calcium channel blockers (*e.g.* nifedipine or diltiazem) have been used when symptoms are more sustained but with limited efficacy. Other drugs that have been used include 5-phosphodiesterase inhibitor (*e.g.* sildenafil, vardenafil) which improve nitric oxide bioavailability, selective serotonin receptor inhibitors and low-dose tricyclic agents (*e.g.* trazadone and nortryptiline) which act in an analgesic capacity for the chest pain [12].

If patients do not respond to pharmacological treatments, pneumatic dilatation may provide relief of dysphagia and regurgitation but their results are not as marked as is seen with achalasia and there is limited evidence for the long-term outcomes of this therapy. Similarly, botox injections could be considered as a second-line treatment but results are variable. The psychological factors, that have been associated with diffuse oesophageal spasm, are perhaps undervalued and may have a greater impact on a patient's response to treatment than we appreciate.

Surgical intervention with a Heller's Myotomy procedure may be offered in intractable cases and should only be reserved for those in whom all other treatment options have failed. A long myotomy, extending the entire length of the thoracic oesophagus may be required and is tailored to the extent of the manometric abnormality [13]. In this scenario, the procedure may require a thoracoscopic approach instead of abdominal and post procedure anti-reflux therapy with medications or a loose partial fundoplication may be required. The new technique, POEM, previously described, has been reported in two cases of diffuse oesophageal spasm with good results but it is still embryonic in its establishment and requires further validation. Oesophagectomy can be considered for patients with intractable symptoms who are unable to derive benefit from other therapies. However, the procedure is more difficult particularly after previous therapeutic attempts and patients have to be fit to withstand the procedure.

Nutcracker Oesophagus

A nutcracker Oesophagus, also known as a hyper contracting oesophagus is characterised by high amplitude (≥ 180 mmHg mean pressure) normal peristaltic contractions in the distal oesophagus on routine manometry. It is a common causes of non-cardiac chest pain with dysphagia and is reported in up to 48%

patients who present with these symptoms. It is more common in females (63%) and the mean age at presentation is 62 years. Its pathogenesis is largely unknown and the literature describes various theories, such as a hyper-cholinergic state affecting the autonomic innervation of the distal oesophagus. The muscularis propria may also be thickened, which manifests as muscular hypertrophy on endoscopic ultrasound [14].

A past medical history of gastro-oesophageal reflux disease is common and up to 77% of patients are on proton pump inhibitors and pH monitoring is used to confirm this. Almost 25% of patients with a nutcracker oesophagus have a co-existing medicated psychiatric disease. In comparison to diffuse oesophageal spasm disease, it does not often occur with regurgitation. A barium swallow is usually normal and reassuringly shows normal peristalsis and no oesophageal pathology. The diagnosis of a nutcracker oesophagus relies upon manometry studies with LOS pressures in excess of 180 mmHg and contractions lasting more than 7.5s. An upper endoscopy should always be done to rule out any obstructing lesions and oesophagitis is a common finding.

Treatment options are variable and once the pain is confirmed as non-cardiac symptoms are usually controlled with drug therapy first. As previously mentioned, gastro-oesophageal reflux is usually treated with a proton pump inhibitor with good results. Anticholinergic drugs, long acting nitrates and calcium channel blockers are of limited value. One study demonstrated that although calcium channel blockers do lower the intra-oesophageal pressures this does not correlate with resolution of symptoms and they have on-going chest pain. Interestingly, the psychosomatic component of a nutcracker oesophagus is an important finding. Studies have suggested that low does tricyclic anti-depressants or cognitive behaviour therapy do provide some symptomatic relief by reducing the sensation of pain. Intermittent pneumatic dilatations may be performed but outcomes are usually unsatisfactory and surgical intervention needs to be carefully thought out and a long oesophageal myotomy can be performed [13].

Vigorous Achalasia

This condition is a variant and more advanced stage of achalasia. It has features of both classic achalasia and diffuse oesophageal spasm. Manometrically, it is characterised by repetitive high amplitude aperistaltic contractions and failure of relaxation of the lower oesophageal sphincter. There is often minimal oesophageal dilatation and prominent tertiary contractions on radiographs. Chest pain is a more prominent feature than in typical achalasia. In addition, the clinical manifestations include dysphagia and regurgitation. Some authorities describe this entity as severe achalasia with more chronic symptoms.

Medical management with long acting nitrates or calcium channel blockers may give some symptomatic relief although the long-term results of this medication are poor. Pneumatic dilatation and botulinum toxin injection also produce temporary relief of dysphagia. However, both PD and Botox injections should be applied to the lower third of the oesophagus as well as the GOJ. Current surgical management consists of a long myotomy from the level of the aortic arch to the gastro-oesophageal junction. This procedure can be performed through a left thoracoscopic approach thus obviating the need for an extensive left postero-lateral thoracotomy. However, the results of this myotomy have been variable. In patients with intractable symptoms, a subtotal oesophagectomy is reported to improve symptoms and nutritional status.

Non-specific Oesophageal Motility Disorders

In non-specific oesophageal motility disorders, a variety of symptoms such as dysphagia, non-cardiac chest pain, regurgitation, heartburn and globus sensation in the absence of an organic disease are reported. The understanding of these motility disorders is still limited, the patients present with a variety of abnormal manometric patterns, but they do not meet the strict criteria of the classical primary oesophageal motility disorders. Therefore, these motor abnormalities have been grouped in a broad category termed non-specific oesophageal motility disorders. The main findings within this group are ineffective (non- propagated) and low amplitude contractions, associated with delayed oesophageal transit of radio-isotopes. Some patients with gastro-oesophageal reflux exhibit these findings, pointing to an association between the two disorders. Whether the motility disorder is the cause or the effect of increased oesophageal acid exposure remains to be determined.

This is a difficult group of patients to diagnosis and treat. Although the motility disorder may be apparent on manometry, there is difficulty in associating the motility disorder with symptoms. Prolonged pH monitoring may isolate a sub-set of patients who might respond to anti-secretory agents. Treatment should be aimed at ameliorating symptoms with medication, which may include sedatives and psychotropic agents.

Chagas' Disease

Chagas disease is a caused by the parasite Trypanosoma Cruzi that is endemic to parts of the Americas, in particular Latin America. Worldwide it affects 6 to 7 million people with a vector borne transmission *via* the triatomine insect. It takes its name from a Brazilian physician, Carlos Ribeiro Justiniano Chagas who first discovered it in 1909. It is a potentially life threatening disease if left untreated. It classically presents with skin lesions and a unilateral purplish swelling of the eyelid and patients may also complain of fevers, headaches, lymphadenopathy and chest or abdominal pain.

Oesophageal involvement is a well-recognized manifestation of the disease and affects up to 25% of patients infested with it. Its pathogenesis is very similar to that of achalasia and thought to be the result of the loss of ganglion cells within the myenteric plexus. Findings on manometry studies show many similarities with achalasia but with a slightly higher LOS pressure in Chagas disease and a shorter contraction period. The proportion of failed contractions seen with Chagas disease is higher and there are less simultaneous contracts than is seen with achalasia [15]. These patients may develop a mega oesophagus and a laparoscopic cardiomyotomy is the treatment of choice with excellent results and long-term resolution of symptoms seen in 95% of sufferers. However, the underlying infection needs to be treated and medications such as Benznidazole or nifurtimox are used to target and eradicate the parasites although there is a lack of structured clinical trials to establish their efficacy in chronic infections. If patient is not fit enough for surgical intervention can be managed with pneumatic dilatation or botulinum toxin therapy.

SECONDARY OESOPHAGEAL MOTILITY DISORDERS

Systemic Sclerosis

This is also known as scleroderma, is the commonest secondary oesophageal motility disorder, however, in itself, it a rare disease affecting 12,000 people in the UK with a prevalence of 88 per million. It is not frequently seen in Asian populations and prevalence varies between world populations (250 per million US and 158 per million in France). Women are affected more frequently than men by approximately 5 times with a peak age in the 5th decade. Systemic sclerosis is an acquired autoimmune disease characterised by thickening of connective tissue as a result of excessive deposition of collagen and other extracellular matrix molecules within the skin and other organs in the body such as the oesophagus [16].

Up to 45% of patients with progressive systemic sclerosis have oesophageal involvement and it develops as a result of smooth muscle atrophy and fibrosis of the distal two thirds of the oesophagus. Deposition of collagen is seen in the lamina propria and submucosal layers of the lower oesophagus, which thins and is often ulcerated. The function of the striated upper segment of the oesophagus and the pharynx is preserved. Almost all of these patients develop a degree of gastro-oesophageal reflux, which can be severe. They demonstrate reduced amplitude or absent peristaltic contractions on motility studies with either a normal or decreased lower oesophageal sphincter pressure. A barium swallow is the principal investigation of choice to identify oesophageal involvement. This shows hypotonia and diminished peristalsis in the lower two thirds of the oesophagus with preservation of the upper third. The longitudinal mucosal folds are lost and oesophagus shows mild to moderate dilatation with a wide-open lower oesophageal sphincter. 17% to 29% of patients develop oesophageal strictures as a result of severe reflux oesophagitis and the literature has reported up to 37% of patients also have Barrett's mucosa. Other features of systemic sclerosis such as those seen in CREST syndrome such as calcinosis, Raynaud's phenomenon, sclerodactyly and telangiectasia, when observed with dysphagia and severe reflux should raise the clinician's suspicion of this diagnosis.

Patients with systemic sclerosis are very difficult to manage and medical therapies with prokinetic agents may be used but with variable outcomes. Surgical management with anti-reflux surgery is an option but results are often unsatisfactory due to the poor calibre of the oesophageal tissue used to suture the wrap to. Patients often complain of post-operative dysphagia as a result of absent peristalsis and even a loose wrap may exacerbate these symptoms. Major surgical resection of the oesophagus with reconstruction of the oesophageal tube using the colon or an isoperistaltic jejunal segment is a theoretical option but is rarely performed and outcomes are of uncertain benefit.

Other less common causes of secondary motility disorders include diabetes, dermatomyositis, lupus erythematosis, rheumatoid arthritis, excessive alcohol consumption and some psychiatric disturbances (*e.g.* anxiety and depression). Management of these patients is targeted at treating the underlying disease rather than the oesophageal symptoms.

GASTROPARESIS

Gastroduodenal motor activity achieves three interrelated digestive functions. First, the stomach is an expansile reservoir, enabling the ingestion of a complete meal without experiencing an uncomfortable sense of fullness. Second, the stomach grinds solids into a fine particulate suspension, liquefying and mixing its contents with saliva, pepsin and hydrochloric acid. This action prepares nutrients for further digestion and absorption from the small bowel. Finally, the stomach and duodenum regulate gastric emptying and entry of nutrients into the small bowel, promoting complete processing and absorption.

There is regional specialization within the stomach with the proximal stomach serving the reservoir function and the body serving the grinding function and the antrum regulating emptying by peristaltic contractions. The antral peristaltic contractions are primarily for solid gastric emptying. Liquid emptying depends on a gastro-duodenal pressure gradient. In response to feeding, the proximal stomach motor activity is in two temporal phases. The first occurs after ingestion of a meal and consists of relaxation reflexes suitable to the reservoir function. The second is a prolonged period of increasing tonic contraction, which maintain the gastroduodenal pressure gradient, and for propelling solids into the body of the stomach for processing. In the distal stomach, the gastric pacemaker stimulates powerful propagating phasic contractions (peristaltic waves), which originate in the mid corpus and proceed to the pylorus. These contractions are responsible for food digestion. Relaxation of the terminal antrum is followed by pyloric opening and emptying of liquids and suspended particles. Larger undigested solids remain trapped ahead of the constricting contractions [17].

Gastroparesis (GP) is a chronic motility disorder of the stomach, which encompasses delayed gastric emptying in the absence of a fixed mechanical obstruction of the pylorus or duodenum. Clinically, this can range from the incidental detection of delayed gastric emptying in an asymptomatic person, to patients with severe nausea, vomiting and malnutrition. Symptoms of GP are nonspecific and may mimic structural disorders such as ulcer disease, partial gastric or small bowel obstruction, gastric cancer, and pancreatico-biliary disorders. A number of conditions can lead to gastroparesis. The most frequent somatic cause is diabetes mellitus. Gastroparesis may also be iatrogenically inflicted by means of surgery or drugs. It may be difficult to discriminate between functional dyspepsia and idiopathic gastroparesis. The condition may have significant consequences for patients with a reduced quality of life, reduced workforce participation and a considerable need for health assistance.

The average prevalence rates of gastroparesis are 30 per 100,000 of population. A gender difference exists with females more commonly affected than males.

Presentation and Clinical Features

Symptoms include early satiety, nausea, bloating, vomiting, abdominal pain and weight loss. Patients often complain of heartburn. Some complain of post-prandial abdominal pain and in severe cases, this may be associated with weight loss. Vomiting is most commonly post-prandial and the vomitus usually contains undigested food. The majority of patients with GP are women. The relationship between upper gastrointestinal symptoms and the rate of gastric emptying is weak. Some patients with markedly delayed gastric emptying are asymptomatic and sometimes, severe symptoms may remit spontaneously. Acute changes in the blood glucose concentration (both hyper-and hypoglycaemia) have a substantial and reversible effect on gastric motility in both healthy subjects and patients with diabetes. Marked hyperglycaemia slows gastric emptying in uncomplicated Type 1 and Type 2 diabetes patients and in diabetic patients with autonomic neuropathy. Changes in the blood glucose concentration within the normal postprandial range can also influence gastric emptying and motility. Conversely, Gastric emptying is a determinant of postprandial glycaemia.

Diagnosis

GP is diagnosed by demonstrating delayed gastric emptying in a symptomatic patient after exclusion of other potential aetiologies of symptoms and obstruction with endoscopy and radiological imaging.

In patients suspected of gastroparesis, diagnostic evaluation requires an initial endoscopy to rule out mechanical causes, followed by a gastric-emptying scintigraphy for diagnosis. Other diagnostic alternatives to scintigraphy would be wireless capsule motility, antro-duodenal manometry, and gastric emptying breath testing (GEBT).

Gastric emptying scintigraphy of a solid-phase meal is considered the gold standard for the diagnosis of GP because this test quantifies the emptying of a physiologic caloric meal. Measurement of gastric emptying in patients with diabetes should be done during euglycaemia. The test involves ingestion of a radioactive labelled meal, either liquid or solid (usually both liquid and solid emptying studies are required). Mathematical processing can then calculate information such as the half emptying time and the fraction of labelled meal that is present in the stomach at different time points. Images should be obtained for up to 4 hours, since retention of greater than 10% of the meal in the stomach at 4 hours is considered abnormal. It is important to note that after gastric surgery, these indices can be misleading as patients often show a fast initial emptying component followed by a slower component [18].

The wireless motility/pH capsule is an orally ingested, non-digestible, data recording device that enables the simultaneous assessment of regional and whole gut transit. Antro-duodenal manometry is a manometric method used for evaluation of stomach and duodenal motility.

The GEBT works by measuring carbon dioxide in a patient's breath over a four-hour period after eating a "test meal." The carbon dioxide measurement is used to calculate the rate at which food is emptied from the stomach.

Pathophysiology

The pathophysiology behind delayed gastric emptying encompasses abnormalities at 3 levels—autonomic nervous system, smooth muscle cells, and enteric neurons. It occurs when the processes of inter-digestive motility, gastric reservoir function or gastric emptying are not controlled.

Several different mechanisms that may cause gastroparesis are as follows:

Fundal hypomotility – the proximal stomach does not stretch when the food is ingested causing early satiety and discomfort. *Antral hypomotility* - where the contractile patterns are not peristaltic or do not flow evenly in a coordinated manner towards the pylorus. *Pyloro-duodenal dis-coordination* causes spasms with material not emptying properly. Gastric pacemaker dysrhythmias in the stomach cause dis-coordinated contractile motility as a result. Excessive inhibitory feedback from the small intestine results in issues with stomach emptying.

Factors that slow gastric emptying include the size and density of the material ingested as well as lipid content. There are also chemical factors including gastric acidity and overall electrolyte tonicity of the ingested material.

Aetiology

Idiopathic Gastroparesis

This may represent the most common form of GP. It usually manifests in patients presenting after an acute viral gastroenteritis-like illness; gastroesophageal reflux disease and non-ulcer dyspepsia; an abdominal-pain-dominated subset; patients who were thought to be depressed or who had received antidepressants in the recent past or were being currently given antidepressants and a subgroup whose symptoms started immediately after a cholecystectomy.

Diabetic Gastroparesis

The true prevalence of digestive symptoms in patients with diabetes and the relationship of these symptoms to delayed gastric emptying are unknown. Delayed gastric emptying is present in up to 58% of patients with type 1 diabetes and 30% with type 2 diabetes. However, highly variable rates of gastric emptying, including acceleration of transit, have been reported in type 1 and 2 diabetes, suggesting that development of GP in patients with diabetes is neither universal nor inevitable. In many diabetics, the magnitude of the delay in gastric emptying is modest and a distinction should be made between the term 'gastroparesis' and 'delayed gastric emptying'. A diagnosis of GP should be restricted to patients in whom gastric emptying is grossly delayed. The delayed gastric emptying in diabetic patients with gastroparesis is probably caused primarily by impaired vagal control [19].

Post-surgical Gastroparesis

GP may occur as a complication of a number of different surgical procedures. Vagal nerve injury may occur in up to 40% of patients who undergo laparoscopic fundoplication for gastroesophageal reflux disease. Some cases of GP have been reported after heart and lung transplantation; this is mostly likely due to vagal nerve injury.

Refractory Gastroparesis

The prevalence of severe, refractory GP is scantily reported in the literature however, it is estimated that the prevalence of severe, symptomatic and refractory GP is around 2 in 10,000 of the population.

Other causes of gastroparesis include metabolic and endocrine disorders, hypothyroidism, electrolyte imbalance, Collagen vascular disease (*e.g.* Scleroderma), medications (anticholinergics, narcotics, levodopa, salbutamol, loperamide), idiopathic and secondary pseudo-obstruction syndromes (amyloidosis, muscular dystrophy, para-neoplastic). In addition, peptic ulcer disease, gastritis and acute viral gastroenteritis can induce temporary gastroparesis.

Complications

Complications of severe gastroparesis include oesophagitis, Mallory–Weiss tear, peptic ulcer disease, and bezoar formation. Severe cases can have severe weight loss and metabolic abnormalities. The majority of these patients have a poor quality of life and are unable to work due to this chronic disabling condition. The different therapeutic modalities provide transient relief from some of the symptoms.

Medical Management of Gastroparesis

Dietary measures (*e.g.,* low fibre, low fat food), prokinetic drugs (*e.g.,* domperidone, metoclopramide, erythromycin) and antiemetic or anti-nausea drugs (*e.g.,* phenothiazines, diphenhydramine, dimenhydrinate, ondansetron, desipramine, nortriptyline, amitriptyline, scopolamine, and hyoscyamine,) are generally effective for symptomatic relief in the majority of patients with GP. Dietary modifications such as small frequent meals with less residue and low fat are encouraged. Liquid meals empty quicker and serum glucose control is important. Medical treatment of severe gastroparesis is a stepwise process beginning with rehydration, followed by progression to soups and finally introduction to more solid food. Fatty foods should be avoided as should red meat, fresh vegetables and fibre which require more electro-contractile work. Behavioural modification/psychiatric treatment may play a role for some patients.

For patients with chronic, symptomatic GP who are refractory to drug treatment, surgical options may include jejunostomy tube feeding, gastrotomy tube for stomach decompression (venting) and pyloroplasty for gastric emptying.

Endoscopy and Gastroparesis

For patients that exhaust all attempts at pharmacotherapy, endoscopic therapy can be considered. Endoscopic treatment of gastroparesis involves the injection of Botox into the pyloric sphincter. Pyloric muscle spasms are believed to contribute to delayed gastric emptying, and these injections offer localized reduction of these contractions however more evidence is required to show the efficacy of Botox in GP. More recently, per oral endoscopic pyloromyotomy has been described. However, it is too early to recommend this emerging therapy until short and long-term outcomes have been evaluated.

Surgery and Gastroparesis

Surgical placement of a jejunostomy tube can be performed in patients with severe refractory gastroparesis. Refractory patients can be managed with gastroenterostomy. Although a number of patients have had considerable improvement in symptoms with a gastroenterostomy, others have not noticed any appreciable improvement. To the contrary, some patients have had additional symptoms related to the gastroenterostomy which they have found more disabling than those related to GP. More recently, surgically inserted gastric electrical stimulation has become a popular mode of treatment for refractory gastroparesis with or without a gastric drainage procedure [20].

Gastric Electrical Stimulation

Treatment with GES is reversible and may be a less invasive option compared to stomach surgery for the treatment of patients with chronic, drug-refractory nausea and vomiting secondary to GP. In theory, GES represents an intermediate step between treatment directed at the underlying pathophysiology and the treatment of symptoms. It is based on studies of gastric electrical patterns in GP that have identified the presence of a variety of gastric arrhythmias. Similar to a cardiac pacemaker, it was hypothesized that GES could override the abnormal rhythms, stimulate gastric emptying and eliminate symptoms [21].

Gastric electrical stimulation (GES) is delivered *via* an implanted system that consists of a neurostimulator and 2 leads (Fig. **11**). The surgical procedure can be performed *via* either an open or laparoscopic approach. An external programmer used by the physician can deliver instructions to the GES, to adjust the rate and amplitude of stimulation. GES may be turned off by the physician at any time or may be removed. The battery life is approximately 4-5 years. For treatment of GP, the GES leads are secured in the muscle of the lower stomach, 10 cm proximal to the pylorus, 1 cm apart and connected to an implantable battery-powered neurostimulator which is implanted subcutaneously in a small pocket in the abdominal wall.

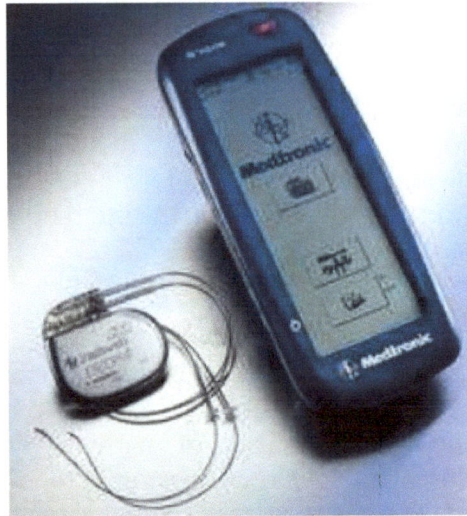

Fig. (11). Gastric Electrical stimulation device and programmer.

Electric stimulation often occurs at a frequency faster than the intrinsic antral flow wave of the stomach. The idea behind gastric stimulation is that theoretically one entrains the gastric slow waves with low frequency (in the sub Hertz range)/long duration pulses (approximately 3 cycles/min.) or high-frequency low-energy, short-duration pulses. The former pacing is called *gastric electrical pacing* and uses low-frequency, high-energy, long-duration pulses to induce propagated slow waves that replace the spontaneous ones. By contrast, most clinical studies examining GES for GP have used high-frequency (4 times the intrinsic slow wave frequency, *i.e.*, 12 cycles per minute), low-energy, short-duration pulses. This type of stimulation does not alter gastric muscular contraction (is unaffected by atropine), and has no effect on slow wave dysrhythmias.

GES improves nausea and vomiting in approx. 50% of patients. It is not however helpful for pain or bloating and is less helpful for those patients on chronic narcotic analgesia. It does not improve gastric emptying scintigraphy and it does not change gastric electrical rhythm. There is a suggestion that it may work better in diabetics than non-diabetics and may improve quality of life. GES should be used more often for symptom control rather than treatment of the motility disorder. However, it should be considered a last resort treatment after all conventional treatments had failed to control symptoms of nausea and vomiting.

There are possible risks associated with the implantation of the device, including the risk of infection that would require the removal of the GES in 5-10% of cases. As such, the use of GES should be restricted to patients who have severe symptoms and are refractory to another less invasive approach such as drugs and diet. A continuous follow-up of the patients is necessary to identify adverse events and effects, assess costs, and study quality of life.

CONSENT FOR PUBLICATION

Not applicable.

ACKNOWLEDGEMENT

Declare none.

CONFLICT OF INTEREST

The authors declare no conflict of interest, financial or otherwise.

REFERENCES

[1]   Fox MR, Bredenoord AJ. Oesophageal high-resolution manometry: moving from research into clinical practice. Gut 2008; 57(3): 405-23.
[http://dx.doi.org/10.1136/gut.2007.127993] [PMID: 17895358]

[2]   Bredenoord AJ, Fox M, Kahrilas PJ, Pandolfino JE, Schwizer W, Smout AJ. Chicago classification criteria of esophageal motility disorders defined in high resolution esophageal pressure topography. Neurogastroenterol Motil 2012; 24 (Suppl. 1): 57-65.
[http://dx.doi.org/10.1111/j.1365-2982.2011.01834.x] [PMID: 22248109]

[3]   Boeckxstaens GE, Zaninotto G, Richter JE. Achalasia. Lancet 2014; 383(9911): 83-93.
[http://dx.doi.org/10.1016/S0140-6736(13)60651-0] [PMID: 23871090]

[4]   Müller M. Impact of high-resolution manometry on achalasia diagnosis and treatment. Ann Gastroenterol 2015; 28(1): 3-9.
[PMID: 25608535]

[5]   Vaezi MF, Pandolfino JE, Vela MF. ACG clinical guideline: diagnosis and management of achalasia. Am J Gastroenterol 2013; 108(8): 1238-49.
[http://dx.doi.org/10.1038/ajg.2013.196] [PMID: 23877351]

[6]   Storr M, Born P, Frimberger E, *et al.* Treatment of achalasia: the short-term response to botulinum toxin injection seems to be independent of any kind of pretreatment. BMC Gastroenterol 2002; 2: 19.
[http://dx.doi.org/10.1186/1471-230X-2-19] [PMID: 12175425]

[7]   Salvador R, Costantini M, Cavallin F, *et al.* Laparoscopic Heller myotomy can be used as primary therapy for esophageal achalasia regardless of age. J Gastrointest Surg 2014; 18(1): 106-11.
[http://dx.doi.org/10.1007/s11605-013-2334-y] [PMID: 24018591]

[8]   Hamer PW, Holloway RH, Heddle R, *et al.* Evaluation of outcome after cardiomyotomy for achalasia using the Chicago classification. Br J Surg 2016; 103(13): 1847-54.
[http://dx.doi.org/10.1002/bjs.10285] [PMID: 27696376]

[9]   Devaney EJ, Lannettoni MD, Orringer MB, Marshall B. Esophagectomy for achalasia: patient selection and clinical experience. Ann Thorac Surg 2001; 72(3): 854-8.
[http://dx.doi.org/10.1016/S0003-4975(01)02890-9] [PMID: 11565670]

[10]   Youn YH, Minami H, Chiu PW, Park H. Peroral endoscopic myotomy for treating achalasia and esophageal motility disorders. J Neurogastroenterol Motil 2016; 22(1): 14-24.
[http://dx.doi.org/10.5056/jnm15191] [PMID: 26717928]

[11]   Achem SR. Diffuse esophageal spasm in the era of high-resolution manometry. Gastroenterol Hepatol (N Y) 2014; 10(2): 130-3.
[PMID: 24803878]

[12]   Burmeister S. Review of current diagnosis and management of diffuse esophageal spasm, nutcracker esophagus/spastic nutcracker and hypertensive lower esophageal sphincter. Curr Opin Otolaryngol Head Neck Surg 2013; 21(6): 543-7.
[http://dx.doi.org/10.1097/MOO.0000000000000002] [PMID: 24157634]

[13]   Shimi SM, Nathanson LK, Cuschieri A. Thoracoscopic long oesophageal myotomy for nutcracker oesophagus: initial experience of a new surgical approach. Br J Surg 1992; 79(6): 533-6.
[http://dx.doi.org/10.1002/bjs.1800790619] [PMID: 1611445]

[14]   Lufrano R, Heckman MG, Diehl N, DeVault KR, Achem SR. Nutcracker esophagus: demographic, clinical features, and esophageal tests in 115 patients. Dis Esophagus 2015; 28(1): 11-8.
[http://dx.doi.org/10.1111/dote.12160] [PMID: 24251375]

[15]   Dantas RO, Deghaide NH, Donadi EA. Esophageal motility of patients with Chagas' disease and idiopathic achalasia. Dig Dis Sci 2001; 46(6): 1200-6.
[http://dx.doi.org/10.1023/A:1010698826004] [PMID: 11414294]

[16]   Ebert EC. Esophageal disease in scleroderma. J Clin Gastroenterol 2006; 40(9): 769-75.
[http://dx.doi.org/10.1097/01.mcg.0000225549.19127.90] [PMID: 17016130]

[17]   Jung HK, Choung RS, Locke GR III, *et al.* The incidence, prevalence, and outcomes of patients with gastroparesis in Olmsted County, Minnesota, from 1996 to 2006. Gastroenterology 2009; 136(4): 1225-33.
[http://dx.doi.org/10.1053/j.gastro.2008.12.047] [PMID: 19249393]

[18]   Stein B, Everhart KK, Lacy BE. Gastroparesis: A review of current diagnosis and treatment options. J Clin Gastroenterol 2015; 49(7): 550-8.
[http://dx.doi.org/10.1097/MCG.0000000000000320] [PMID: 25874755]

[19]   Marathe CS, Rayner CK, Jones KL, Horowitz M. Novel insights into the effects of diabetes on gastric motility. Expert Rev Gastroenterol Hepatol 2016; 10(5): 581-93.
[http://dx.doi.org/10.1586/17474124.2016.1129898] [PMID: 26647088]

[20]   Davis BR, Sarosiek I, Bashashati M, Alvarado B, McCallum RW. The long-term efficacy and safety of pyloroplasty combined with gastric electrical stimulation therapy in gastroparesis. J Gastrointest Surg 2017; 21(2): 222-7.
[http://dx.doi.org/10.1007/s11605-016-3327-4] [PMID: 27896652]

[21]   Wo JM, Nowak TV, Waseem S, Ward MP. Gastric electrical stimulation for gastroparesis and chronic unexplained nausea and vomiting. Curr Treat Options Gastroenterol 2016; 14(4): 386-400.
[http://dx.doi.org/10.1007/s11938-016-0103-1] [PMID: 27678506]

CHAPTER 3

Oesophageal Neoplasms

Pradeep Patil[*] and **Sami M. Shimi**

Department of Surgery, Ninewells Hospital and Medical School, Dundee, Scotland, UK

Abstract: Oesophageal cancer is the eighth most common cancer and the sixth most common cause of death from cancer. Histologically, oesophageal cancers are composed mainly of two variants: squamous cell cancer and adenocarcinoma of the oesophagus. Benign tumours are rare. The aetiology of squamous cell cancer is largely unknown but adenocarcinoma progresses from Barrett's oesophagus. Diagnosis is by endoscopy and staging is done by a combination of CT, EUS and PET/CT. Many tumour markers have been elucidated and their potential importance in diagnosis and treatment is actively pursued. Endoscopic therapy is appropriate for node negative patients with early cancers limited to the mucosa. Less than 30% of all patients with oesophageal cancer are suitable for curative treatment. Surgical treatment by oesophagectomy is appropriate for medically fit patients with T<4, N<3 and M<1 tumours. Neoadjuvant therapy (chemoradiotherapy or chemotherapy) is advocated for all tumour types. The management of patients with locally advanced or metastatic oesophageal cancer and patients with poor general medical condition must be individualised based on stage, characteristics of the tumour, patient's medical condition and patient preference. The aim of palliative treatment is to achieve rapid and sustained relief of dysphagia. Chemotherapy alone or in combination with radiotherapy should be considered with other palliative measures. Canalisation of the tumour and restoration of swallowing is best achieved using self-expanding metallic stents. Best supportive care may be appropriate in frail patients with advanced disease at presentation.

Keywords: Adenocarcinoma, Cancer of oesophago-gastric junction, Non-surgical treatment, Oesophagectomy, Palliation of oesophageal cancer, Pathology, Squamous cell cancer, Staging.

GENERAL FEATURES OF OESOPHAGEAL TUMOURS

Oesophageal cancer is the eighth most common cancer and the sixth most common cause of death from cancer. Oesophageal cancers are composed mainly of two histological variants: squamous cell cancer and adenocarcinoma of the oesophagus. The incidences of these cancers vary between the eastern and western hemispheres of the globe. Squamous cell carcinomas are dominant in Asia

---

[*] **Corresponding author Pradeep Patil:** Department of Surgery, Ninewells Hospital and Medical School, Dundee DD1 9SY, Scotland, UK; Tel/Fax: +44 1382 660111; E-mail: pradeeppatil@nhs.net

especially china and along the southern belt of Russia including Iran and Afghanistan. Adenocarcinoma is predominantly seen in the western hemisphere and Australia. Oesophageal cancer is predominantly a male disease with squamous cancer being two to four times common and adenocarcinomas being four to eight times common in males.

Tumours of the oesophagus are predominately malignant. Symptomatic benign tumours are rarely encountered in clinical practice and account for less than 1% of all oesophageal neoplasms.

Aetiology and Risk Factors

The aetiology of oesophageal cancer remains unknown but is currently thought to be multifactorial. The biology and aetiology of squamous cell cancer of the oesophagus and adenocarcinoma of the oesophagus are different. The important factors for squamous cell cancer of the oesophagus include the following:

1. Excess alcohol intake.
2. Smoking
3. Absence of protective substances in fruits and green vegetables.
4. Ingestion of exogenous carcinogens and promoting factors.

Various epidemiological surveys have shown a good correlation between excess alcohol intake and smoking with the incidence of oesophageal cancer. Alcohol is thought to act as a promoter rather than a direct carcinogen. Tobacco however, is considered a direct carcinogen. Certain vitamins (A, B^{12}, C, E, folic acid and riboflavin) and trace elements (iron, zinc, selenium and molybdenum) are thought to be protective. Deficiency of these substances either from inadequate ingestion of green vegetables and fruits or as a consequence of soil depletion (in the case of trace elements), is associated with a high incidence of oesophageal cancer. The carcinogenic compounds and promoters, which have been implicated in endemic areas are nitrosamines, tannins (polyhydrophenyls), alcohol and phorbol esters (present in herbal/medicinal teas).

Risk factors linked to oesophageal squamous carcinoma are tobacco smoking, alcohol and hot beverages and food intake. Diets high in fruit and vegetables have been shown to be protective against cancer.

Risk factors for adenocarcinoma include white race and male gender, smoking, obesity, gastro oesophageal reflux disease and Barrett's oesophagus [1]. Adenocarcinomas of the distal oesophagus or gastro oesophageal junction typically affect patients (males) more than 50 years with the highest incidence between 55 and 65 years of age. In addition, there are certain disorders, which are known to predispose to the development of cancer of the oesophagus.

Tylosis palmaris et plantaris is a hereditary autosomal dominant disorder transmitted by a single autosomal gene. It is characterised by the development of hyperkeratosis of the skin of the palms and feet during the first and second decades and the subsequent development of cancer of the oesophagus in virtually all affected individuals by the seventh decade.

The risk of oesophageal cancer in patients with *achalasia* is not reduced by myotomy. When carcinoma develops in this condition and in patients with long standing strictures, it is usually diagnosed late and therefore carries a poor prognosis. The slightly increased risk in patients with *scleroderma* is secondary to gastro-oesophageal reflux rather than the condition itself. There is controversy as to whether infection with the human papilloma virus predisposes to squamous cell cancer of the oesophagus. Other high-risk diseases include *Plummer-Vinson syndrome*, strictures associated with Lye ingestion and the human papilloma virus infection.

For adenocarcinoma of the oesophagus, case control studies indicate that smoking, obesity and a history of chronic gastro-oesophageal reflux are significant factors. There is a clear racial, gender, and site predilection for oesophageal adenocarcinoma. Approximately 95% of patients are white, men outnumber women 5:1, and approximately 80% of patients have tumours in the distal third of the oesophagus or gastro-oesophageal junction.

Presentation

The commonest presenting feature of oesophageal cancer is progressive dysphagia. Patients report difficulty in swallowing and pain with swallowing, particularly when eating meat, bread, or raw vegetables. As the tumor grows, it can block the thoroughfare to the stomach. Even liquid may be painful to swallow. In this scenario, patients are not able to swallow their saliva. Other patients report pressure or burning in the chest akin to indigestion or heartburn. Some complain of chest (mediastinal), throat or referred pain to the shoulders when the oesophagus is distended with food material. Some complain of choking on food items with spontaneous or induced regurgitation or vomiting. Some describe this choking as recurrent episodes of coughing or hiccups. Cervical cancers can present with hoarseness of the voice or stridor in advanced cases. Obstructing gastro oesophageal junctional cancers can occasionally present with features of achalasia (pseudo-achalasia). Patients can also have features of malnutrition such as weight loss, anorexia, lethargy, tiredness and anaemia. Metastatic cancers can present with liver or lung signs or bone pain suggestive of bony metastases. In advanced cases, cancer cachexia is evident.

The majority of patients in the west present with advanced stages of the disease. Dysphagia may not become apparent until two thirds of the oesophageal lumen has been obliterated. Oesophageal obstruction will result in malnutrition, weight loss, regurgitation and occasionally aspiration. Some patients may have palpable cervical lymph nodes and hepatic or cutaneous metastases at presentation.

Diagnosis

The key investigation for establishing the diagnosis in patients with progressive dysphagia with or without weight loss is endoscopy with biopsy (cytology). Endoscopy gives precise information on the site and extent of circumferential involvement of the oesophagus by the tumour. For best results, a biopsy protocol should be adopted and should include biopsy forceps with adequate tissue retrieval and a mandatory minimum number of biopsies at primary endoscopy. Contrast radiology gives a good assessment of the length of stenotic lesions, which do not allow complete endoscopic assessment. However, this information is more readily obtained from three-dimensional imaging. Resectability and cure rates decline sharply for lesions longer that 5 cm. As such both endoscopy and 3-D radiology are essential and complimentary. Endoscopy is the most reliable modality for screening in high-risk areas and in individuals with known predisposing conditions.

The advanced stages of this disease are associated with non-resectability and poor survival even after resection. Detecting the disease at an early stage is proven to increase the resectability and survival rates. The most sensitive and cost effective screening method is endoscopy. However, screening can only be justified in areas of high prevalence and in individuals with predisposing conditions such as Barrett's oesophagus. Although the area of biomarkers has received a lot of recent research interest, serum markers have not so far been shown to be useful in the detection of early oesophageal tumours. However, progress in this area is expected and would be appreciated.

PATHOLOGY, HISTOLOGY AND BIO-MARKERS

Benign Tumours

The commonest benign tumour of the oesophagus is leiomyoma (smooth muscle tumour). They occur most commonly in the lower oesophagus (Fig. **1**) and may be multiple.

Fig. (1). A CT scan slice through the upper abdomen showing lower oesophageal leiomyoma.

The majority are small and asymptomatic but larger ones can be seen as uniform oval swellings, which project in to the lumen of the oesophagus and are covered by an intact mucosa. Some lesions may calcify. The most common presentation is with dysphagia. Bleeding, due to ulceration is less common than with gastric leiomyomas although it is well documented. Malignant transformation can occur but is rare. As the tumours are well encapsulated, they can be removed by enucleation without oesophageal resection. Endoscopic removal is suitable for small pedunculated lesions. Localised resection is indicated if the lesion is large, adherent to the mucosa or at the gastro-oesophageal junction.

The next common benign tumours in the oesophagus are fibrous or fibro- vascular polyps. They occur commonly in the upper third of the oesophagus and are covered by squamous epithelial lining, which may be ulcerated. Inflammatory polyps, also called oesophago-gastric polyps are encountered at the gastro-oesophageal junction, and are covered by both gastric and oesophageal epithelium and are associated with chronic oesophagitis. Adenomatous polyps are usually encountered at the lower end of the oesophagus and may be sessile or pedunculated. Most adenomatous oesophageal polyps arise as a consequence of reflux oesophagitis or columnar metaplasia.

Squamous cell papillomas (caused by the human papilloma virus) may occur anywhere in the oesophagus. They are usually single, multi-lobulated with a granular or warty surface and can vary in size. Granular cell tumours, which are rare, arise from Schwann cells. They effect middle-aged women and are usually found in the distal oesophagus. Haemangiomas are rare in the oesophagus and are usually discovered incidentally. Neurofibromas are also rare and occur as a manifestation of neurofibromatosis.

Malignant Oesophageal Neoplasms

Malignant oesophageal neoplasms are mostly carcinomas and carry a poor prognosis with an overall five-year survival of 5%. In the west, cancer of the oesophagus is predominantly a disease of elderly (more than 60 years) men with an overall incidence of 10-20 per hundred thousand of population per annum. The highest incidence in the Western Hemisphere is found in France, followed by Scotland where the frequency of the disease has more than doubled in the last 30 years. Carcinoma of the oesophagus is some 20 to 30 times more common in China, Iran and the Transkei region of South Africa than in the west. The endemic cancers in these high incidence countries occur at a younger age and the male predominance of the disease is not as marked as in western countries. Throughout the world, the incidence of cancer of the oesophagus is increasing in both sexes with a trend towards a greater increase in women. In contrast, there is a clear declining trend in Finland, with a decrease in incidence and mortality of about 10% every 5 years for both sexes.

The vast majority of malignant neoplasms of the oesophagus are carcinomas. Typical squamous cell carcinoma (SCC) and adenocarcinoma (AC) account for 95% of oesophageal cancers. The remaining cases include unusual histologic variants of squamous cell carcinoma such as verrucous carcinoma, basaloid squamous carcinoma (adenoid cystic carcinoma), pseudosarcomatous squamous cell carcinoma (carcinosarcoma), variants of adenocarcinoma such as adenosquamous carcinoma and mucoepidermoid carcinoma, and a variety of other tumour types including choriocarcinoma, gastrointestinal stromal tumours (leiomyosarcoma), liposarcoma, malignant fibrous histiocytoma, synovial sarcoma, rhabdomyosarcoma, small cell carcinoma and melanoma. In addition, the oesophagus can be involved in metastatic cancer primarily from the lung and breast.

The predominant histological type throughout the world is squamous but adenocarcinomas especially of the lower oesophagus and gastro-oesophageal junction are increasing particularly in the west. Adenocarcinoma of the oesophago-gastric junction can behave biologically similar to adenocarcinoma of the oesophagus. These are however classified separately into three types. In the west, the peak incidence of the disease is found over the age of 60 years and predominantly in males although in the past decade there has been an increased incidence in the younger age group (30-50 years), and the male to female sex predominance is narrowing.

Macroscopically tumours assume one of three forms:

1. Polyploid (fungating, protruded) (60%) (Fig. **2**).

2. Stenosing (scirrhous, flat, diffuse, infiltrative) (15%) (Fig. **2**).
3. Ulcerative (excavated) (25%) (Fig. **2**).

Growth of oesophageal cancer (SCC or AC) occurs by intra-oesophageal spread, direct extension and lymphatic or haematogenous metastasis. SCC more typically invades adjacent structures than AC. Distant metastasis may be present in 25 – 30% of patients at the time of diagnosis and in up to 50% of patients at autopsy. The liver (32%), lungs (21%), and bones are the most frequent sites.

Early cancer of the oesophagus (confined to mucosa/submucosa) is rarely encountered in the west because of the absence of screening programmes. The transition between severe dysplasia to carcinoma-in-situ and invasive adenocarcinoma of the oesophagus is well documented. The results of surgical treatment for early oesophageal cancer are extremely favourable with a very low operative mortality and a five-year survival of 80-85%. There is an increasingly stronger argument for screening programmes, particularly in areas of high incidence and in patients with known predisposing conditions. The increased incidence of adenocarcinoma in the west and its relationship to columnar metaplasia has prompted structured surveillance programmes for patients with metaplasia and dysplasia.

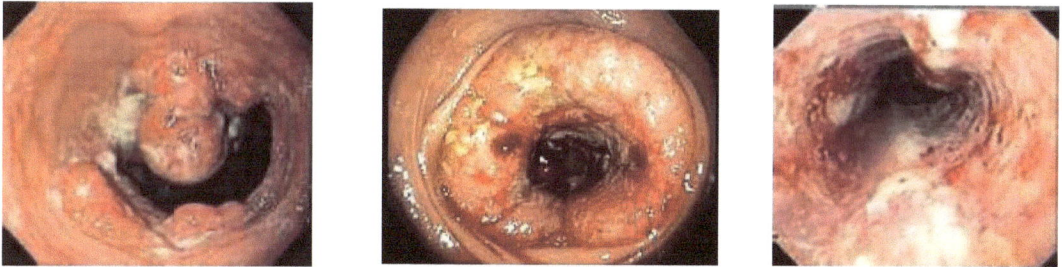

Fig. (2). Endoscopic photographs of polypoidal (left), stenosing (centre) and ulcerative adenocarcinomas of the oesophagus (right).

Histology

The histological types of oesophageal cancer include Squamous cell carcinoma, Adenocarcinoma, squamous cell cancer variants, adenocarcinoma variants and other less prevalent tumours.

Squamous Cell Carcinoma (OSCC)

This accounts for 90% of oesophageal cancers (excluding gastric cardia cancers). Squamous cell cancers occur throughout the length of the oesophagus and are equally common in the middle and lower thirds but are less frequent in the upper third. Early lesions appear as small, grey-white, plaque-like thickenings or elevations of the mucosa. Depending on the degree of keratinization and cytological atypia, the histological appearance can be well, moderate or poly-differentiated. The degree of differentiation does not seem to correlate with the extent of the disease, the presence of metastases or the prognosis. Two histological variants are occasionally seen. These are the verrucous carcinoma and the carcino-sarcoma, which has a mixture of squamous and spindle cells and is less aggressive. The carcinoma invades the muscle walls of the oesophagus and the adjacent mediastinal structures, particularly nerves (recurrent laryngeal, phrenic) and/or the major bronchi and trachea and pericardium. Lymph node spread from tumours of the upper third is predominately to the supraclavicular, cervical and upper mediastinal nodes; from middle third neoplasms may involve all the mediastinal nodes and those along the left gastric and coeliac vessels, whereas neoplasms in the lower third usually spread preferentially to the lower mediastinal and sub-diaphragmatic nodes. Metastatic spread is preferentially to the liver, lungs and bones. Most symptomatic tumours are quite large by the time they are diagnosed and have already invaded mediastinal structures and metastasised. Squamous cell carcinoma of the oesophagus is sensitive to radiotherapy.

Adenocarcinoma (OAC)

The majority of adenocarcinomas of the oesophagus usually originate from Barrett's epithelium following long-standing gastro oesophageal reflux. Consequently, they are usually located in the distal oesophagus and may invade the adjacent gastric cardia. A few adenocarcinomas may arise from ectopic gastric epithelium or from the oesophageal sub-mucus glands.

The sequence of progression from intestinal metaplasia through dysplasia to carcinoma *in situ* and invasive carcinoma is well documented. The time interval between each of the phases however is unknown. The lesion initially appears as a flat or raised patch of an otherwise intact mucosa. It can then assume one of the three macroscopic features. Microscopically most tumours are mucin producing glandular tumours. The tumours may exhibit intestinal-type features or less often are made up of diffusely infiltrative signet-ring cells of a gastric type. Occasionally squamous cells, adenosquamous cells and adenocarcinoid cells can be found within the tumour. The mode of spread of adenocarcinoma is similar to that of squamous tumours. The prognosis of oesophageal adenocarcinoma is poor and these tumours are relatively insensitive to radiotherapy.

Squamous Cell Variants

These include verrucous carcinoma, basaloid squamous carcinoma (adenoid cystic carcinoma), and pseudosarcomatous squamous cells carcinoma (carcinosarcoma).

Verrucous carcinoma is a tumour with a low-grade malignancy however prognosis can be fairly poor. Oesophageal resection is the treatment of choice. Carcinosarcoma is a polypoid tumour with squamous cells as well as spindle cell components. The tumour behaves biologically like squamous cell carcinoma and the treatment is similar. Adenoid cystic carcinomas are histologically and biologically identical to adenoids cystic carcinoma of the salivary gland. They are intramural tumours and are believed to arise from oesophageal submucosal glands. The tumours are slow growing indolent lesions. Basaloid squamous carcinoma is a locally aggressive malignant lesion, which generally metastasises late in its course. Oesophageal resection is indicated for these tumours.

Adenoma Carcinoma Variants

Mucoepidermoid carcinoma and adenosquamous carcinoma have oesophageal squamous cell cancer with a mucin-secreting component. They are uncommon and are thought to arise from oesophageal submucosal glands. The tumours behave biologically similar to primary oesophageal squamous cell carcinoma. Oesophageal resection is the treatment of choice.

Other Tumours

Leiomyosarcoma of the oesophagus arise from the muscularis propria or more rarely from the muscularis mucosa. They consist of irregular whorls of neomorphic spindle cells. They appear more frequently in the lower third of the oesophagus, with the remainder equally distributed in the middle and upper thirds. These tumours are slow growing, of a low grade and uncommonly metastasise. The treatment of choice is wide surgical resection. Although these tumours are considered radio resistant, radiotherapy can be considered for some patients with co-morbid disease.

Liposarcoma, malignant fibrous histiocytoma, synovial sarcoma, and rhabdomyosarcoma are rare in the oesophagus and should be treated by radical resection when possible. Primary lymphomas are very uncommon and most of the reported cases have been of the non-Hodgkin's type [2].

Peptide-secreting malignant oesophageal tumours are rare, but are well documented. Most, but not all, have been instances of oat cell type tumour with secretory granules but others are histologically squamous cell carcinomas. Inappropriate secretion of ACTH, calcitonin, parathyroid hormone and VIP has been reported.

Tumour Biomarkers

Cancer biomarkers may provide some promising therapeutic targets for the diagnosis, treatment, and prognosis of oesophageal cancer. They provide an important potential in the development of treatment strategies, which can be integrated with diverse clinical characteristics [3].

Immunohistochemical Biomarkers

Immunohistochemistry (IHC) is the most widely applied pathological technique in determining the expression of tumor-associated proteins and in studying the prognostic and clinical relevance of biomarkers. Several investigators have demonstrated that many immunohistochemical markers have potential diagnostic, prognostic, or predictive indicators in oesophageal cancer. The role of IHC is important in elucidating pathways for epidermal growth, angiogenesis, and apoptosis. Several biomarkers have been studied in detail including: epidermal growth factor receptor (EGFR), p53, vascular endothelial growth factor (VEGF), and estrogen receptor (ER).

EGFR is a transmembrane protein with intrinsic tyrosine kinase activity. It is associated with specific ligands, such as EGF and TGF-α. Elevated levels of EGFR or increased expression levels of the EGFR gene have been reported in a number of human cancers of epithelial origin including oesophageal cancer. Increased EGFR expression is associated with advanced disease, tumor metastases, and poor prognosis. A member of the EGFR family, epidermal growth factor receptor 2 (HER2) has become a therapeutic target for some tumors including oesophageal cancer. HER2, a transmembrane receptor tyrosine kinase family member, is involved in cell regulation, cell growth, survival, differentiation, and migration of important substances.

Decrease in the expression of the three proteins E-cadherin, α-catenin, and β-catenin is associated with a decrease in the survival of patients with oesophageal adenocarcinoma.

p53 was found to play a supplementary role in the diagnosis of dysplasia and can be used as a predictor of disease progression. VEGF is a potent source of angiogenesis, and it is responsible for the development and maintenance of a vascular network that promotes tumor growth and metastasis for a wide range of human tumors. In clinical specimens, the expression of VEGF-C in oesophageal cancer tissues is higher than that in noncancerous tissues. Positive expression of VEGF-C may be closely related to the progression of the disease.

Oestrogen receptor types ORa and ORb were detected in the nuclei in cases of OSCC. There are suggestions that ORb can be used as an indicator of prognosis. In addition, MEKK3/MAP3K3, SOX2 (sex determining region Y-box 2) and AGR2 (Anterior gradient 2) overexpression was found in a large series of OAC and OSCC.

Blood-based Biomarkers

In the early stages of carcinogenesis, the antigen immune response is believed to occur during cancer immune surveillance, in which the antigen is recognized by the immune system, which destroys the invading pathogen and host cell of the cancer. Antibodies against tumor-associated antigen (TAA), which is present in the serum of patients with various types of cancers, can be used as a biomarker for early diagnosis of oesophageal cancer. These antibodies are complex and are not yet fully understood in the theory of carcinogenesis. Numerous studies have indicated that TAAs in the blood circulation of cancer patients can be detectable several years earlier than the positive imaging findings, so they can be used as novel screening markers. Thus, TAAs produced by autoantibodies can be biomarkers for the early detection of malignant transformation criteria for preclinical studies, which can be used as a biomarker for early detection.

Anti-p53 induced by mutant p53 protein in serum is one of the most frequently tested antibodies and has a promising potential diagnostic value in oesophageal cancer. However, it has low sensitivity. However, s-p53-antibody may be useful for monitoring residual tumor cells and for aiding in the selection of candidates for less invasive treatment procedures because of its high specificity.

Four antibodies (*i.e.,* SURF1, HOOK2, LOC146223, and AGENCOURT_ 7565913) are highly specific for oesophageal cancer, in comparison with other common cancers. Microarrays can be used to identify the combination of Fas ligand and anti-NY-ESO-1, with a high sensitivity and specificity for the detection of OAC. Autoantibody markers and a combination of antibodies and other proteins can be detected using a combination of antibody markers and conventional tumor markers, such as CEA, CA199, CYFRA211 or SCC-Ag.

mRNA-based Biomarkers

MicroRNA (miRNA) is a group of evolutionary conserved single chain non-coding RNAs that can participate in physiological processes, such as cell differentiation, proliferation, metabolism, and apoptosis. Some miRNAs play an important role in the tumor gene or tumor suppressor gene in the development of tumors. Circulating plasma and serum miRNAs are potential markers for noninvasive cancer diagnosis, which can be used in the diagnosis, prognosis, and targeted therapy of oesophageal cancer.

Increasing evidence suggested that miR-129 has the potential to become a companion diagnostic biomarker along with clinical histopathological diagnosis. SOX4 (sex determining region Y-box 4) is a transcription factor closely related to several critical pathways in the process of tumorigenesis, such as TGF-β (transforming growth factor-beta), Notch, and hedgehog signaling. It may play an important role in tumor metastasis and progression.

The role of miR-200 in tumor progression, invasion, metastasis, and drug resistance has also been described. Its interactions with E-cadherin and vimentin, the two surrogate markers of the epithelial–mesenchymal transition (EMT), integrin β1-AKT pathway *via* targeting kindlin-2 and the PI3 K-AKT signaling pathway have been described.

Various studies reported that other miRNAs are involved in the onset, development, progression and response to treatment of oesophageal cancer. These include miR-31, miR-196a, ANXA1 (can mediate cell apoptosis and inhibit cell proliferation), miR-21, miR-106b-25 (can inhibit the expression of target genes p21 and Bim and promote the transformation from Barrett to OAC), miR-205 (can inhibit the expression of ZEB (Zinc finger E-box binding homeobox), thereby blocking the epithelial-to-mesenchymal transition-EMT, GNG7 (guanine nucleotide binding protein (G protein), gamma 7), miR-375 and miR-27a (may affect the multidrug resistance of oesophageal cancer).

In addition to miRNA, long non-coding RNAs (lncRNAs), another type of RNA molecule, are steadily becoming the next frontier of cancer research. Recent findings confirmed that lncRNA is a key regulator of tumor development and progression in the oesophagus. lncRNA can be easily and rapidly extracted from serum and tissue, as well as in the gastric juice in oesophageal cancer patients. It is expected to be a useful biomarker and therapeutic target in clinical practice.

Gene Expression Profiling Biomarkers

Currently, gene expression microarray, which generates quantitative expression data for thousands of genes, has been considered as a powerful tool for understanding the biological characteristics of cancers and in particular response to therapeutic agents. Studies suggest that gene expression profiling is a powerful tool to identify gene sets for selection of optimal and personalized therapy for patients with oesophageal cancer.

STAGING OF OESOPHAGEAL CANCER

Once a diagnosis of oesophageal cancer is made, staging of the disease is essential to choose the best therapeutic option for the patient, and for assessing tumour resectability. Staging should ideally be carried out for all patients with malignant tumours of the oesophagus. However, in a small subset of patients who at presentation are unfit for any type of management, and are unlikely to improve and become fit, staging is unnecessary and these patients should be offered end of life care or best supportive care depending on the clinical situation. The stage of the disease at the time of diagnosis is the single most important prognostic factor. However, the fitness of the patient at the time of diagnosis should be taken into consideration in recommending the appropriate management. The most common clinical staging system used is the TNM classification, which is based on independent measures of the depth of oesophageal wall penetration, regional lymph node involvement and the presence or absence of distant metastatic disease [4] (Table 1). Currently, all the TNM staging criteria could be provided by a combination of CT, PET CT and endoscopic ultrasound.

Table 1. T, N, and M status and histologic grade definitions for esophagus and oesophago-gastric junction cancer in the 7th edition of the American Joint Committee on Cancer (AJCC) Cancer Staging Manual [4].

T Status	
Tis	High-grade dysplasia
T1	Invasion into the lamina propria, muscularis mucosa, or submucosa
T2	Invasion into muscularis propria
T3	Invasion into adventitia
T4a	Invades resectable adjacent structures (pleura, pericardium, diaphragm)
T4b	Invades unresectable adjacent structures (aorta, vertebral body, trachea)
N Status	
N0	No regional lymph node metastases
N1	1 to 2 positive regional lymph nodes
N2	3 to 6 positive regional lymph nodes
N3	7 or more positive regional lymph nodes
M Status	
M0	No distant metastases
M1	Distant metastases
Histologic Grade	
G1	Well differentiated
G2	Moderately differentiated
G3	Poorly differentiated
G4	Undifferentiated

This staging system offers a reasonable correlation to prognosis but underestimates the importance of the length of the tumour. For comparative purposes between patients included in different clinical trials, stage groupings are provided (Table 2).

Table 2. AJCC 7th edition stage groupings [5].

Stage	Adenocarcinoma				Squamous Cell Carcinoma				
	T	N	M	Grade	T	N	M	Grade	Location
0	is	0	0	1	is	0	0	1	Any
IA	1	0	0	1-2	1	0	0	1	Any
IB	1	0	0	3	1	0	0	2-3	Any
	2	0	0	1-2	2-3	0	0	1	Lower
IIA	2	0	0	3	2-3	0	0	1	Upper, Middle
					2-3	0	0	2-3	Lower
IIB	3	0	0	Any	2-3	0	0	2-3	Upper, Middle
	1-2	1	0	Any	1-2	1	0	Any	Any
IIIA	1-2	2	0	Any	1-2	2	0	Any	Any
	3	1	0	Any	3	1	0	Any	Any
	4a	0	0	Any	4a	0	0	Any	Any
IIIB	3	2	0	Any	3	2	0	Any	Any
IIIC	4a	1-2	0	Any	4a	1-2	0	Any	Any
	4b	Any	0	Any	4b	Any	0	Any	Any
	Any	3	0	Any	Any	3	0	Any	Any
IV	Any	Any	1	Any	Any	Any	1	Any	Any

Cancer location definitions: upper thoracic, 20-25 cm from incisors; middle thoracic, 25-30 cm from incisors; lower thoracic, 30-40 cm from incisors.

For the assessment of oesophageal wall depth of invasion, computed tomography (CT) with both oral and intravenous contrast and endoscopic ultrasonography (EUS) are the standard investigations. The accuracy of CT is poor with medium sensitivity and good specificity. This is due to limitations in determining the primary tumour stage (T) and regional lymph node stage (N). In contrast, CT scanning is highly sensitive and specific for detecting metastatic disease to the lung, liver, and adrenal glands. Magnetic resonance imaging (MRI) has shown similar limitations in sensitivity and specificity as CT and currently offers no additional advantage in the pre-operative staging of patients with oesophageal cancer. Positron emission tomography (PET) has proved very helpful for the detection of previously unsuspected metastases (15 – 20%) and confirmation of distant and regional lymph node metastasis as well as organ metastasis seen previously on CT. PET /CT is now accepted as a standard staging test for oesophageal neoplasms. Endoscopic ultrasound (EUS) using a radial scanning echoendoscope, provides detailed examination of five ultrasonographic layers in the wall of the oesophagus. Local structures around the oesophagus can also be identified and the local lymph nodes are seen. The T staging of the primary tumour with EUS has an accuracy of 80-90% but is largely operator dependent. EUS is also reported to be 80-90% accurate in detecting mediastinal lymph node metastasis [6]. Intervention EUS using a curved linear echoendoscope can provide aspirates (FNA) of suspect lesions (lymph nodes) around the oesophagus for cytological confirmation. The main difficulty with EUS is the slow acquisition of experience to confidently analyse the images. The introduction of higher frequency probes with better imaging may overcome the initial difficulties. The other main difficulty is in assessment of stenotic tumours. Slim echo probes, which pass over a guide-wire introduced endoscopically, have been developed to overcome this difficulty. Oesophageal ultrasound is limited to evaluation of the oesophagus and peri-oesophageal structures but have no utility in the detection of visceral metastasis. EUS and CT are complimentary in providing the TNM stage of the disease, which may be modified after PET/CT. The above staging modalities establish the pre-treatment clinical stage, which can be used to guide subsequent treatment.

Bronchoscopy should be performed for proximal oesophageal tumours to determine bronchial involvement, which is considered a contra-indication to curative treatment strategies. CT and EUS can be suggestive of airway involvement but are not as accurate as direct visual inspection of the airway. Mediastinal lymph node assessment and cytological sampling can also be carried out using endoscopic bronchial ultrasound (EBUS). Vocal cord paralysis determined by ENT examination and phrenic nerve paralysis (diaphragmatic screening by fluoroscopy or ultrasound) are indications of inoperability as is distant organ metastasis. Minimally invasive tests (thoracoscopy and laparoscopy) are unnecessary in the vast majority of patients but should be considered for select patients considered to have a high risk of treatment related complications. Staging laparoscopy in particular may have a valuable role for patients with adenocarcinoma of the oesophago-gastric junction.

There is controversy over the optimal treatment approach to adenocarcinoma of the Oesophagogastric junction (OGJ). These tumors are centered in an area ranging from 5 cm above and below the OGJ. The seventh edition of the American Joint Committee on Cancer (AJCC) TNM staging manual, categorized all adenocarcinomas of the OGJ as esophageal cancers, irrespective of the Siewert type [7]. This new staging system for adenocarcinomas of the OGJ and stomach was based on a consensus of Eastern and Western countries, utilising large databases from the East and West, which analyzed gastric cancer outcomes [8]. The move to classify all OGJ tumors as esophageal cancers was justified on the basis that tumors located in the proximal stomach and OGJ were noted to have a much worse prognosis (similar to oesophageal adenocarcinomas) than tumors located in the distal stomach and different molecular pathology [9].

Currently, there is momentum to reclassify different types of OGJ tumors as oesophageal or *gastric* cancers (depending on the epicenter of the tumor) in the 8th edition of the AJCC staging manual but this remains uncertain. There is consensus at least amongst surgeons to continue adoption of the Siewert Classification. Siewert type I tumors are treated like esophageal cancer and Siewert type III cancers are treated like gastric cancers. The main controversy remains focused on how to treat true adenocarcinomas of the GOJ (Siewert type II tumors).

Siewert *et al.* proposed a very pragmatic classification system for GOJ tumors based purely on their topographic anatomy and the location of the epicenter of the tumor [10] (Fig. **3**).

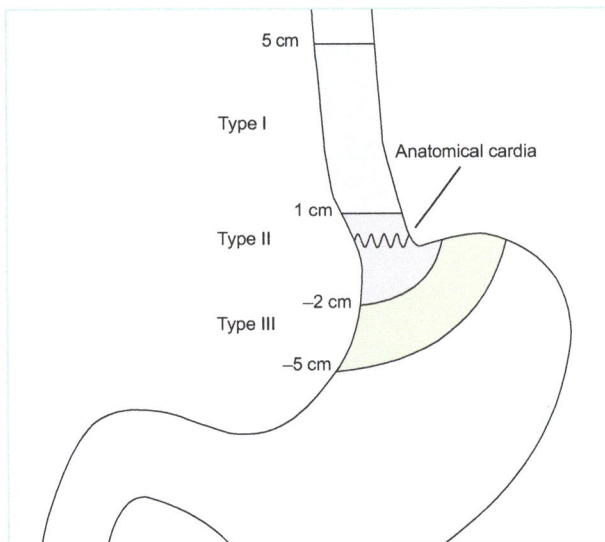

Fig. (3). Siewert classification. Topographic-anatomic classification of adenocarcinomas of the oesophago gastric junction (OGJ) based on the relationship to the endoscopic gastric cardia. *Type I*: adenocarcinoma of the distal esophagus; *Type II*: true adenocarcinoma of the cardia; *Type III*: sub-cardia gastric carcinoma infiltrating the oesophago gastric junction. (*Adapted from*: Siewert JR and Stein HJ [11]).

Adenocarcinoma of the GOJ was defined as a tumor whose epicenter was within 5 cm above or below the oesophago gastric junction. A Siewert type I tumor was defined as an adenocarcinoma of the distal esophagus in which the epicenter of the tumor was located 1-5 cm above the OGJ and which typically arises from an area of intestinal metaplasia of the esophagus (*i.e.*, Barrett esophagus). A Siewert type II tumor was defined as a true carcinoma of the cardia arising immediately at the OGJ (tumor epicenter located from 1 cm above to 2 cm below the OGJ). Lastly, a Siewert type III tumor was defined as a sub-cardia gastric carcinoma that infiltrates the OGJ and/or distal esophagus from below (tumor epicenter located 2-5 cm below the OGJ).

Many surgeons have continued to use this classification system to select the surgical approach for adenocarcinomas of the OGJ, typically treating type I tumors as esophageal cancers and type III tumors as gastric cancers. This is based on tumor biology, the frequency and distribution of nodal metastasis and the location and pattern of recurrence [12]. The difficulty remains in selecting the appropriate surgical approach for Type II tumors. With uncertainty about the optimal extent of prophylactic lymph node dissection for this tumor, both subtotal oesophagectomy and extended total gastrectomy have been advocated. The former is favorable in terms of guaranteeing the proximal resection margin, while the latter focuses on the complete clearance of abdominal lymph nodes much more than mediastinal dissection. These two procedures are extremely different in terms of the surgical approach, extent of resection, and, more importantly, the type of reconstruction. Therefore, mortality, morbidity and quality of life after surgery are deemed to not be equivalent. Since the survival rate based on the extents of resection are comparable, conclusive evidence as to which procedure should be recommended is currently lacking [13, 14]. One pragmatic approach is to consider type II tumors as oesophageal as per AJCC staging manual 7th edition. The surgical approach would consist of an Ivor Lewis or trans-hiatal oesophagectomy depending on the patient's condition, the surgeon's preference and aptitude for mediastinal lymphadenectomy. However, in either case, an upper abdominal prophylactic lymphadenectomy is carried out during gastric mobilisation.

MANAGEMENT OF OESOPHAGEAL CANCER

All suitable patients diagnosed with oesophageal cancer should be discussed by a dedicated multidisciplinary team which includes oncologists, nutritionists, specialist nurses, physiotherapists, trained theatre, intensive care and surgical ward nurses in addition to specialised surgeons and anaesthetists. The treatment of patients with oesophageal cancer depends on the stage of the disease and the condition of the patient. Some patients with resectable lesions are unfit for surgery by virtue of significant co-morbid disease. The role of the surgeon includes selection of patients, optimisation of pre-existing deficiencies, technical surgery and making appropriate assessments and management decisions in the immediate post-operative course. Clear protocol driven care greatly improves patient outcomes and the quality of their experience. Since the majority of patients usually undergo neoadjuvant chemotherapy or chemo radiotherapy, there is potential to utilise this time of approximately three months to educate the patient and family and to optimise their health, nutrition, medical co morbidities and increase their cardiovascular and respiratory reserves to help them tolerate a major operation involving at least two or sometimes three body compartments.

General Considerations

Nutrition

All patients should be seen and assessed by a dedicated nutrition team. They are advised on healthy and high protein diets. Protein supplements are prescribed if necessary. Dysphagia can be significant in some patients. Enteral feeding can be improved in such patients by the use of removable fully covered oesophageal stents or absorbable stents preoperatively. Other enteral routes can be in the form of a fine bore naso-gastric feeding tube or a laparoscopic feeding jejunostomy. The nutritional management also includes biochemical, vitamin and trace element assessment and these can be replaced by vitamin supplements preoperatively. All patients should be reviewed regularly by the dietetic team to optimise the patient outcomes. Appropriate advice on food texture and consistency should be given at each consultation and preferably by a leaflet itemising food substances, their calorific value and any modifications required to make them more easily ingested.

Physical Fitness

All patients should be advised to undergo a strict exercise regime. Examples include brisk walking twice a day for a total of three miles or swimming up to 6 swimming pool's length (incrementally). With the easy availability of pedometers and smartphone accessories they can be given a target of steps to achieve each day - typically 10,000 steps. All patients should be given incentive spirometers and trained on their daily use. Spirometers with clearly visible markings and targets are ideal as patient compliance and improvement can be monitored.

Respiratory and Cardiovascular Optimisation

All patients are strongly advised to stop smoking. Providing easy access to nicotine patches or chewing gum facilitates smoking cessation. Many specialist centres do not operate on patients if they do not stop smoking. Patients are advised that continuing smoking puts them at increased risk of major respiratory complications and mortality. Cardiovascular function is optimised by the above measures and specialist cardiology input should be made available for patients with pre-existing cardiovascular conditions. Patients should be regularly reviewed by the surgical team and the specialist nurses to ensure that all goals are achieved before finally finalising the timing of surgery.

Anatomical Considerations

The oesophagus extends from the pharynx in the neck through the thoracic cavity to the stomach in the abdomen. It is intimately related to the membranous trachea, recurrent laryngeal nerves and thyroid in the neck. In the upper mediastinum, it lies behind the trachea till the carina. In the lower mediastinum, it lies behind the inferior pulmonary vein and the left atrium. The descending thoracic Aorta lies posteriorly and the parietal pleura on either side of the lower thoracic oesophagus before it passes into the abdomen through the diaphragmatic hiatus of the right crus at the level of the tenth thoracic vertebra. These close relationships to adjoining structures make treatment decisions for oesophageal pathologies especially challenging.

The epithelial lining of the oesophagus is non-keratinized stratified squamous epithelium (M1). This changes to columnar epithelium at the junction with the stomach. Underneath the non-keratinized stratified squamous epithelium is the lamina propria (M2). There is a muscularis mucosa (M3) at the boundary of the mucosa and submucosa. This is thicker than that in the stomach and intestine, and includes only longitudinal muscle fibres. This layer is more fibrous and less cellular than the lamina propria of the mucosa and is the strongest layer of the oesophageal wall. The submucosa consists of connective tissue with mucous glands, blood vessels, lymphatics and the submucosal nerve plexus of Meissner. The submucosal lymphatics are longitudinal and continuous along the length of the oesophagus. The submucosa is divided into deep and superficial parts (SM1 and SM2). The submucosa is covered by muscularis propria. This consists of an inner circular and outer longitudinal muscle fibres. The myenteric plexus of Auerbach is contained between the two muscle layers. A fine lymphatic plexus is also present in this layer. The two lymphatic systems are densely interconnected and this creates little or no barrier for lymphatic spread of cancer. The upper third of the oesophagus has striated muscle in the muscularis propria. The lower third of the oesophagus has smooth muscle and the middle third contains both types. Most of the oesophagus lacks serosa and is covered by a thin adventitial layer, which merges with the connective tissue of the surrounding structures (Fig. **4**).

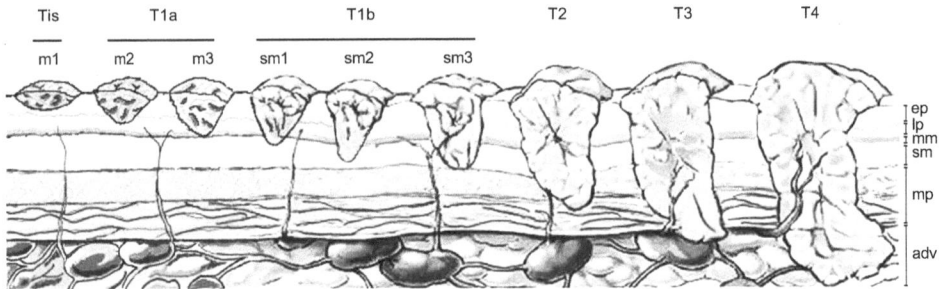

Fig. (4). A schematic diagram illustrating the layers of the oesophageal wall and the T classification of tumours with different levels of invasion into the wall of the oesophagus.
Ep: Epithelium, lp: Lamina propria, mm: Muscularis mucosa, mp: Muscularis propria, adv: Adventitia.

The arterial supply to the oesophagus is by the inferior thyroid artery, oesophageal and bronchial branches of the thoracic aorta and left gastric and left phrenic arteries. Venous blood from the oesophagus drains into a submucosal system. From here, it drains to the peri-oesophageal venous plexus. Oesophageal veins arise from the peri oesophageal plexus and drain segmentally according to the arterial supply. This includes the inferior thyroid vein in the neck, portal vein *via* the left gastric vein in the abdomen and the thoracic oesophagus drains into the azygos and hemi-azygos systems, intercostal, and bronchial veins.

The intimate relationship of the oesophagus to its surrounding structures, lack of serosa and convergence of the connective tissues around it provides no effective barrier for spread of oesophageal cancer. In addition, the longitudinal venous and lymphatic plexuses do not pose any opposition to spread. The lack of serosa makes oesophageal anastomoses rely on the strength of the submucosa. In addition to all these, the passage of the oesophagus through three anatomical areas makes surgical management complex.

Treatment Strategy

Surgery is the gold standard option to obtain loco regional control and has the best overall survival rate but comes with major risks of complications and reduced quality of life. The aim of surgery in these patients should be an R0 resection (complete macroscopic and microscopic removal of tumour) and an appropriate dissection of involved and predicted lymph nodes (prophylactic lymphadenectomy) for cure. Although palliation of dysphagia is an important objective, there is no place for resection surgery purely for the palliation of dysphagia.

In general, some 30-40% of oesophageal tumours are resectable (20% for T4a, 50% for T3, and 80-90% for T1-T2), however, not all these patients are medically fit to have surgery. With advanced staging modalities used nowadays, very few patients should be found to have inoperable disease at operation. Mortality rate of oesophagectomy should be less than 5% in specialised centres and approximates 1 – 2% in high volume centres. The most frequent complications are anastomotic leakage and broncho pulmonary complications. Recent favourable reports suggest that the 5-year survival of all resected patients is 24% and those patients resected with a curative intent (R0) is approximately 40% independent of the histology. These favourable results are thought to be due to lower operative mortality, increased surgical radically, better staging and selection of patients and multimodality treatment.

Treatment depends on the stage of the cancer and patient fitness. In node negative patients with early cancers limited to the mucosa (T1a) – ultrasonographic M1,M2 and M3, endoscopic therapy in the form of either endoscopic mucosal resection (EMR) or endoscopic submucosal dissection (ESD) is recommended with subsequent endoscopic surveillance [15]. Those superficial cancers involving part of the submucosa SM1 can be managed with EMR or ESD with caution since a considerable proportion (up to 50%) may have occult lymph node metastases.

Node positive T1-T3 cancers should be considered for surgery based on the number of involved lymph nodes. Involvement of 8 or more lymph nodes (N3) has been shown to have a very high incidence of systemic spread and the role of surgical management for loco regional control is controversial. Therefore, T2-4a tumours with N0, N1 and N2 disease should be considered for surgery. Patients with T4b tumours or N3 disease are best treated with radical chemo radiotherapy.

For tumours localised in the oesophageal segment below the tracheal bifurcation (T1 to T3), with only limited nodal disease, neoadjuvant chemo or chemo-radiotherapy followed by oesophagectomy with loco-regional lymphadenectomy should be considered and may be regarded as potentially curative. Junctional tumours (Siewert Type I and II) can be removed by transthoracic partial or trans hiatal oesophagectomy with one or two-field regional lymphadenectomy. More proximal tumours require a transthoracic oesophagectomy with a two-field lymphadenectomy. Pre-operative chemoradiotherapy may incur a survival benefit and post-operative chemo radiation is recommended for the more advanced lesions with residual disease or involved lymph nodes. Patients who are unfit for surgery should be managed by radical chemoradiotherapy.

The management of patients with locally advanced or metastatic oesophageal cancer and patients with poor general medical condition must be individualised based on stage, characteristics of the tumour, patient's medical condition and patient preference. The aim of palliative treatment is to achieve rapid and sustained relief of dysphagia with minimal hospital stay. Chemotherapy alone or in combination with radiotherapy should be considered with other palliative measures.

For squamous cell carcinoma with its multi-focal potential, sub-total oesophagectomy with a cervical anastomosis remains to be the treatment of choice. However, the benefit of surgical resection in improving survival compared to definitive chemo radiation for esophageal squamous cell carcinoma has been questioned. Several randomized trials have suggested that definitive chemo radiation could offer equivalent survival to treatment that involves surgery for locally advanced, non-metastatic esophageal SCC. Currently, most treatment guidelines recommend definitive chemo radiation for patients who are unfit for surgery and those who decline surgery. For adenocarcinoma, curative resection should include adequate proximal and distal margins, and must include the part of the oesophagus lined with columnar metaplasia. Circumferentially, the dissection should aim to resect the tumour with surrounding tissue planes (meso-oesophagectomy).

For tumours in the upper oesophagus (cervical oesophagus and proximal part of the thoracic oesophagus above the tracheal bifurcation) virtually all of these are squamous cell cancers. Pharyngolaryngectomy is the treatment of choice for T1 and T2 tumours of the cervical oesophagus and radiotherapy is advocated for more advanced lesions.

Surgical Resection
(a). Tumours of the Cervical Oesophagus

The majority of proximal tumours arise from the hypopharyngeal area (pyriform fossa, posterior wall of the pharynx and postcricoid region) and tumours of the cervical oesophagus are rare. They carry a poor prognosis and survival beyond one year after treatment is uncommon. Radiotherapy is the treatment of choice for these tumours since the majority are advanced at presentation. Pharyngolaryngectomy is indicated for early lesions (T1, T2). These patients have a permanent tracheostomy [16]. Until recently, reconstruction was achieved with colon (brought up retrosternally or subcutaneously), stomach or myocutaneous flaps. Viscus transposition increases the operative mortality in this group of patients while myocutaneous flap repairs have a high incidence of complications mainly stricture and fistulae. However, the best results in terms of swallowing, voice production and early hospital discharge are achieved with free revascularised jejunal or greater curve gastric grafts which are interposed between the proximal pharynx and the distal oesophagus after the blood supply has been restored to the graft by anastomosis of the artery and vein to the superior thyroid artery and facial vein (Fig. **5**).

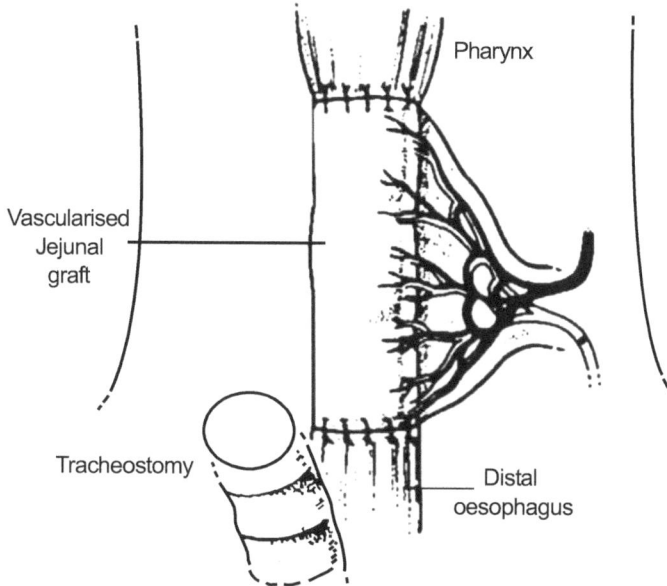

Fig. (5). Free revascularised jejunal graft reconstruction after pharyngo-laryngectomy.

(b). Tumours of the Thoracic Oesophagus

Surgical approach to the oesophagus can be transthoracic or through the mediastinum (trans-hiatal). In general, transthoracic operations have a higher degree of operative mortality and morbidity and reduced post-operative quality of life [17].

The procedure may consist of a subtotal oesophagectomy with a cervical anastomosis or a partial oesophagectomy with a mid-thoracic anastomosis. Because of the multifocal potential of squamous cell carcinoma, subtotal oesophagectomy is carried out, the anastomosis for reconstruction being carried out in the neck. For adenocarcinoma, curative resection should include 10 cm proximal and distal margins as part of the en-bloc resection, and the entire columnar lined oesophagus.

Some surgeons prefer partial oesophagectomy (Lewis-Tanner operation) as the routine procedure for tumours of the lower two-thirds of the oesophagus and reserve sub-total oesophagectomy for high thoracic oesophagus tumours. The advantages of sub-total oesophagectomy are better tumour clearance and an easier anastomosis in the neck, dehiscence of which is rare and less life threatening in this situation. The important complication of intra-thoracic oesophageal anastomosis is leakage with the development of empyema. This complication is the major cause of post-operative mortality after oesophageal resection. Careful attention in the performance of this anastomosis to ensure mucosa-to-mucosa coaptation, experience and avoidance of any tension are the most important factors in the prevention of anastomotic dehiscence. Management of an anastomotic leak is similar to the management of a perforation (see chapter 6).

Partial Oesophagectomy

The two-stage Lewis-Tanner (Ivor-Lewis) procedure was the standard operation for resection of tumours of the lower two-thirds of the oesophagus and junctional tumours. It achieves better clearance than the left thoracotomy approach, which is seldom used nowadays. The abdominal or first stage of the Lewis-Tanner operation is usually performed through an epigastric incision (transverse or midline). The entire stomach is mobilised and its vascular supply maintained through the right gastro-epiploic and occasionally the right gastric vessels. The short gastric vessels are individually controlled (ligated or coagulated). The left gastric artery is ligated at its origin through the coeliac axis. The duodenum and head of pancreas are mobilised sufficiently to expose a long segment of the vena cava and to enable their reflection to the midline or beyond. Proximal, the peritoneum over the gastro-oesophageal junction and the phreno - oesophageal membrane are divided. The abdominal oesophagus is mobilised, the vagal trunks are sectioned and blunt dissection of the lower posterior mediastinum around the oesophagus performed. In lower third lesions, the tumour should become palpable at this stage. Gastric outlet drainage pyloromyotomy or pyloroplasty is unnecessary but some surgeons advocate intra-operative injections of Botox into the pyloric muscles. This is based on the premise that adequate drainage in the early post-operative period reduces the incidence of gastric retention and consequently aspiration and or anastomotic leakage.

The thoracic or second stage is performed through a right posterolateral thoracotomy carried out through the bed of the fifth rib. The oesophagus is eminently accessible through this approach and the only overlying structure is the azygos vein. A minimum of 5 cm proximal clearance from the upper margin of the tumour is necessary because of the submucosal spread of oesophageal cancer. The stomach is pulled into the posterior mediastinum after the oesophagus and the tumour have been mobilised (Fig. **6**). The distal resection margin is at the cardio-oesophageal junction or upper third of the stomach depending on the lower extent of the disease. The gastric end is closed and the stomach then anastomosed to the intrathoracic oesophagus either manually or using a stapler. In transecting the oesophagus, the muscle coat should be divided all the way around to expose the mucosal tube which is then transected 1.0 cm further distally (Fig. **10**). This prevents retraction of the oesophageal mucosa inside the muscular layers and therefore facilitates and ensures the safety of the anastomosis. A tension free anastomosis can be carried out with a single layer technique using interrupted sutures or preferably using a mechanical stapler.

Sub-total Oesophagectomy

For squamous cell cancer and for proximal lesions and for individual surgeon's preference sub-total oesophagectomy with anastomosis of the mobilised stomach or colon to the cervical oesophagus can be carried out. This is achieved either by means of a three-stage operation (McKeown's oesophagectomy) or by the technique of trans-hiatal oesophagectomy without thoracotomy, popularised by Orringer. Endoscopic oesophagectomy also achieves subtotal oesophagectomy without thoracotomy.

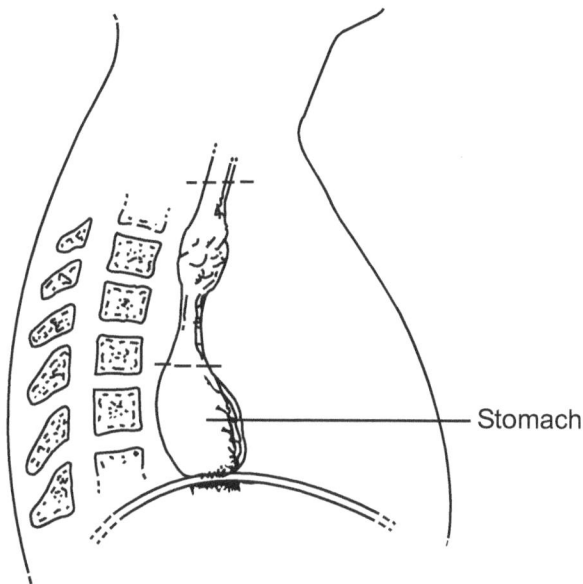

Fig. (6). Schematic diagram of the posterior mediastinal position of the gastric tube reconstruction after oesophagectomy.

The first stage of the McKeown's procedure is identical to that of the Lewis Tanner oesophagectomy. The second stage differs in that it entails mobilisation of the thoracic oesophagus up to and including the thoracic inlet. The chest is then closed and the patient is re-positioned in the supine posture. A variant of the described McKeown's procedure is 'en-bloc oesophagectomy'. This aims to remove an envelope of tissue surrounding the tumour-bearing oesophagus, including adjacent pleura and pericardium and the posterior mediastinal tissues anterior to the vertebral bodies, including the azygos vein and the thoracic duct.

The cervical or third stage is conducted through an oblique or transverse incision on the left side of the neck 2.0 cm above the clavicle. After mobilisation of the cervical oesophagus, the distal gullet with tumour is pulled up into the neck until the cardia appears. The gastro-oesophageal junction and the lesser curvature, together with associated lymph nodes are then clamped, divided and closed, and the oesophagus then resected. The anastomosis is performed in the neck between the proximal cervical oesophagus and the fundus of the stomach tube.

Trans Hiatal Oesophagectomy

In oesophagectomy without thoracotomy, the stomach is skeletonized as described previously. The thoracic oesophagus is mobilised by manual dissection through the hiatus, which may be divided to facilitate the procedure. The cervical and upper thoracic oesophagus are mobilised through an approach along the anterior border of the left sternomastoid. The cervical oesophagus is then transected and a long rubber tube is attached to the distal end. The thoracic oesophagus with the tumour is then withdrawn into the abdomen; the gastro-oesophageal junction is transected and closed. The oesophagus is then detached from the rubber tube and removed. The tube is anchored to the fundus of the stomach. Traction at the cervical end of the rubber tube is used to pull up the stomach through the posterior mediastinum into the neck for anastomosis to the cervical oesophagus (Fig. **7**). The advantage of this procedure is the avoidance of a thoracotomy, especially in elderly patients and patients with significant broncho-pulmonary disease.

A variant of the trans hiatal oesophagectomy is the vagal-sparing oesophagectomy. This operation is described for proven severe dysplasia in patients with intestinal metaplasia of the oesophagus. A vein-stripper is advanced through a limited gastrotomy into the cervical oesophagus. The cervical oesophagus is then divided after securing the vein stripper in the distal segment. The stripper is then pulled through the gastrotomy to strip the oesophagus from surrounding structures preserving the vagal nerves in the process. The stripped oesophagus is then divided from the stomach and the gastrotomy wound closed. An isoperistaltic colon segment is then passed retrosternally or in the posterior mediastinum. The colon is anastomosed proximally to the oesophagus and distally to the stomach. The advantages of this procedure include those of the trans hiatal oesophagectomy in addition to excellent functional results.

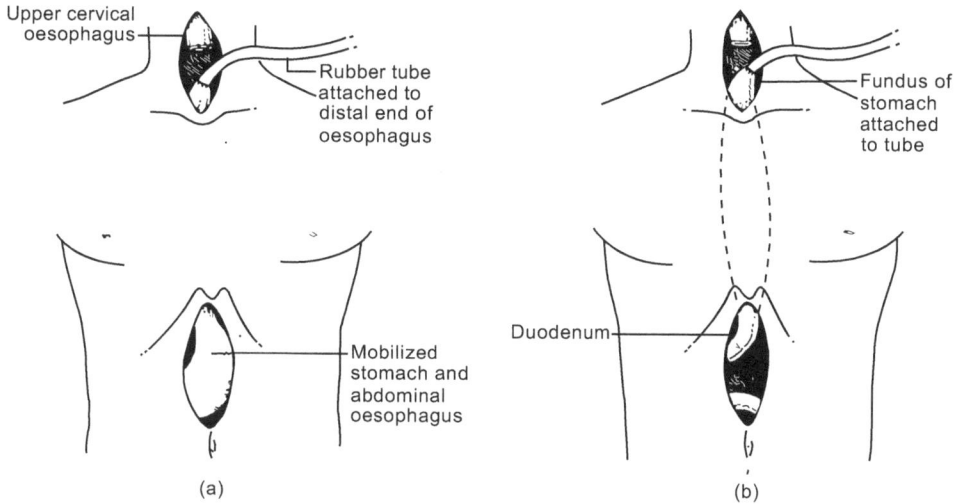

Fig. (7). Reconstruction after trans hiatal oesophagectomy. (a) The stomach and duodenum have been mobilised with preservation of right gastroepiploic and right gastric vessels. The thoracic oesophagus is mobilised by hand dissection through the hiatus. The cervical oesophagus is mobilised through a cervical incision. The oesophagus is transected and the distal end attached to a Ryle's tube. The tumour-bearing oesophagus is withdrawn into the abdomen until the Ryle's tube is encountered. The oesophagus is removed, the stomach tube fashioned and attached to the Ryle's tube. (b) The Ryle's tube is pulled from the cervical incision and the stomach trails it. The oesophago-gastric anastomosis is fashioned in the neck.

Endoscopic Oesophagectomy

Endoscopic oesophagectomy is a recent advance on blunt trans hiatal oesophagectomy. The principle benefit of both approaches is the avoidance of a thoracotomy, which is particularly relevant in oesophageal cancer as the majority of patients suffering from this disease are above the age of 60 years. The advantages of the endoscopic procedure over the blunt trans hiatal resection include a precise visually guided dissection, with minimum blood loss and less risk of injury to the azygos vein, left bronchus and recurrent laryngeal nerves.

There are two techniques for dissecting the oesophagus endoscopically (minimal access); the mediastinascopic approach described by Buess and the right thoracoscopic technique first introduced by Cuschieri. The mediastinascopic dissection is performed using a special operating rigid mediastinascope, which is introduced through a left cervical incision along the anterior margin of the sternomastoid. It allows perivisceral mobilisation of the intra-thoracic oesophagus up to the abdominal hiatus. After the oesophagus is resected and removed through the abdomen by the abdominal operator (operating synchronously), the mobilised stomach or gastric tube is brought up through the mediastinum for anastomosis to the proximal cervical oesophagus. The main disadvantage of the mediastinascopic approach is the difficulty of dissection and removal of the para-oesophageal lymph nodes, which are often left behind. In this respect, the resection is usually non-curative but in view of the advanced nature of most oesophageal cancers this is acceptable in most instances. The dissection of the lower thoracic oesophagus is also difficult with this technique due to the bulge and pulsation of the aorta on which the operating mediastinascope tends to impinge.

The right thoracoscopic operation is conducted using a double lumen endobronchial tube for isolating the left lung in order to achieve collapse of the right lung. The procedure is identical to the thoracic stage of the McKeown operation and permits precise visually guided dissection of the oesophagus and the regional para-oesophageal and tracheo-bronchial lymph nodes with little blood loss. In tumours of the lower third, the azygos vein is simply mobilised from the oesophagus but in middle third lesions, the vein is ligated and divided. Another advantage of the procedure is the ability to perform the dissection of the lower cervical oesophagus through the right chest by extending the mobilisation beyond the thoracic inlet. After the endoscopic mobilisation is completed, the patient is turned in the supine position for the second stage. The neck is opened through an oblique or transverse incision. The mobilised cervical oesophagus is then transected. At the same time, the abdominal surgeon performs the standard gastric mobilisation and after resection of the oesophagus, the stomach tube is pulled up to the neck for proximal anastomosis to the cervical oesophagus. The results of right thoracoscopic oesophagectomy for cancer to date have been excellent in a few centres with appropriately selected patients. The procedure entails single lung anaesthesia for 90 to 120 minutes. Patients with inadequate respiratory reserve cannot tolerate this intra-operatively and tend to develop more respiratory problems post-operatively. The haemodynamic upset caused by single lung ventilation may be misinterpreted as over infusion. In addition, shunting tends to occur with subsequent lung damage, which becomes apparent 48 hours post-operatively. The main advantages of this procedure are; minimizing blood loss, abolition of post-thoracotomy pain, and reduction in post-operative ventilatory difficulty and early discharge from hospital [18].

(c). Tumours of the Oesophago-gastric Junction

Resection of the tumour with an adequate lymphadenectomy of the field surrounding the tumour is the goal of surgical resection [19]. This can be achieved by oesophago-gastrectomy or partial oesophagectomy with resection of the proximal margin of the stomach. Oesophago-gastrectomy can be carried out through the abdominal route, removing an oncologically safe margin of the oesophagus with the upper third of the stomach. The lower oesophageal dissection can be carried out through the trans hiatal route or by transthoracic dissection and anastomosis. Partial oesophagectomy is more appropriate for type 1 and some type 2 oesophago-gastric junction tumours with an oesophago-gastrectomy being more appropriate for some Type 2 and Type 3 tumours.

Lymphadenectomy

The goal of extensive lymphadenectomy is to remove all regional lymph node groups with potential metastatic deposits in order to improve the pathological staging of the disease. A *one-field* lymphadenectomy involves the dissection of the diaphragmatic, right and left para cardiac, lesser curvature, left gastric, coeliac and common hepatic nodes. A *two-field* lymphadenectomy includes the para-aortic (mediastinal nodes) together with the thoracic duct, the right and left pulmonary hilar nodes, the para-oesophageal nodes and the para-tracheal bronchial nodes. *Three-field* lymphadenectomy additionally includes the brachio-cephalic, deep lateral and external cervical nodes including the right and left recurrent nerve lymphatic chains (deep anterior cervical nodes). Approximately 75% of patients with lower third cancers have involved lymph nodes in the coeliac trunk, left gastric and common hepatic territories. These will be removed in a single field (abdominal) lymphadenectomy. Approximately 60% of patients with middle and lower oesophageal tumours have mediastinal and sub-diaphragmatic lymph node involvement. This would be covered by a two-field lymphadenectomy. Due to the lower incidence of cervical node metastases in patients with cancer of the sub-carina oesophagus and due to the little difference in five-year survival between patients undergoing a three- or a two- field dissection, dissection of cervical nodes in these patients is questionable. In addition, a three-field lymphadenectomy incurs an additional morbidity and mortality even in experienced centres. For patients with upper third tumours, three-field lymphadenectomy should be considered in clinical trial protocols. In addition, for a sub-set of patients in which lymph node metastases are detectable only by cervical ultrasound, three-field lymphadenectomy should be considered, especially for low risk patients. This may necessitate referral to a Specialist Centre, which practices this type of surgery in the context of clinical trials. To date, there is little evidence to suggest that extensive lymphadenectomy carries a survival benefit or improves loco-regional control in western oesophageal surgical practice. This is in contrast to the favourable survival results with more extensive lymphadenectomy in Japanese patients.

Reconstruction

The standard reconstruction of the alimentary tract after oesophagectomy is performed using the gastric pull-up (Fig. **8**).

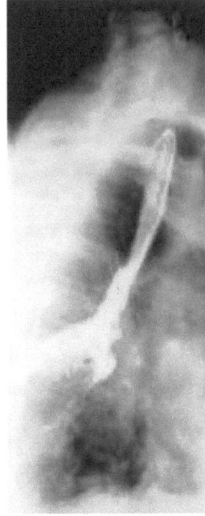

Fig. (8). Radiograph showing gastric tube reconstruction after a partial oesophagectomy.

This guarantees good functional results with a safe and quick operation. If the stomach is unsuitable due to previous surgery or concurrent disease, an isoperistaltic colonic segment on a vascular pedicle should be considered with the left colon being preferred to the right colon. This is claimed to reduce post-operative reflux oesophagitis, which occurs in 30% of patients after a partial oesophagectomy and in 15% of patients after a subtotal oesophagectomy. After a lower third oesophagectomy or oesophago-gastrectomy a pedicled isoperistaltic jejunal loop would suffice. The transposition path of choice is the posterior mediastinum as it is the most direct, and guarantees less morbidity and better post-operative functional results. The alternative retrosternal transposition route is preferred for by-pass purposes and in patients in whom residual disease is left behind. The retrosternal route would avoid involvement of the transposed viscus either by local recurrence or by post-operative irradiation.

Technical Steps in Oesophagectomy

Cervical Stage

Access

- The patient is supine with a soft towel role or jelly pad is placed behind the shoulders to extend the neck. The neck is turned to the right for access to the left neck. The clavicle is marked. A line from the sternum to the mastoid process marks the anterior border of the sternocleidomastoid muscle. The cricoid cartilage should be palpated and marked.

- A horizontal skin crease incision, which is better for cosmetic results, or a vertical incision along the sternocleidomastoid, which is better for exposure, can be used. The horizontal skin incision is located two fingerbreadths above the clavicle or just below the level of the cricoid. The incision extends from the midline to the lateral border of the muscle.

Exploration

- The platysma is incised and sub-platysma flaps are developed on both sides to achieve a good exposure.
- The fascia covering the sternocleidomastoid muscle is incised along its length and the muscle is retracted posterolaterally to give good exposure, which can be maintained with self-retaining retractors.
- The omohyoid muscle traverses the wound and the tendon is divided to expose the omohyoid fascia (middle layer of deep cervical fascia). Division of this fascial layer vertically brings the internal jugular vein into view.
- The middle thyroid vein is ligated and divided. Further dissection exposes the carotid artery.
- The carotid is retracted laterally and the thyroid medially to stretch the sheath between the laryngo-tracheal complex and the carotid which is carefully divided to expose the inferior thyroid artery which is ligated and divided. This prevents the left recurrent laryngeal nerve from being pulled out of the trachea-oesophageal groove during lateral traction.
- The left lobe of the thyroid is retracted anteriorly and medially to expose the oesophagus with the naso-gastric tube which can be palpated as an aid.

Dissection

- The oesophageal fascia is incised vertically or the fascia dissected bluntly on the posterior aspect to expose the oesophagus at the level of the skin incision, which is just below the cricoid. Once the sub-fascial layer is reached the dissection is kept close to the oesophageal muscular layer and a circumferential plane developed by blunt dissection.
- The oesophagus is then encircled by a sling and blunt dissection continued with right angle forceps or cotton swabs to mobilise the oesophagus, which is delivered into the wound.
- The oesophagus can then be transected at the desired level. The caudal end of the divided oesophagus is tied to a tape or the tip of a fresh sterile tube and pulled back into the abdomen.
- The tip of the preformed stomach conduit is then tied to the same tube and slowly delivered through the chest in its correct orientation by simultaneously manoeuvring the gastric tube into the chest cavity from the abdomen and slowly pulling on the other end of the tube to deliver the gastric conduit to the neck in

preparation for the oesophago gastric anastomosis.

- Once this is complete, haemostasis is checked, the wound is cleaned with an antiseptic solution, a small bore suction drain inserted and the bound closed in two layers - the platysma and the skin.

Abdominal Stage

Access

- This is achieved by a roof top transverse abdominal incision or a midline laparotomy that extends to just below the umbilicus.
- The roof top incision along with the use of fixed retractors gives excellent access to the oesophageal hiatus and lower mediastinum, which is needed to perform a meso-oesophagectomy.

Exploration

- Once access is established, an exploratory laparotomy is conducted to identify anatomical abnormalities or occult metastases not previously detected. The stomach is also inspected for its suitability as an oesophageal replacement conduit.
- The left triangular ligament of the liver is divided and the left lobe of the liver retracted to completely expose the hiatus.

Dissection

- The principle of meso-oesophagectomy involves the resection of the lower oesophagus with the tumour completely surrounded by structures such that the muscular fibres of the oesophagus are not visible and are completely enclosed by adventitia or surrounding tissue.
- This starts by dividing the pars flaccida as laterally as possible to expose the right crus of the diaphragm. The left phrenic vein is seen crossing above the hiatus and the left crus should be visualised. These are the main anatomical landmarks for starting the dissection.
- No attempt should be made to enter the normal anatomical planes around the oesophagus. Non anatomical planes are dissected to enclose the oesophageal specimen with surrounding structures that include a cuff of the right crus of diaphragm along with the right pleura, cuff of left crus with left pleura, rim of diaphragm with left phrenic vein and all pericardial fat (including lymph nodes) and all para aortic fascia.
- The first step of this dissection is to incise the right crus away from the oesophagus. This incision is extended cranially until the right pleural cavity is entered.

- The lung with inferior pulmonary ligament is dissected off the pleura keeping the pleura attached to the oesophagus.
- The dissection is carried as high as possible into the right pleural cavity. Attention should then turn to the left side and a similar dissection of the left crus and pleura achieved.
- The next step is anterior mobilisation of the oesophagus. The diaphragm is incised all along the left phrenic vein and joined to the two lateral dissection points. The phrenic vein is ligated at both lateral ends and should form part of the resection. The diaphragmatic incision is then deepened to reach the pericardium. All the pericardial fat is swept down towards the oesophagus and the dissection is carried cranially to expose all of the pericardium visible and taking all the pericardial fat with the resection.
- Attention is then turned to the Aorta. The incisions in the right and left crura of the diaphragm are then extended medially to reach the lateral edges of the Aorta. The Aorta is then completely exposed taking all para aortic tissue with the resection. This dissection is carried along the aorta as far cranially as possible.
- The dissection in all four areas should go cranial to the top of the palpable tumour if possible. This provides a lower oesophageal tumour that is enclosed by a cuff of diaphragm, right and left pleural membranes, pericardial and para aortic fat. No part of the oesophagus is visualised making the possibility of a circumferentially positive margin very low.
- Once this is achieved, attention can be turned to creation of the gastric tube and left gastric and coeliac lymphadenectomy. The right gastro epiploic artery is given off at the lower border of the pylorus from the gastro duodenal artery and damage to this artery should be avoided. The gastro epiploic vein joins the accessory right colonic vein and drains into the superior mesenteric vein *via* the trunk of Henle and should be carefully protected. It is critical that all members of the surgical team handle the gastric tube with the right gastro-epiploic vessels with the utmost care (Fig. **9**).
- The lesser sac is reached by opening the gastro colic omentum at least 2 cm away from the gastro epiploic vessels. A safe area to approach this is to the left of the midline. The stomach is handled gently and the dissection carried towards the pyloric end freeing the stomach from its adhesions to the anterior surface of the pancreas. As dissection nears the antrum, the two leaves of omentum must be carefully separated to enter the space.
- Dissection is usually stopped here and attention turned towards the right lateral area to free the hepatic flexure from adhesions to the gall bladder and duodenum.
- The duodenum can be Kocherised at this stage. It is easier to enter the plane between the two leaves of omentum on the right lateral side above the second part of the duodenum and the pancreatic head. Care should be taken to enter the

plane between the two leaves here and avoid pulling or tearing the right accessory colonic vein, which can damage the drainage of the right gastro epiploic vein.

- Once the 'bubble' plane is reached, the colon is mobilised away and the bubble plane to the left reached.
- The dissection is carried towards the gastro epiploic vein. Care should be taken not to take the dissection too close to the vein as this makes it prone for tearing when the stomach is transposed. Adequate tissue should be left around the vein to protect it.
- Next, mobilisation of the greater curvature and fundus of the stomach is completed. The incision in the gastrocolic omentum is extended cranially to reach the short gastric vessels. A leaf of omentum is preserved with the greater curvature, which will later be used to cover the anastomosis.
- The dissection can then be kept close to the fundus to reach the hiatal dissection.
- The entire stomach is carefully retracted cranially to expose the superior border of the pancreas, splenic artery, the left gastric vessels and the medial border of the Hepato-duodenal ligament to start the lymphadenectomy.

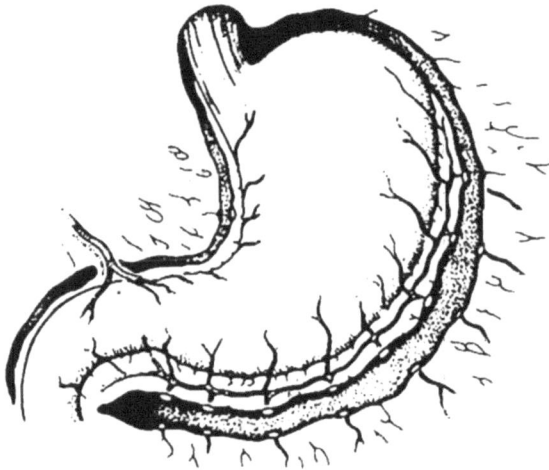

Fig. (9). Gastro-duodenal mobilisation with preservation of the right gastric and right gastro-epiploic arteries.

Creation of the Gastric Tube

- The stomach, especially the greater curvature along with the gastro epiploic vessels should be handled gently. The starting point of the creation of the gastric tube is on the lesser curve just distal to the second branch of the right gastric artery. A linear stapler with a closed staple height of between 1.5 mm (blue cartridge) or 2 mm (green) is used for the first one or two firings followed by the blue cartridge for the rest of the tube.
- The site of the tumour and the final site for the anastomosis determine the

creation of the gastric tube including its length, breadth and distance from the gastro oesophageal junction. Ideally the tube should not be less than 2 cm wide and not more than 4 cm width.

- The tip can be left attached to the gastro oesophageal junction if a thoracic anastomosis is planned. If, however a cervical anastomosis is planned the tube is completely separated from the oesophageal specimen.
- Orientation of the gastric tube should be maintained and checked before closing the abdominal incision.

Lymphadenectomy

- All tissue cranial to the superior border of the pancreas and medial to the hepato-duodenal ligament is dissected en-bloc with the pathological specimen. Dissection is started along the superior border of the pancreas to expose the splenic artery and the common hepatic artery.
- All lymphatic tissue is separated of these vessels and the left gastric vein and artery ligated and divided as close to the portal vein (or splenic vein) and the origin of the artery.
- Dissection is then continued along the medial border of the common hepatic artery up the hepato-duodenal ligament. Care should be taken to avoid damage to the gastro duodenal artery and the right gastric arteries, which are important to the survival of the gastric tube.
- The medial border of the portal vein is freed from fascia.
- The dissection is the continued cranially to meet the previously exposed anterior surface of the Aorta. This completes the entire lymphadenectomy in the abdomen.

Pyloric Drainage

- Attention can now be turned to do a pyloric drainage procedure and a feeding jejunostomy.
- Two drains are necessary. One is placed *via* the abdomen into the left chest and another is placed in the gastric bed at the area of the lymphadenectomy.
- Haemostasis is checked and finally the orientation of the gastric tube confirmed before closing the laparotomy incision.

Right Posterolateral Thoracotomy

Access

- The patient is intubated with a double lumen endotracheal tube so that the right lung can be collapsed to facilitate this stage of the operation.
- The patient is placed in right lateral position with the right arm stretched over

the head and it should lie comfortably on a rest. Patient positioning is important on the table so that the table can be adjusted to increase the lateral extension of the thoracic cavity to help access and visualisation. Once the final position is confirmed and all bony and vulnerable areas are protected the patient should be secured to the table preferably with soft straps. Care must be taken not to compress the abdomen with the support so as to allow good respiratory movement and not increase the ventilation pressures.

- The lower end of the scapula marks the seventh intercostal space and an incision is made from the anterior axillary line along the lower border of the scapula and then extended posteriorly and cranially. The posterior extent can be increased to get better access.
- The latissimus dorsi muscle is divided. The serratus anterior muscle can either be divided or retracted medially to expose the sixth rib.
- The exposed part of the sixth rib is resected and the parietal pleura opened to enter the chest cavity.

Exploration

- The thoracic cavity is inspected for metastatic disease, anatomical variants and lung adhesions can be divided.
- The right lung is deflated by the anaesthetist to allow proper exposure of the cavity. The lung is retracted anteriorly to expose the thoracic oesophagus, which is crossed by the azygos vein.

Dissection

- If the abdominal part has already been completed, the lower thoracic oesophagus with its surrounding structures will already have been mobilised. The pleural dissection margins can then be extended on both sides to above the azygos vein. If this is the first stage, dissection usually begins by releasing the right inferior pulmonary ligament of its attachments to the pleura.
- The next step is to clarify the anatomy by identifying the azygos vein, the oesophagus, the Aorta, the right main bronchus and the inferior pulmonary vein. The aim is to resect the oesophagus with surrounding structures to above the azygos vein for a two-stage oesophagectomy or to mobilise the entire thoracic oesophagus for a three-stage oesophagectomy.
- The next step is to identify the area where the right main bronchus enters the lung. The pleura in incised one cm proximal to this point at the border of the lung. The dissection is then bluntly extended to reach the posterior surface of the pericardium.
- The dissection is extended caudally and all pericardial and para-oesophageal tissue is dissected towards the oesophagus gradually exposing and baring the entire posterior aspect of the pericardium exposing the inferior pulmonary vein.

This plane is extended to reach the plane from the abdominal stage or to the right diaphragmatic crus.

- The pleura overlying the oesophagus on the proximal and distal parts of the azygos vein are then dissected. The part of the vein with pleura overlying the oesophagus should be resected still attached to the oesophagus.
- The incision is now deepened behind the oesophagus to reach the aorta. All tissue is mobilised towards the oesophagus skeletonising the azygos vein and the descending thoracic aorta. This tissue includes the thoracic duct, which is excised with the resection.
- This dissection is progressed caudally to either meet the abdominal stage of the dissection or the diaphragmatic hiatus. At this point the incision on the pleura is turned towards the oesophagus to meet the pleural dissection from the right side.
- The cut end of the thoracic duct is identified in the area near the crus next to the aorta and double ligated or clipped.
- The oesophagus is now lifted up with an instrument and the two dissection planes are joined on top of the aorta. The oesophagus can now be encircled with a sling to help retraction and dissection is continued caudally along the aorta resecting all para aortic tissue with the oesophagus.
- With the oesophagus retracted by a sling, attention is turned towards the carina. The pleural incision along the right main bronchus is extended towards the carina mobilising all the carinal lymph nodes towards the oesophagus. Care must be taken not to injure the membranous part of the bronchus or carina.
- The dissection is then continued along the left main bronchus and all lymph nodes mobilised towards the oesophagus to completely expose both the right and left main bronchi and the carina.
- The oesophagus is then dissected of the membranous part of the trachea above the azygos vein.
- For a two-stage oesophagectomy dissection is brought towards the oesophagus sparing the bronchial branch of the vagus nerve. The oesophagus can be transected just above the azygos vein to deliver the resection into the chest and plan the oesophago gastric anastomosis (Fig. **10**).
- For a three-stage oesophagectomy, dissection continues cranially to mobilise the oesophagus and complete the superior mediastinal lymphadenectomy.
- The pleural incision at the medial end of the ligated azygos vein is incised along the superior vena cava towards its origin at the confluence of the two brachiocephalic veins.
- All lymphatic tissue underneath this triangular flap of pleura from the superior edge of the right main bronchus upwards is mobilised towards the oesophagus.
- The vagus nerve is carefully followed till the origin of the right recurrent laryngeal nerve near the caudal side of the right subclavian artery. The vagus nerve is divided caudal to the origin of the recurrent laryngeal nerve.

- The right recurrent nodal chain begins here and forms a continuous chain that extends into the neck. This chain of lymph nodes is resected either en-bloc or separately and named as right recurrent laryngeal lymph nodes.
- The superior mediastinal oesophagus is then carefully dissected off the membranous part of the trachea before turning attention to the left recurrent laryngeal lymphadenectomy.
- The posterior pleural incision at the left main bronchus is extended along the superior intercostal vein towards the arch of the aorta.
- The trachea is gently retracted anteriorly to mobilise all the intervening tissue towards the oesophagus.
- The left vagus nerve is carefully followed to the aortic arch to identify the origin of the left recurrent laryngeal nerve. The left bronchial artery should be identified and preserved. The vagus nerve is divided below the origin of the left recurrent laryngeal nerve. The left recurrent lymphatic chain is resected either en-bloc or separately and labelled.
- The remainder of the thoracic oesophagus with its surrounding areolar tissue is mobilised till the thoracic inlet. This completes the superior mediastinal dissection.
- Haemostasis is checked. Before closure of the thoracotomy, two chest drains are inserted into the thoracic cavity, one apical and one basal.
- The fifth and seventh ribs are approximated with non-absorbable sutures. A mechanical drill is used to drill holes through the seventh rib. The suture passes through these holes and above the fifth rib to approximate them. This avoids crushing the neurovascular bundle that is situated at the lower border of the rib.
- The lung is fully inflated again before full approximation and closure of the muscle and skin layers.

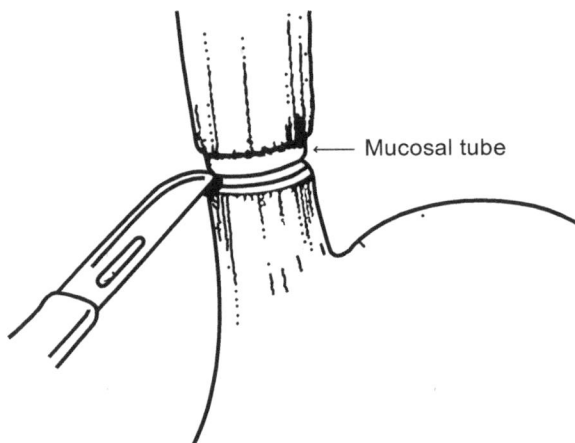

Fig. (10). The oesophageal muscular coat is divided down to the mucosal tube which in turn is transected 1.0 Cm lower down. This prevents retraction of the mucosa inside the muscular layer.

Oncological Management

Radiotherapy

Treatment by super voltage external beam radiotherapy may be curative (radical) or palliative to relieve dysphagia and metastatic bone pain in patients with advanced disease. It can also be given as an adjunct to surgical treatment either in the form of multi-modality treatment or after oesophagectomy to improve loco regional control. In many institutions, complete surgical resection has been the 'gold standard' against which other therapies are compared. It is difficult to make a meaningful comparison between surgery and radical radiation therapy for the primary treatment of resectable oesophageal cancer in the absence of comparative clinical trials between these two modalities in otherwise fit patients with early (resectable) oesophageal cancer. An analysis of retrospective series indicates that patients selected for radical treatment with radiotherapy have similar overall results to surgery except that the mortality of radical radiotherapy is small and its morbidity is significantly lower than that accrued by surgery. In general, radiotherapy achieved relief of dysphagia and local control of the disease but remote failure was common. There are, however, certain definite contraindications to radical radiotherapy. These include large tumours (more than 9.0 cm) and the presence of a tracheal broncho-oesophageal fistula. The main disadvantages of radical radiotherapy are the development of a fibrous stricture in half the patients treated. A variety of radiation therapy regimens have been described (40 to 70 Gy in 20 to 30 fractions) but no survival benefit was detected between them. Accelerated fractionation regimes that decrease the overall time of treatment may enhance local control at the expense of increased stricture rate.

Brachytherapy (intra-cavity irradiation) with caesium or iridium pellets loaded into an applicator and placed in the lumen of the oesophagus is another technique for delivering radiotherapy locally. The main limitation of this technique is the effective treatment distance, which in the case of iridium is one cm. Larger tumours would be irradiated in the centre but not peripherally. As such this technique is useful for palliation of dysphagia but not for radical treatment unless combined with external-beam super-voltage radiotherapy.

Radiotherapy is the treatment of choice for patients with cervical oesophageal cancer and for some patients with upper thoracic oesophageal cancer. Squamous carcinomas are considered radiosensitive and adenocarcinomas are considered relatively radio-resistant. For patients considered healthy enough to receive radical radiation therapy, concomitant chemotherapy is the preferred option.

Palliative treatment to relieve dysphagia is usually administered by external-beam super-voltage radiotherapy using a dose of 45 to 50 Gray. Dysphagia may temporarily worsen during the course of treatment and may take up to two months before effective palliation of dysphagia is realised. In addition, the duration of palliation after radiation therapy is variable but is generally poor and can be accompanied by the development of fibrotic strictures in 30% of patients. Combined chemo/irradiation produces better palliation of dysphagia at the expense of a higher rate of toxicity. Brachytherapy as a palliative measure is reported to give excellent results with relief of dysphagia in 65%.

Chemotherapy

In view of the metastatic rate of oesophageal cancer the disease should be regarded as systemic in the majority of patients, regardless of the stage of the disease at presentation. Systemic chemotherapy is advocated to address this problem. Several agents have been identified which can be used in combination treatment regimens for oesophageal cancer. These include 5-fluoro uracil (5-FU), cisplatin, vindesine, mitomycin C, paclitaxel and etoposide. Paclitaxel is one of the new group of taxanes with a high response rate in metastatic oesophageal cancer, which also acts as a radiation sensitiser and as such a useful adjunct to radiotherapy. Combination regimens are preferred to single agent use to increase the response rate using agents with different mechanisms of action and different toxicity profiles. Most combination regimens have the antimetabolite 5-fluorouracil in bolus injections or low dose continuous infusions with or without leucovorin. The second commonest agent used in combination regimens is cisplatin. The combination of cisplatin and 5-FU has consistently produced a complete pathological response rate of around 10% and a partial response rate (regression) of 50 – 60% but with significant toxicity, which can be up to 60%. Adding a third agent, such as bleomycin, has only fractionally improved the response rate at the expense of universally worse toxicity.

Multi-Modality Treatment

The majority of patients with oesophageal cancer present with advanced stages of the disease, which jeopardises the chances of a curative resection. This has led to the use of various multi-modality treatment schedules with or without surgery. The combined use of chemotherapy and radiotherapy is based on the rationale that different tumour cell sub-populations may be resistant to one modality but sensitive to another. In addition, apart from activity against micro metastases, some chemotherapeutic agents have radio-sensitising properties. In early resectable disease, it seems that survival rate is not significantly influenced by multi-modality regimens compared to surgery alone. However, in locally advanced disease, the potential benefit of the regimens becomes more evident with substantial numbers of patients having the stage of their disease lowered and becoming eligible for resection [20].

The combined use of chemotherapy and radiation therapy for the primary treatment of oesophageal cancer has produced better response rates in terms of tumour and metastatic disease response with improved survival, than either modality alone. One popular regimen, which is used in the treatment of patients with metastatic disease, is the Herskovic regimen. This consists of 50 Gy of radiation delivered over six weeks (25 fractions) with cisplatin and 5-FU given on weeks 1, 5, 8, and 11 (two courses of chemotherapy during and two after radiation).

Since residual disease after standard oesophagectomy is between 35-67%, radiotherapy has been commonly used with surgical resection for loco regional control. Theoretically, pre-operative radiotherapy is potentially advantageous from the radiobiology viewpoint. The dissected post-operative field is ischaemic and likely to be hypoxic. Tumour cell hypoxia is one mechanism of radio-resistance. In practice however, pre-operative radiotherapy does not appear to have a significant effect on loco regional control or on survival. However, post-operative radiotherapy seems to improve loco regional control (disease free interval) in node negative patients but has no impact on overall survival.

Pre-operative chemotherapy or chemoradiotherapy (neoadjuvant) followed by surgery is primarily used to improve survival although it can rarely be used to downstage advanced tumours in order to increase the resectability rate. Giving the treatment pre-operatively should result in better drug delivery to the tumour, as the local blood supply has not been disturbed by operative dissection. Distant control should also be enhanced as micro metastases are treated early without having to wait for post-surgical recovery. In addition, pre-operative treatment allows for the identification of responders who may benefit from additional post-operative therapy. Results from the UK MRC trial using 5-FU and cisplatin in two courses pre-operatively *vs* surgery alone suggest a 9% two-year survival benefit in patients who received pre-operative chemotherapy. The response seems to be similar for adenocarcinoma and squamous cell cancer.

The Chemoradiotherapy for Oesophageal Cancer Followed by Surgery Study (CROSS) trial provided definitive evidence for the benefit of preoperative CRT compared with surgery alone for patients with operable squamous cell carcinomas and adenocarcinomas of the esophagus and OJG. However, there has been no study to date, which has conclusively demonstrated the benefit of preoperative CRT over preoperative chemotherapy alone for oesophageal tumors [21].

Postoperative CRT is another standard of care, particularly in the West, for the adjuvant treatment of lymph node or margin positive tumors and for recurrent disease. However, approximately 30-40% of patients are not able to complete the post-operative course.

Intra-operative radiotherapy using mobile and custom-built delivery devices initially produced encouraging results. However, the technique was cumbersome, involved relatively large machinery and shields, added to intra-operative time and thus became unpopular for the majority of routine clinical use.

Despite the early enthusiasm, immuno-therapy with biological response modifiers (interferon, interleukin-2 and LAK cells) has not been successful in oesophageal and other gastrointestinal tumours.

Palliation of Oesophageal Cancer

Despite recent improvements in the diagnosis, staging and treatment of oesophageal cancer, around 50% of patients have advanced disease at presentation and can only have palliative measures. Although cancer cachexia is a frequent feature in these patients, dysphagia is the most troublesome complaint. The survival of these patients is short and every effort should be focussed on restoring the ability to swallow. These patients should be advised from the outset that no measure is likely to restore their pre-disease swallowing ability for a substantial period. However, patients should be able to swallow fluids and some solid or semi-solid food. A variety of interventional methods have evolved over the years to alleviate dysphagia including surgical bypass, laser canalisation, tumour necrosis (electro-coagulation, alcohol injection, arterial occlusion, radio-frequency ablation) and intubation [22].

Surgical Bypass

These are less popular than intubation procedures because they carry a high mortality, which averages around 30% and are major operations, which do not seem justified in patients with advanced disease or poor general condition with very limited survival. Gastro-oesophageal anastomosis warrants a thoracotomy and for this reason is seldom performed electively. In the presence of facilities for intubation using self-expanding metallic stents, surgical bypass is not justified.

Laser Canalisation

Laser photocoagulation used to be an effective method of oesophageal canalisation in patients with obstructive, advanced oesophageal cancer. In most instances the Nd:YAG laser was used as it produced good destruction of malignant tissue and its energy is not absorbed by blood. Currently, with the widespread use of self-expanding metallic stents, laser canalisation is seldom used and only when stenting was not possible.

Photodynamic therapy was another form of palliative re-canalisation of the oesophagus using Laser light energy for advanced oesophageal neoplasms. The principle entails a prior intravenous administration of a photosensitiser usually haematoporphyrin derivative, (HpD) or oral administration of 5-Aminolevulinic acid (5-ALA). These photosensitisers are taken up and retained by the tumour. After 6 – 24 hours the tumour is irradiated by light (wave length of 630 nm). This type of light energy excites the photosensitiser in the tumour to the triplet state with the production of highly reactive species such as singlet oxygen, which induced necrosis of the tumour (largely by occlusion of the tumour circulation). This modality is no longer in use due to mechanical difficulties of producing and transmitting the light, because of cutaneous sensitisation to sunlight and due to lack of effectiveness data in comparison with stents.

Electrocoagulation

Endoscopic guided fulguration of advanced oesophageal neoplasm is possible with the BICAP probe. This is passed over a guide wire to the proximal margin of the tumour, which is coagulated under endoscopic control. The procedure continues with antigrade coagulation of the tumour until the lower end of the lesion is reached when the probe is rotated 180° and retrograde coagulation applied creating a sizeable channel through the neoplastic mass. This technique is mainly used for ablation of tumour overgrowth and ingrowth through stents.

Ethanol Injection

Absolute alcohol can be injected under endoscopic control *via* a variceal injection needle into the obstructing tumour tissue to induce necrosis. This method, though cheap, quick and painless, has had limited application. The technique can be applied for lesions anywhere in the oesophagus and may be useful when the oesophageal lumen is completely obstructed by tumour. It is generally used as an adjunct to other methods such as stenting when it can be used to manage tumour overgrowth and tumour ingrowth through the stents.

Intubation

This is the most popular method of palliation of dysphagia for inoperable oesophageal cancer. Traction intubation entails surgical intervention to railroad the tube in position and anchor it to the stomach. The most common types of traction tube used are the Mousseau-Barbin and Celestin tubes. Increasingly, pulsion intubation is preferred since this avoids a laparotomy. Pulsion tubes, which can be placed through the lesion by means of a flexible introducer inserted over a guide wire, are very rarely used nowadays (Atkinson's pulsion tubes). A preliminary dilatation is usually necessary before insertion of pulsion tubes. Intubation is more effective for distal than proximal lesions. The main disadvantages of the rigid tubes included the small diameter necessitating liquidised food, perforation of the oesophagus at the time of insertion, erosion of the tube through the tumour and dislodgement with upper airway obstruction.

Self-expanding metallic stents are the gold standard used for the palliation of advanced oesophageal cancer. They provide excellent palliation of dysphagia. They are relatively easy to insert by practicing endoscopists and interventional radiologists. The stents are introduced with the deployment device over a guide wire and positioned across the marked malignant stricture in the oesophagus. The guide wire can be introduced endoscopically or radiologically. Fluoroscopy is necessary to mark the limits of the stricture. Preliminary dilatation of the stricture up to 12 mm (depending on the type of stent) is required. This reduced extent of dilatation has reduced the risk of perforation markedly with consequent reduction in hospital mortality. Once the stent is expanded, the large lumen achieved (16-20 mm) and the flexibility of the stent allow for restoration of swallowing with little dietary modification (Fig. **11**).

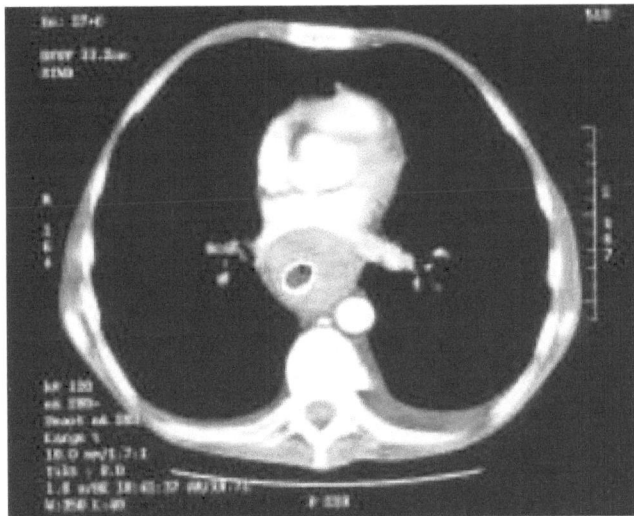

Fig. (11). CT scan slice through the chest showing a bulky lower oesophageal tumour with a self-expanding metallic stent keeping the lumen open.

The stents can be used for proximal and distal oesophageal obstruction but have had limited success in oesophago-gastric junction tumours due to angulation and migration. Several types are available (Fig. **12**) with varying diameters and lengths. Some have a polyethylene coating over the mesh of the stent (covered stents) and some have distal antireflux valves. Delayed stent failure however can occur in a number of patients due to migration of the stent in up to 29% of patients, tumour ingrowth through the mesh of uncovered stents in up to 36% of patients, tumour overgrowth above or below the stent (15%), symptomatic gastro-oesophageal reflux after stenting across the oesophago-gastric junction, stent related haemorrhage (6-9%), and post stenting chest pain requiring opiate analgesia in up to 10% of patients. The major limitation of self-expanding metallic stents is their cost.

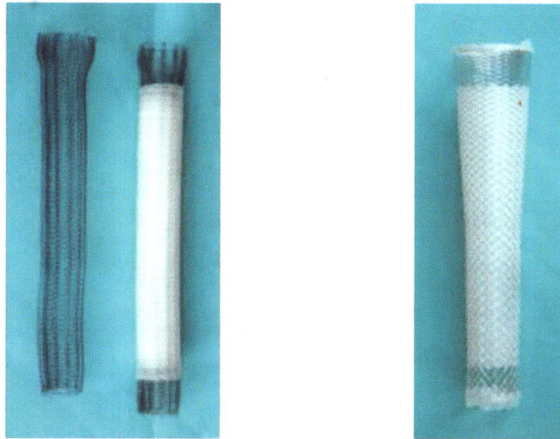

Fig. (12). Ultraflex stents covered and uncovered (left) and covered Flaming stent (right).

The most difficult patients to palliate are those who develop a malignant tracheo-oesophageal fistula either spontaneously (5%) or as a result of radiotherapy. Some fistulae arise as a result of pressure necrosis caused by a plastic prosthesis or a stent or as a result of a canalisation procedure. Supportive care provides a median life expectancy of about three weeks and death usually results from pulmonary complications. The aim of palliation therapy is to seal the fistula rapidly in order to improve the quality of life for this group of patients. The conservative method of management, with cessation of oral intake and providing nutritional support is indicated for a short period as a temporary measure to improve the patient's condition. Surgical closure or bypass surgery is associated with high morbidity and mortality. Closure by means of cyanoacrylates and fibrin, have had varying degrees of success. Placement of plastic balloon endoprosthesis is associated with considerable morbidity and mortality without consistent closure of the fistula. Covered self-expanding metallic stents are reported to have a success rate of sealing tracheo/broncho oesophageal fistulae in 67-100%. Despite their cost, covered stents are the most reliable and cost effective method in the management of these patients.

CONSENT FOR PUBLICATION

Not applicable.

ACKNOWLEDGEMENT

Declare none.

CONFLICT OF INTEREST

The authors declare no conflict of interest, financial or otherwise.

REFERENCES

[1]   Huang FL, Yu SJ. Esophageal cancer: Risk factors, genetic association, and treatment. Asian J Surg 2016; (Dec): 13.
        [PMID: 27986415]

[2]   Tripathi M, Swanson PE. Rare tumors of esophageal squamous mucosa. Ann N Y Acad Sci 2016; 1381(1): 122-32.
        [http://dx.doi.org/10.1111/nyas.13108] [PMID: 27310830]

[3]   Tan C, Qian X, Guan Z, *et al.* Potential biomarkers for esophageal cancer. Springerplus 2016; 5: 467.
        [http://dx.doi.org/10.1186/s40064-016-2119-3] [PMID: 27119071]

[4]   Berry MF. Esophageal cancer: staging system and guidelines for staging and treatment. J Thorac Dis 2014; 6 (Suppl. 3): S289-97.
        [PMID: 24876933]

[5]   UICC. Oesophagus including oesophagogastric junction, TNM classification of malignant tumours. New York: Wiley-Blackwell 2009.

[6]   Crabtree TD, Yacoub WN, Puri V, *et al.* Endoscopic ultrasound for early stage esophageal adenocarcinoma: implications for staging and survival. Ann Thorac Surg 2011; 91(5): 1509-15.
        [http://dx.doi.org/10.1016/j.athoracsur.2011.01.063] [PMID: 21435632]

[7]   Rice TW, Blackstone EH, Rusch VW. 7th edition of the AJCC Cancer Staging Manual: esophagus and esophagogastric junction. Ann Surg Oncol 2010; 17(7): 1721-4.
        [http://dx.doi.org/10.1245/s10434-010-1024-1] [PMID: 20369299]

[8]   Rice TW, Rusch VW, Ishwaran H, Blackstone EH, Worldwide Esophageal Cancer C. Worldwide Esophageal Cancer Collaboration. Cancer of the esophagus and esophagogastric junction: data-driven staging for the seventh edition of the American Joint Committee on Cancer/International Union Against Cancer Cancer Staging Manuals. Cancer 2010; 116(16): 3763-73.
        [http://dx.doi.org/10.1002/cncr.25146] [PMID: 20564099]

[9]   Lehmann K, Schneider PM. Differences in the molecular biology of adenocarcinoma of the esophagus, gastric cardia, and upper gastric third. Recent Results Cancer Res 2010; 182: 65-72.
        [http://dx.doi.org/10.1007/978-3-540-70579-6_5] [PMID: 20676871]

[10]   Siewert JR, Stein HJ. Classification of adenocarcinoma of the oesophagogastric junction. Br J Surg 1998; 85(11): 1457-9.
        [http://dx.doi.org/10.1046/j.1365-2168.1998.00940.x] [PMID: 9823902]

[11]   Siewert J, Stein H. Carcinoma of the gastroesophageal junction-classification, pathology and extent of resection. Dis Esophagus. Dis Esophagus 1996; 9: 173-82.

[12]   Dresner SM, Lamb PJ, Bennett MK, Hayes N, Griffin SM. The pattern of metastatic lymph node dissemination from adenocarcinoma of the esophagogastric junction. Surgery 2001; 129(1): 103-9.

[http://dx.doi.org/10.1067/msy.2001.110024] [PMID: 11150040]

[13]   Mullen JT, Kwak EL, Hong TS. What's the best way to treat GE junction tumors? approach like gastric cancer. Ann Surg Oncol 2016; 23(12): 3780-5.
[http://dx.doi.org/10.1245/s10434-016-5426-6] [PMID: 27459983]

[14]   Rüdiger Siewert J, Feith M, Werner M, Stein HJ. Adenocarcinoma of the esophagogastric junction: results of surgical therapy based on anatomical/topographic classification in 1,002 consecutive patients. Ann Surg 2000; 232(3): 353-61.
[http://dx.doi.org/10.1097/00000658-200009000-00007] [PMID: 10973385]

[15]   Galey KM, Wilshire CL, Watson TJ, *et al.* Endoscopic management of early esophageal neoplasia: an emerging standard. J Gastrointest Surg 2011; 15(10): 1728-35.
[http://dx.doi.org/10.1007/s11605-011-1618-3] [PMID: 21811883]

[16]   Tong DK, Law S, Kwong DL, Wei WI, Ng RW, Wong KH. Current management of cervical esophageal cancer. World J Surg 2011; 35(3): 600-7.
[http://dx.doi.org/10.1007/s00268-010-0876-7] [PMID: 21161656]

[17]   Hulscher JB, van Sandick JW, de Boer AG, *et al.* Extended transthoracic resection compared with limited transhiatal resection for adenocarcinoma of the esophagus. N Engl J Med 2002; 347(21): 1662-9.
[http://dx.doi.org/10.1056/NEJMoa022343] [PMID: 12444180]

[18]   Cuschieri A, Shimi S, Banting S. Endoscopic oesophagectomy through a right thoracoscopic approach. J R Coll Surg Edinb 1992; 37(1): 7-11.
[PMID: 1573620]

[19]   Kakeji Y, Yamamoto M, Ito S, *et al.* Lymph node metastasis from cancer of the esophagogastric junction, and determination of the appropriate nodal dissection. Surg Today 2012; 42(4): 351-8.
[http://dx.doi.org/10.1007/s00595-011-0114-4] [PMID: 22245924]

[20]   Castoro C, Scarpa M, Cagol M, *et al.* Complete clinical response after neoadjuvant chemoradiotherapy for squamous cell cancer of the thoracic oesophagus: is surgery always necessary? J Gastrointest Surg 2013; 17(8): 1375-81.
[http://dx.doi.org/10.1007/s11605-013-2269-3] [PMID: 23797888]

[21]   Smyth EC, Waddell TS, Cunningham D. Optimal management of esophageal adenocarcinoma: should we be CROSS? J Clin Oncol 2014; 32(27): 3080-1.
[http://dx.doi.org/10.1200/JCO.2014.55.5243] [PMID: 25071100]

[22]   Mao A. Interventional therapy of esophageal cancer. Gastrointest Tumors 2016; 3(2): 59-68.
[http://dx.doi.org/10.1159/000447512] [PMID: 27904858]

CHAPTER 4

Gastric Neoplasms

Sami M. Shimi[*]

Department of Surgery, Ninewells Hospital and Medical School, Dundee, Scotland

Abstract: Neoplasms of the stomach may be benign or malignant. Gastric cancer is the fourth most commonly diagnosed cancer and the second most common cause of cancer-related death worldwide. Gastric carcinogenesis is probably a multi-step process based on a model referred to as the Correa Cascade. It progresses mainly from *H. pylori* induced chronic gastritis. Diagnosis is by endoscopy and biopsy. CT and laparoscopy are required for adequate staging. Endoscopic mucosal resection or surgery, are the standard treatment options for Tis, T1 early gastric cancer. No further treatment is necessary if there is no residual or nodal disease. Subtotal or total gastrectomy with regional lymphadenectomy is the standard surgical treatment for early stage gastric cancer with lymph node metastases. In many parts of the world, multi-modality treatment using chemotherapy or chemoradiotherapy (either following surgery or combined pre-operative and post-operative administration) is the preferred treatment strategy. In very advanced cases, a number of clinical trials have produced evidence that chemotherapy improves survival in comparison to best supportive care in selected patients. Gastro-intestinal stromal tumours are responsible for 2.2% of malignant gastric tumours without any gender preference. They have a much better prognosis than adenocarcinoma of the stomach. The incidence of gastric neuro-endocrine tumours is constantly rising. The majority of gastric NETs have a benign course and asymptomatic behaviour. Primary gastric lymphoma originates from the gastric wall or from the adjacent lymph nodes. The primary treatment is oncological.

Keywords: Benign gastric tumours, Cancer of oesophago-gastric junction, Gastrectomy, Gastric adenocarcinoma, Gastric lymphoma, Gastro-intestinal stromal tumours, Neuroendocrine tumours, Non-surgical treatment, Palliation of gastric cancer, Pathology, Staging.

TUMOURS OF THE STOMACH

Neoplasms of the stomach may be benign or malignant. Benign neoplasms include gastric polyps, which are usually regenerative hyperplastic polyps. Malignant neoplasms include gastric adenocarcinoma (the commonest variety) and gastric MALTomas (low grade B-cell lymphomas derived from Mucosa

[*] **Corresponding author Sami M. Shimi:** Department of Surgery, Ninewells Hospital and Medical School, Dundee DD1 9SY, Scotland, UK; Tel: +44 1382 383550; E-mail: s.m.shimi@dundee.ac.uk

Associated Lymphoid Tissue). High grade non-Hodgkins B-cell lymphomas also occur in the stomach. Mesenchymal neoplasms are described as spindle cell tumours and include benign leiomyomas, malignant leiomyosarcomas and Gastro intestinal stromal tumours (GISTs) (with a spectrum from benign to malignant).

Benign Tumours of the Stomach

The majority of gastric polyps are regenerative *hyperplastic polyps*. They are usually asymptomatic and are discovered incidentally. They account for up to 75% of gastric polyps and can occur anywhere in the stomach but predominantly in the antrum of the stomach. These polyps usually arise on the background of inflammation and are usually associated with gastritis, *Helicobacter pylori* and peptic ulcer disease. The polyps appear as smooth nodules of varying sizes and consist of proliferating glands with hyperplasia. Once discovered, the polyps can be observed and require no intervention unless they grow in size or display unusual surface features or start to bleed. If suspicion arises, they can be removed or biopsied endoscopically.

Inflammatory fibroid polyps (eosinophilic granulomas, haemangiopericytomas) are rare. They are usually found in the gastric antrum and can be sessile or pedunculated. The polyps consist of vascular stroma containing numerous capillaries and arterioles, fibroblasts and inflammatory cells with an abundance of eosinophils. These polyps are not associated with systemic eosinophilia or eosinophilic gastroenteritis.

Myoepithelial hamartomas arise from the sub-mucosal layer of the gastric antrum and appear as smooth sessile masses usually in the gastric antrum. The polyps are composed of glands surrounded by smooth muscle. Peutz-Jeghers hamartomatous polyps are a rare variety.

Fundic gland polyps are usually small, multiple and found in the fundus of the stomach. They consist of micro cysts lined by fundic epithelium including oxyntic cells. They are associated with long-term proton pump inhibitor therapy. While sporadic fundic gland polyps and fundic gland polyps in association with long-term proton pump inhibitor therapy are without risk, somatic APC mutations are detectable in >70% of fundic gland polyps associated with polyposis syndromes. Patients with >20 fundic gland polyps, young onset of the polyps (<40 years), additional duodenal adenomas and fundic gland polyps in other regions than the gastric corpus are under suspicion for familial adenomatous polyposis.

Gastric adenomas are rare and the majority, are found in the antrum of the stomach. They may be single or multiple and appear sessile, villous, pedunculated or lobulated. Due to their malignant potential, all gastric adenomas should undergo endoscopic resection and follow-up. Rarely, they progress to adenocarcinoma and endoscopic resection is advisable.

Malignant Tumours of the Stomach

Malignant adenomas are rare, occur predominantly in the antrum of the stomach and are either sessile or pedunculated. They consist of typical glands with pseudo-stratified epithelium showing nuclear abnormalities and mitotic figures. They also contain endocrine cells positive for serotonin or other peptide hormones. They are categorized as tubular, tubulovillous and villous. These adenomas have a low malignant potential (5% within 5 years) which is size dependent. Endoscopic removal and surveillance is recommended.

Hypertrophic gastropathy (Menetrier's disease) appear as large hypertrophic gastric mucosal folds and can be associated with a protein losing enteropathy. The large folds are usually centred along the greater curvature with sharp demarcation of the abnormal and normal gastric mucosa. Histologically, they show marked foveolar hyperplasia with an inflamed and oedematous stroma. Although the volume of gastric secretions is high, the acid content is low. Bleeding can occur from the giant folds and the patient may present with anaemia. Patients can also present with hypoproteinaemia. Rarely, this condition can lead to gastric malignancy. At biopsy, it is important to ensure that these folds do not represent gastric varices. Management depends on the presentation and may have to include gastrectomy.

GASTRIC ADENOCARCINOMA

Gastric cancer is the fourth most commonly diagnosed cancer and the second most common cause of cancer-related death worldwide. While the intestinal type of gastric cancer is often related to environmental factors such as *Helicobacter pylori* infection, diet, and life style, the diffuse type is more often associated with genetic abnormalities. The incidence of gastric cancer in the world is decreasing and the disease carries a poor prognosis. The incidence is highest in Japan, Korea, China, Latin America and Eastern Europe.

The incidence of gastric cancer is decreasing. The sharpest decline in the incidence of gastric cancer of around 60% has been reported in Finland. In contrast to the overall decline in the incidence of gastric cancer, tumours of the upper third of the stomach including the oesophago-gastric junction have increased and now account for approximately 40% of gastric cancer. Today, the incidence of early gastric cancer has reached above 50% in Japan while in the west two thirds of gastric cancers are at an advanced stage at the time of diagnosis

The disease is rarely seen below 40 years of age and the incidence rises sharply beyond the fourth decade. The male preponderance (2:1) is observed throughout the world. Gastric cancer is more common in lower socio-economic classes. The overall 5-year survival is around 10%. The exact reasons for this are not clear. Currently, the only potentially curative option for gastric cancer is surgery, which involves complete resection (R0), although the extent of regional lymphadenectomy has been a matter of debate.

Gastric carcinogenesis is probably a multi-step process based on a model referred to as the Correa Cascade (Fig. **1**). Chronic gastritis either de novo or precipitated by *Helicobacter pylori* leads to atrophy and intestinal metaplasia which progresses to dysplasia. The mechanism for the stepwise carcinogenesis is brought about by a series of unknown genetic changes which culminate in a clone of neoplastic cells devoid of growth control checks and able to proliferate and disseminate. Different gene mutations and growth factors are involved in this cascade.

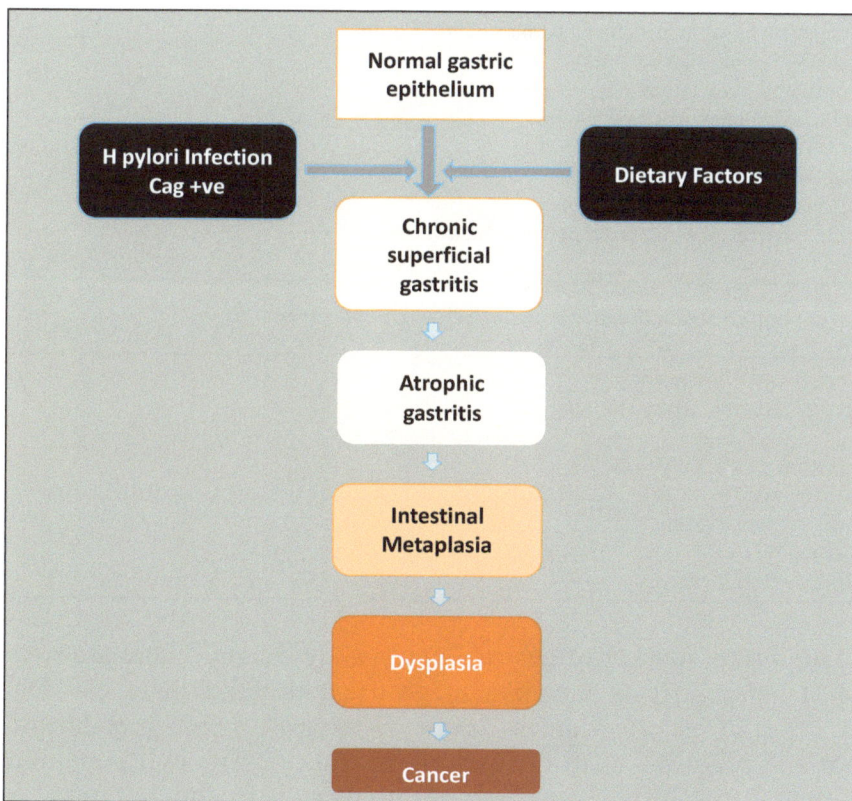

Fig. (1). Flow chart of a model of gastric carcinogenesis.

A number of factors have been implicated in carcinogenesis, although causality remains unproven (Table **1**). The most recognized risk factor in carcinogenesis is *H. pylori* through induction of gastritis and gastric atrophy. The next commonly recognized factor is atrophic gastritis. The incidence of gastric atrophy increases with age and is frequently encountered in patients above 60 years in the Western. In addition to *H. pylori*, other factors can cause primary damage of the gastric mucosa leading to the development of atrophic gastritis. There is evidence for progression from gastric atrophy to intestinal metaplasia, dysplasia and carcinoma *in situ*.

Other recognized risk factors in the development of gastric cancer are mentioned in Table **2**.

Table 1. Factors implicated in gastric carcinogenesis.

• *H. Pylori* gastritis
• Spiced, salted or pickled food
• Polycyclic hydrocarbons, especially those generated by high temperature pyrolysis of animal fat and aromatic amino acids in grilled and barbecued meat.
• Inorganic dust (miners and potters)
• High consumption of animal fat
• High salt consumption (causing osmotic damage to gastric mucosa)
• Protein malnutrition (*via* achlorhydria)
• Excess alcohol consumption
• Tobacco smoking
• Dietary nitrates (in drinking water and vegetables)
• Refluxed bile acids

Table 2. Factors implicated in the development of gastric carcinogenesis.

• Persistent *H. pylori* infection.
• Atrophic gastritis and pernicious anaemia
• Previous gastric surgery
• Adenomatous gastric polyps
• Familial polyposis
• Hypogammaglobulinaemia
• Blood group A
• Type III intestinal metaplasia

The most important marker of gastric cancer is dysplasia. There are two types of dysplasia. Type A affects metaplastic gastric epithelium and can lead to the intestinal type of gastric cancer. Type B arises in non-metaplastic gastric epithelium and predisposes to diffuse gastric cancer. The cell population of the glands in type B dysplasia is largely made up of undifferentiated round cells with a clear or amphophillic cytoplasm lacking a brush border. Dysplasia is graded histologically into mild, moderate and severe. The morphometric grading is based on architectural parameters such as volume and surface densities of glands and epithelium, which describe the arrangement and shape of the nuclei and nucleolar size. Severe dysplasia is recognized as *in situ* gastric cancer. Whereas mild and moderate dysplasia may progress slowly, severe dysplasia progresses to invasive cancer in the majority of patients. Thus, mild and moderate dysplasia, merit endoscopic surveillance. However, severe dysplasia proven on two biopsies merits gastrectomy. In up to 50% of patients, invasive gastric cancer will be found in the resected stomach on pathological examination.

Whereas genetic factors are considered important in diffuse gastric cancer, there is no evidence for familial predisposition in the development of intestinal type gastric cancer. Diffuse gastric cancer is more common in people with blood group A, in relatives of patients with diffuse gastric cancer, and in familial hypogammaglobulinaemia. This is a genetically determined disorder, which is characterized by defective production of IgG antibodies and is usually accompanied by pernicious anaemia. These patients have a 50-fold increased risk in developing gastric cancer.

Presentation and Clinical Features

Men are more frequently affected by gastric cancer than women (male: female ratio; 2:1) and the median age at diagnosis is 70 years of age. Early gastric cancer is usually asymptomatic and the diagnosis is usually made at endoscopy carried out for screening (in high prevalence countries) or incidentally. Typically, lesions near the cardia can give rise to dysphagia and prepyloric lesions can give rise to gastric outlet obstructive symptoms, which may be initially intermittent. Overt bleeding is not a usually feature of early gastric cancer however, early lesions can ooze and the patient may present with iron deficiency anaemia due to chronic blood loss. Advanced gastric cancer may however present with overt bleeding which can be troublesome and difficult to stop. The cardinal symptoms of malignancy in the upper gastrointestinal tract include dysphagia, unintentional weight loss, persistent vomiting, iron deficiency anaemia (or suspicion of GI bleeding) and the presence of an epigastric mass on examination. The symptom of dyspepsia is so common and vague making it unreliable as an indication for endoscopy. However, persistent dyspepsia of recent onset in a person over 55 years of age is a strong indication for endoscopy. This is particularly so, if dyspepsia is combined with any of the cardinal symptoms of malignancy in the upper GI tract. In addition, unexplained symptoms such as early satiety, post-prandial fullness, loss of appetite or malaise, require investigations by endoscopy as a minimum when they are persistent, worsening or combined with one or more of the cardinal symptoms (Tables **3** and **4**).

Table 3. Indications for urgent referral to endoscopy.

Patients aged 55 years and older with unexplained and "persistent" recent-onset dyspepsia.
Patients of any age with dyspepsia when presenting with any of the following: • Chronic gastrointestinal bleeding   • Progressive unintentional weight loss   • Progressive difficulty swallowing (dysphagia)   • Persistent vomiting   • Iron deficiency anaemia or other evidence of GI bleeding   • Epigastric mass or suspicious barium meal   • Epigastric pain severe enough for hospitalisation
Patients presenting with any of the following (<u>even in the absence of dyspepsia</u>):   • Dysphagia   • Unexplained upper abdominal pain and weight loss, with or without back pain   • Upper abdominal mass   • Obstructive jaundice (depending on clinical state).
In patients over 55 years old, when symptoms persist despite *Helicobacter pylori* (*H. pylori*) testing (or eradication if positive), acid suppression therapy, and when patients have one or more of the following: • Previous gastric ulcer or surgery,   • Continuing need for NSAID treatment or   • Raised risk of gastric cancer or   • Anxiety about cancer
Patients with unexplained worsening of chronic dyspepsia and any of the following risk factors: • Known Barrett's oesophagus   • Known dysplasia on previous biopsies   • Known atrophic gastritis (pernicious anaemia)   • Known intestinal metaplasia on previous biopsies   • Peptic ulcer surgery more than 20 years ago   • Previous proven achalasia (with or without prior treatment).

Table 4. Indications for routine endoscopy.

• Patients with liver disease, to detect oesophageal varices   • Patients with resistant *H. pylori* infection with worsening dyspepsia   • Patients with dyspepsia who have not responded to treat and test policy   • Patients diagnosed with gastric ulcer or bleeding duodenal ulcer after a course of treatment.   • Surveillance of patients with Barrett's oesophagus.   • Patients suspected of having coeliac disease (for biopsy confirmation).   • Patients with a known oesophageal ulcer after a course of treatment

The common presenting symptoms in advanced gastric cancer (AGC) include dysphagia, early satiety, epigastric pain, weight loss, anaemia, anorexia, nausea, vomiting and melena. However, advanced gastric cancer can present with any of the cardinal symptoms with weight loss being a significant feature. Dysphagia is frequently associated with proximal tumours, and early satiety can be caused by distal tumours or tumours with linitis plastica appearance due to gastric outlet obstruction or loss of stomach distensibility. The symptom duration is less than 3 months in nearly 40% of patients and longer than 1 year in only 20%. Presenting symptoms and signs also depend on the presence or absence of distant metastasis. These patients may show an enlarged abdominal mass or abdominal swelling due to tumour metastasis to the liver or malignant peritoneal effusion (ascites). The presence of a palpable epigastric mass, jaundice, hepatomegaly or ascites also indicate advanced incurable disease with limited survival. Occasionally, the non-regional lymph node metastasis to the supraclavicular area can be superficial and palpable (Virchow's lymph node). Metastases in or around the umbilicus (Sister Mary Joseph node), in the pelvic cul-de-sac (Blumer's shelf on pelvic examination) on the ovaries (Kruckenberg's tumour) and in the left axilla (Irish's node) are uncommonly encountered. Although often stressed, these nodes are a rare physical finding in gastric cancer. However, when present, in the context of gastric cancer, they indicate advanced incurable disease.

Peritoneal metastatic spread may be evident as a palpable mass(s) in the abdomen, palpable ovary on pelvic examination (Krukenberg tumour) or metastasis to the pouch of Douglas on rectal examination (Blumer's shelf sign). Rarely, women may present with vaginal bleeding due to metastasis to the endometrium. Patients with AGC may present with Para neoplastic syndromes such as diffuse seborrheic keratosis, acanthosis nigricans, microangiopathic haemolytic anaemia, and Trousseau's syndrome.

Given the common and often vague nature of the presentations of early gastric cancer, some patients will already have self-medicated with over the counter medications to control their symptoms. Equally, it is not unreasonable for primary care practitioners to treat vague symptoms by prescribing symptom control medicines with a "wait and watch" strategy. The exceptions to this policy are if patients have any of the cardinal symptoms or if the symptoms have been chronic despite self-medication. If patient's symptoms persist despite the medication or after cessation of a course of medication, then early referral for establishing a diagnosis is indicated (Tables **3** and **4**).

Diagnosis of Gastric Cancer

White-light, conventional upper gastrointestinal endoscopy with biopsy for histological confirmation is the gold standard tests for the detection of gastric cancer. Recent innovations in equipment used for upper gastrointestinal endoscopy have contributed to finding increased numbers of early-stage gastric cancers. Chromoendoscopy using indigo dye spraying played an important role in identifying early lesions. Magnifying endoscopy with narrow-band imaging (NBI) has undergone technological improvements, to make it accurate and reliable for the diagnosis of early gastric cancer. Magnifying endoscopy with NBI allows observation of the micro vascular architecture of the mucosa and micro surface pattern of the lesion, and is useful for assessing the area of the lesion and the depth of tumor invasion. Furthermore, endocytoscopy, a technique allowing microscopic visualization of the mucosal surface, has been developed. Endocytoscopic visualization of nuclei might allow pathological diagnosis without the need for biopsy. This novel technology is expected to play a major role in the diagnosis of early gastrointestinal cancer in the near future. Another diagnostic innovation is virtual endoscopy, which uses multi-detector-row computed tomography (CT). With further development, it is anticipated that this noninvasive diagnostic modality will be established as a screening tool for gastrointestinal disease. However, the radiation burden will have to be addressed.

Although double-contrast upper gastrointestinal radiology can be cost-effective, with a low risk of side effects, the differentiation between a benign ulcer from a malignant one or gastric lymphoma can be very challenging. The diagnostic accuracy rate of endoscopy with biopsy for upper gastrointestinal cancers is more than 95%. The diagnostic accuracy of the biopsies usually increases with the increased numbers of sample taken. It is recommended that between six and eight biopsies should be obtained from any lesion with one from each quadrant and two from the centre of the lesion, using jumbo biopsy forceps. Biopsy should be taken from the edge of an ulcerative lesion and not from the base, which contains mainly necrotic tissue. Gastric forceps biopsy may have limitation for the proper diagnosis and determination of degree of differentiation in some cases. Hence, endoscopic features should be considered together with the biopsy diagnosis to determine the appropriate treatment strategy for the lesions.

Staging of Gastric Cancer

Once a diagnosis of gastric carcinoma has been made, endoscopic ultrasonography, Multi-Detector Computed Tomography (MDCT) scan and laparoscopy with peritoneal cytology are usually employed for tumour staging. EUS carried out by an experienced practitioner is particularly useful to estimate the depth of tumour invasion for local staging. Accuracy of EUS for T staging in gastric carcinoma is approximately 82%, with a sensitivity and specificity of over 70% and 87%, respectively. However, differentiating T2 and T3 gastric carcinoma may be difficult in some cases due to associated fibrosis in T2 mimicking T3 lesions. EUS is best for differentiating T1a and T1b lesions, which is important for selection of endoscopic and submucosal resection respectively. EUS can also sample adjacent lymph nodes for confirmation of involvement. MDCT is not as accurate for early gastric cancer (EGC) but is equal if not superior to EUS in differentiating T2, T3 or T4 tumours. CT scanning of chest abdomen and pelvis in the prone position with appropriate gastric distension should provide information on enlarged lymph nodes and distant metastasis [1]. Accuracy for T staging of gastric carcinoma by spiral CT is approximately 64%, lower than that of EUS. Detection of lymph node involvement by spiral CT scan is not reliable with low sensitivity rates ranging from 24% to 43%, because lymph node size is not a good parameter for determining nodal metastasis. CT scan has been used for identifying distant metastasis to lung, liver, bone, *etc*. Peritoneal dissemination, which has been difficult to identify using conventional diagnostic imaging techniques, is the most frequent non-curative manifestation of gastric cancer. In some patients, peritoneal dissemination cannot be found before surgery, and laparotomy becomes an exploratory procedure after dissemination is discovered. Staging laparoscopy (SL) is a minimally invasive, brief procedure that only requires a small incision. The advantages of SL include providing an accurate diagnosis of peritoneal dissemination and extraserosal invasion, and the ability to perform peritoneal lavage for cytology. In patients with advanced gastric cancer for which imaging does not yield a diagnosis, peritoneal lavage cytology obtained before treatment can be very important for treatment planning. Negative findings on peritoneal lavage cytology can confirm the treatment intent as curative and aid in the decision to perform resection after neoadjuvant chemotherapy [2]. Gastric cancer patients with positive findings on peritoneal lavage cytology are considered to have stage IV disease, and the treatment intent is palliative. Carcinomatous peritonitis occurs at a relatively high rate even without overt dissemination in patients who are found to have free intraperitoneal cancer cells on peritoneal lavage cytology. Therefore, staging laparoscopy should be applied to patients with advanced gastric cancer with potential peritoneal dissemination. SL is probably useful for patients with the following: (1) endoscopic or CT findings suggesting extraserosal invasion, (2) scirrhous gastric cancer, which tends to disseminate throughout the peritoneum, and (3) CT findings suggesting peritoneal dissemination or a small amount of ascites.

Magnetic Resonance Imaging (MRI) is comparable to CT scan for staging of AGC and useful to confirm a liver metastasis in equivocal cases. However, MRI is less sensitive, has longer scanning times and a higher cost than CT scan. MRI is not currently recommended for the staging of gastric cancer.

There have been several reports on the effectiveness of PET for staging gastric cancer. However, very little additional information can be gained from PET/ CT over and above multi-detector helical CT in gastric cancer patients. Bony metastases are uncommon in patients with gastric cancer. Bone scintigraphy is the gold standard examination to detect bone metastasis in suspicious cases. Early detection of bone metastasis is important as it changes the treatment intent and directs additional measures to alleviate bone pain and prevent pathologic fractures. In addition to bone scintigraphy, FDG-PET/CT is also useful for early detection of bone metastasis. PET has also been reported to be useful for assessing response to chemotherapy; changes in the metabolism of glucose by tumour cells have been reported to appear early during chemotherapy. Recent studies have shown that uptake of tracer in the primary tumor and nodes is an independent and significant prognostic factor for predicting cancer recurrence or non-curable operations.

With the benefit of all staging investigations a reasonably accurate clinical stage could be established (Tables **5** and **6**).

Table 5. TNM Classification of Gastric Cancer (TNM 7th edition) [3].

Primary tumour (T)	
TX	Primary tumour cannot be assessed
T0	No evidence of primary tumour
Tis	Carcinoma *in situ*: intraepithelial tumour without invasion of the lamina propria
T1	Tumour invades lamina propria, muscularis mucosa, or submucosa
T1a	Tumour invades lamina propria or muscularis mucosa
T1b	Tumour invades submucosa
T2	Tumour invades muscularis propria
T3	Tumour penetrates subserosal connective tissue without invasion of visceral peritoneum or adjacent structures
T4	Tumour invades serosa (visceral peritoneum) or adjacent structures
T4a	Tumour invades serosa (visceral peritoneum)
T4b	Tumour invades adjacent structures
Regional lymph nodes (N)	
NX	Regional lymph node(s) cannot be assessed
N0	No regional lymph node metastasis
N1	Metastasis in 1-2 regional lymph nodes
N2	Metastasis in 3-6 regional lymph nodes
N3	Metastasis in seven or more regional lymph nodes
N3a	Metastasis in 7-15 regional lymph nodes
N3b	Metastasis in 16 or more regional lymph nodes
Distant metastasis (M)	
M0	No distant metastasis
M1	Distant metastasis

Table 6. Staging of Gastric Cancer.

Stage	T	N	M
0	Tis	N0	M0
IA	T1	N0	M0
IB	T2	N0	M0
	T1	N1	M0
IIA	T3	N0	M0
	T2	N1	M0
	T1	N2	M0
IIB	T4a	N0	M0
	T3	N1	M0
	T2	N2	M0
	T1	N3	M0
IIIA	T4a	N1	M0
	T3	N2	M0
	T2	N3	M0
IIIB	T4b	N0	M0
	T4b	N1	M0
	T4a	N2	M0
	T3	N3	M0
IIIC	T4b	N2	M0
	T4b	N3	M0
	T4a	N3	M0
IV	Any T	Any N	M1

Serological Biomarkers of Gastric Cancer

No specific biologic tumour marker, have been verified for gastric cancer. Serum markers are not useful for the diagnosis of early gastric cancer, but they are useful for detecting recurrence and distant metastasis, predicting patient survival, and monitoring after surgery or chemotherapy [4]. Tumour marker monitoring may be useful for patients after surgery because the positive conversion of tumour markers usually occurs 2-3 months before imaging abnormalities. CEA, CA19-9 and CA72-4 are probably the most significant in gastric cancer. The positive rates are 21.1% for CEA, 27.8% for CA19-9, and 30.0% for CA72-4. The serum levels of these three markers taken together are significantly associated with tumour stage and patient survival. Monitoring a combination of CEA, CA19-9, and

CA72-4 may be useful for detection of recurrence or evaluation of response.

Classification of Gastric Cancer

Gastric carcinoma is clinically classified as early or advanced stage to help determine appropriate management, and histologically into subtypes based on major morphologic component (Table **7**). For the anatomic classification, difficulty often arises when the tumour is located at proximal stomach or cardia, especially when the tumour also involves the gastroesophageal junction (GEJ). The scheme endorsed by the International Gastric Cancer Association separates gastric cancers into type I, type II and type III, to represent the tumours at distal oesophagus, at cardia and at the stomach distal to cardia, respectively. This is the classification used by surgeons. The 7th Edition of the TNM classification by the American Joint Committee on Cancer (AJCC) has simplified the classification of proximal gastric cancer based on the location of tumour epicentre and the presence or absence of GEJ involvement [5]. The tumour is to be stage grouped as oesophageal carcinoma if its epicentre is in the lower thoracic oesophagus or GEJ, or within the proximal 5 cm of stomach (*i.e.*, cardia) with the tumour mass extending into GEJ or distal oesophagus. If the epicentre is >5 cm distal to the GEJ, or within 5 cm of GEJ but does not extend into GEJ or oesophagus, it is stage grouped as gastric carcinoma. Pathologists have adopted this scheme (Fig. **2**). Some surgeons and oncologists have found this classification controversial although it was based on a consensus of Eastern and Western clinical opinion [6]. There is momentum in the clinical community to reclassify different types of OGJ tumours as oesophageal or *gastric* cancers (depending on the epicentre of the tumour) in the 8th edition of the AJCC staging manual but this remains uncertain. There is consensus at least amongst surgeons to continue adoption of the Siewert Classification. Siewert type I tumours are treated like oesophageal cancer and Siewert type III cancers are treated like gastric cancers. The main controversy remains focused on how to treat true adenocarcinomas of the GOJ (Siewert type II tumours).

Siewert *et al.* proposed a very pragmatic classification system for GOJ tumours based purely on their topographic anatomy and the location of the epicentre of the tumour (Fig. **2**). Adenocarcinoma of the GOJ was defined as a tumour whose epicentre was within 5 cm above or below the oesophagogastric junction [7]. A Siewert type I tumour was defined as an adenocarcinoma of the distal oesophagus in which the epicentre of the tumour was located 1-5 cm above the OGJ and which typically arises from an area of intestinal metaplasia of the oesophagus (*i.e.*, Barrett oesophagus). A Siewert type II tumour was defined as a true carcinoma of the cardia arising immediately at the OGJ (tumour epicentre located from 1 cm above to 2 cm below the OGJ). Lastly, a Siewert type III tumour was defined as a sub-cardial gastric carcinoma that infiltrates the OGJ and/or distal oesophagus from below (tumour epicentre located 2–5 cm below the OGJ) [8].

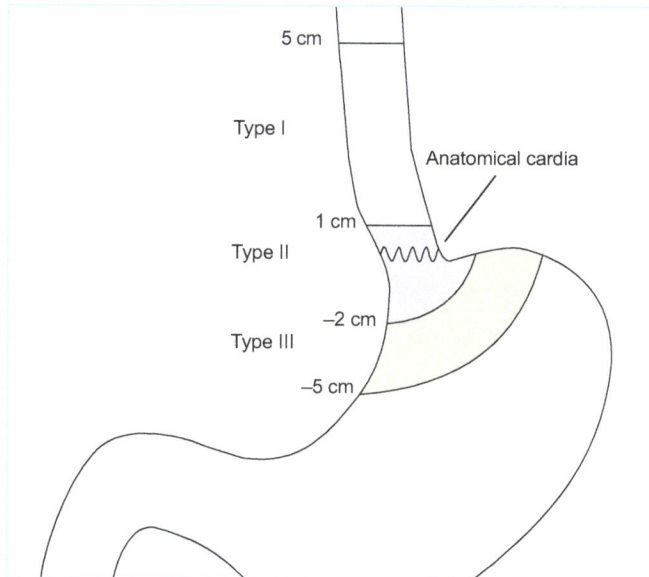

Fig. (2). Classification of tumours arising at the oesophago-gastric Junction (OGJ) [7].

Many surgeons have continued to use this classification system to select the surgical approach for adenocarcinomas of the OGJ, typically treating type I tumours as oesophageal cancers and type III tumours as gastric cancers. This is based on tumour biology, the frequency and distribution of nodal metastasis and the location and pattern of recurrence. The difficulty remains in selecting the appropriate surgical approach for Type II tumours. With uncertainty about the optimal extent of prophylactic lymph node dissection for this tumour, both subtotal oesophagectomy and extended total gastrectomy have been advocated. The former is favourable in terms of guaranteeing the proximal resection margin, while the latter focuses on the complete clearance of abdominal lymph nodes much more than mediastinal dissection. These two procedures are extremely different in terms of the surgical approach, extent of resection, and, more importantly, the type of reconstruction. Therefore, mortality, morbidity and quality of life after surgery are deemed to not be equivalent. Since the survival rate based on the extents of resection are comparable, conclusive evidence as to which procedure should be recommended is currently lacking. One pragmatic approach is to consider type II tumours as oesophageal as per AJCC staging manual 7th edition.

Various methods of pathological classifications exist for stomach cancer, including microscopic, macroscopic, biological behaviour, lesion depth and TNM classification. The gross appearance of advanced gastric carcinomas can be exophytic, ulcerated, infiltrative or combined. Based on Borrmann's classification, the gross appearance of advanced gastric carcinomas can be divided into type I for polypoid growth, type II for fungating growth, type III for ulcerating growth, and type IV for diffusely infiltrating growth which is also referred to as linitis plastica in signet ring cell carcinoma when most of gastric wall is involved by infiltrating tumour cells (Table **7**) [9].

Table 7. Morphological Classification of Gastric Cancer [9].

Type 0	Superficial polypoid, flat/depressed, or excavated tumours	EGC
Type 1	Polypoid carcinomas, usually attached on a wide base	AGC
Type 2	Ulcerated carcinomas with sharply demarcated and raised margins	
Type 3	Ulcerated, infiltrating carcinomas without definite limits	
Type 4	Non-ulcerated, diffusely infiltrating carcinomas	
Type 5	Unclassifiable advanced carcinomas	

Histology

Gastric carcinoma demonstrates marked heterogeneity at both architectural and cytological level, often with co-existence of several histologic elements. Several histological classifications have been used.

Over the past half century the histologic classification of gastric carcinoma has been largely based on Lauren's criteria, in which intestinal type and diffuse type adenocarcinoma are the two major histologic subtypes, plus an indeterminate type as an uncommon variant [10]. The relative frequencies are approximately 54% for intestinal type, 32% for the diffuse type, and 15% for the indeterminate type. There are indications that the diffuse type gastric carcinoma is more often seen in female and young individuals while the intestinal type adenocarcinoma is more often associated with intestinal metaplasia and *Helicobacter pylori* infection.

The 2010 the World Health Organisation (WHO) classification recognizes four major histologic patterns of gastric cancers: tubular, papillary, mucinous and poorly cohesive (including signet ring cell carcinoma), plus uncommon histologic variants [11]. The classification is based on the predominant histologic pattern of the carcinoma which often co-exists with less dominant elements of other histologic patterns. In addition to the above four major histologic subtypes, WHO classification also endorses other uncommon histologic variants, such as adenosquamous carcinoma, squamous carcinoma, hepatoid adenocarcinoma, carcinoma with lymphoid stroma, choriocarcinoma, parietal cell carcinoma, malignant rhabdoid tumour, mucoepidermoid carcinoma, Paneth cell carcinoma, undifferentiated carcinoma, mixed adeno-neuroendocrine carcinoma, endodermal sinus tumour, embryonic carcinoma, pure gastric yolk sac tumour and oncocytic adenocarcinoma [12].

Gastric carcinoma with lymphoid stroma (medullary carcinoma) is one of the uncommon subtypes. It occurs more commonly in the proximal stomach and generally follows a less aggressive clinical course. Histologically, this type of carcinoma is characterized by a sharply demarcated advancing margins composed of irregular nests or sheets of polygonal tumour cells associated with a prominent lymphoid infiltrate in a non-desmoplastic stroma.

Micro papillary carcinoma of stomach is a newly recognized histologic variant characterized by small papillary clusters of tumour cells without a distinct fibrovascular core. The micro papillary features are often noted in the deep advancing edge of the tumour, surrounded by an empty space mimicking retraction artefact. Micro papillary carcinoma of stomach, as its counterpart at other organs, tends to form endolymphatic tumour emboli and metastasize to lymph nodes. Because of the high incidence of lymphatic invasion and nodal metastasis (up to 82%), endoscopic resection should not be used for gastric carcinoma with invasive micro papillary components.

Spread of Gastric Cancer

In striving to achieve a surgical cure for gastric cancer it is essential to understand the modes of spread of gastric cancer. The metastatic pathways include direct extension into neighbouring organs, lymphatic spread *via* subserosal and submucosal lymphatic plexuses depending on the depth of invasion, peritoneal (transcoelomic) spread, and haematogenous spread primarily to the liver *via* the portal drainage system but subsequently to other organs.

Direct Extension

The diffuse type of gastric cancer spreads by direct extension through the submucosal and subserosal lymphatic plexuses to penetrate the gastric wall rapidly. The intestinal type, remains localized for a relatively longer period and disseminates less readily. Once a lesion has extended beyond the gastric wall, a multitude of organs and structures can be involved, dependent on lesion location within the stomach. For proximal lesions, organs or structures that may be involved with superior or anterior extra gastric extension include the left diaphragm, anterior abdominal wall, or unusually the under surface of the liver, while with posterior extension, the coeliac artery, body of pancreas (anterior, superior), aorta, or diaphragmatic crura may be involved. For body of stomach lesions, anterior extension may involve the anterior abdominal wall or liver; lateral extension-the gastrosplenic ligament or spleen; posterior extension-the pancreas (tail, body); superior extension-the gastrohepatic ligament or lesser omentum; and inferior extension--the transverse colon or mesocolon, or greater omentum. With distal gastric lesions, posterior extension may involve the head of pancreas or porta hepatis structures; inferior extension-the transverse mesocolon and colon.

Lymphatic Spread

This occurs *via* subserosal and submucosal lymphatic plexuses depending on the depth of invasion. The lymphatic drainage of the stomach follows the arterial supply. Spread to recognized lymph node stations is dependent on the anatomical site of the primary tumour in the stomach (Fig. **3**). Although most lymphatics ultimately drain into the celiac nodal area, lymph drainage sites can include the splenic hilum, suprapancreatic nodal groups, porta hepatis, and gastroduodenal areas. Abundant lymphatic channels are present within both the submucosal and subserosal layers of the gastric wall. Microscopic or subclinical spread well beyond the visible gross lesion, occurs *via* these lymphatic channels (intramural spread), and gives a misleading impression of the margins. The submucosal lymphatic plexus is also prominent in the oesophagus and the subserosal plexus in the duodenum, allowing both proximal and distal intramural tumour spread. Although a so-called "duodenal block" occurs with the mucosa scarcely ever being involved for more than 1-2 mm beyond the pylorus, the existence of a prominent subserosal plexus allows distal spread in as high as 30% to 40% of patients. In the stomach, as in other organs, the very presence of cancer can alter the normal lymphatic drainage. Obstructed vessels can divert the drainage so that metastases appear in unexpected nodes. Collateral lymphatics can form, producing a shift in the drainage pattern.

Peritoneal Spread

Because stomach is a peritoneal organ once the tumour cells have extended beyond the stomach wall to the serosal surface peritoneal (transcoelomic) spread may happen. Peritoneal spread may initially be a localized process confined to the surrounding ligaments. This appears as haziness of the surrounding fatty structures on CT scans. Subsequently, overt peritoneal spread is evident with multiple tumour nodules throughout the peritoneal cavity as well as in the pelvis (Krukenberg tumour). In the initial stages some of these nodules may not be demonstrable on CT imaging.

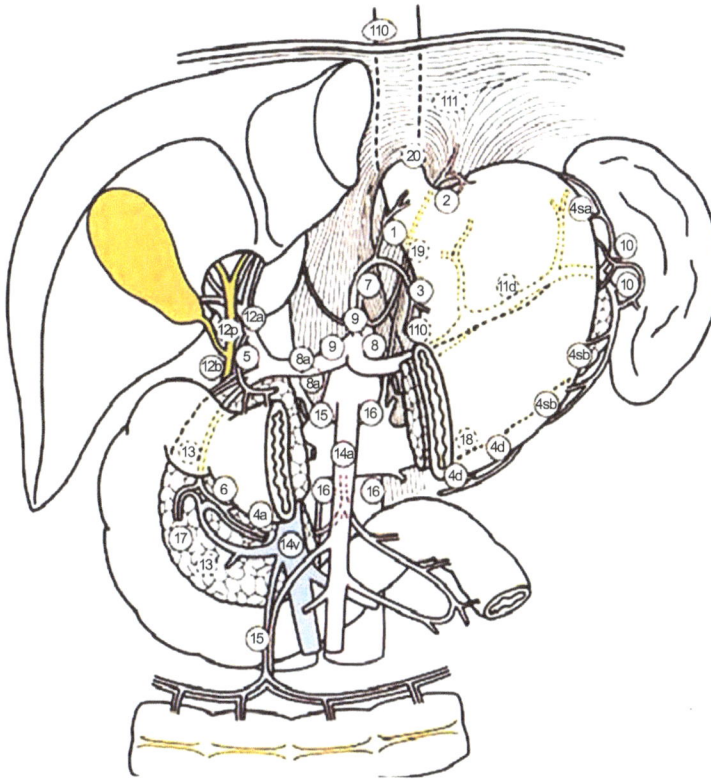

Fig. (3). Lymph node stations around the stomach.

Haematogenous Spread

For gastric cancer confined to the stomach the venous drainage is to the liver, which proves an effective filter. As the neoplasm invades beyond the stomach wall into adjacent organs, haematogenous spread through the lymphatics and venous system of the involved organs occurs and metastasis to other organs manifest.

Early Gastric Cancer

Early gastric carcinoma (EGC) is defined as invasive carcinoma confined to mucosa and/or submucosa, irrespective of the presence or absence of lymph node metastasis. Most early gastric carcinomas are small, measuring up to 5 cm in size, and often located at the lesser curvature around the incisura angularis. It accounts for around 5% of newly diagnosed gastric cancer in the West but can be up to 40% of newly diagnosed gastric cancer in high prevalence countries, which have screening programs. The prognosis of EGC is excellent with a 5-year survival rate of over 90%.

Two major factors associated with the prognosis of patients with early gastric cancer are the depth of wall invasion and status of lymph node metastasis with the latter being the more important. Although the depth of wall invasion (mucosa *vs.* submucosa) is associated with survival, it is not an independent prognostic factor.

According to the PARIS classification of superficial (type 0) neoplastic lesions in the digestive tract (Table **7**), type 0 is divided into three categories corresponding to protruding lesions (0-I), non-protruding and non-excavated lesions (0-II), and excavated lesions (0-III). Type 0-I is subdivided into pedunculated (0-Ip) and sessile (0-Is) lesions. Type 0-II is divided into three subtypes, a, b, and c, corresponding to slightly elevated, flat, and depressed lesions. Type 0-III is all ulcer. Mixed patterns with elevation and depression also occur (Fig. **4**). The combined patterns of excavation and depression are termed 0-III+IIc or 0-IIc+III, depending on the respective surface of the ulcer and of the depressed area. The highest risk of invasion is seen in protruding (0-I) or depressed (0-IIc) lesions. When the invasion is less than the cut-off limit of 500 μm, the proportion of involved lymph nodes is around 5%; beyond this limit the proportion increases to around 20%. The distinction between intramucosal carcinoma and carcinoma *in situ* or high-grade dysplasia is important, as the intramucosal carcinoma of stomach, unlike the intramucosal carcinoma in the colon, does metastasize.

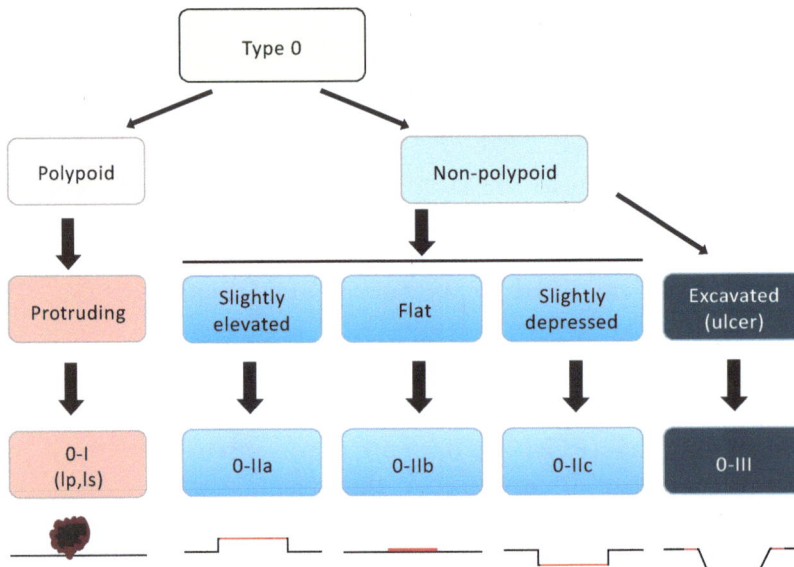

Fig. (4). Superficial neoplastic lesions in the upper digestive tract (Paris Classification).

Endoscopic Diagnosis

Unlike advanced cancer, which is easy to detect endoscopically, early gastric cancer often appears as subtle changes in the mucosal surface. To avoid missing the presence of cancer on endoscopy, the characteristics of early stage disease must be well understood and gastric observation must be thorough and detailed. The diagnosis is usually based on conventional white light endoscopy findings. However, the use of dye-based image-enhanced endoscopy (chromoendoscopy), equipment-based image-enhanced endoscopy (narrow band imaging—NBI), and endoscopic ultrasonography (EUS) can contribute to improved diagnostic capabilities for early gastric cancer.

White Light Endoscopy

Accurate diagnosis of early gastric cancer relies on having a good grasp of the characteristics of early stage disease. It is important to pay attention to points such as slight colour changes in the mucosa (pale redness or fading of colour), loss of visibility of underlying submucosal vessels, thinning of and interruptions in mucosal folds, and spontaneous bleeding. These findings are often subtle and require meticulous observation and verification skills. When a lesion is observed, the endoscopist should make a comprehensive diagnostic judgment considering mural thickness and hardness, colour, fold concentration, depression depth, and protrusion length. The accuracy of conventional endoscopy to discriminate between intramucosal carcinoma and submucosal carcinoma is reported to be 72%–84%. When subtle mucosal changes such as those described are observed, detailed observation using chemoendoscopy or NBI is an effective aid to diagnosis. In order to quantify the depth of invasion, endoscopic ultrasound is essential.

Chromoendoscopy

This is a dye-based image-enhanced endoscopy. Typically, 0.1% indigo carmine is sprayed directly *via* the forceps channel. Early gastric cancer is diagnosed through comparison with the surrounding mucosa. This method highlights subtle differences in elevation of the mucosal surface and changes in the surface structure and colour and helps to improve qualitative diagnosis and diagnosis of the extent of invasion.

Narrow Band Imaging

NBI is a common type of equipment-based image-enhanced endoscopy that enhances the superficial surface structure and vascular architecture of the mucous layer by illuminating blue and green narrowband lights. Magnified endoscopy with NBI makes it possible to observe micro vascular and micro surface patterns on the gastric mucosa in detail to discriminate between small gastric cancer and benign abnormalities (*e.g.*, gastritis) accurately in many cases. In addition, the utility of NBI magnification helps in margin determination prior to endoscopic therapy.

However, NBI is not suitable for identifying lesions within the stomach. Furthermore, while it is very useful for margin determination with differentiated cancers, it has only limited utility with undifferentiated cancers.

Endoscopic Ultrasonography

With more endoscopic procedures being performed for early gastric cancer, it has become necessary to determine preoperative invasion depth more accurately. Although conventional endoscopic observation has an accuracy of around 80%, diagnosing invasion depth can be difficult in many cases. Furthermore, as such diagnosis with conventional endoscopic observation is subjective, EUS can be used to make a more objective diagnosis. Normally, the main objective of EUS for early gastric cancer is to determine whether the patient can undergo endoscopic therapy, and small diameter lesions are often targeted. Therefore, while the procedure is more often conducted using 20 MHz catheter-based miniprobes than with the 12 MHz catheter-based miniprobes, the latter are concomitantly used for large type 0-I lesions. The accuracy of depth diagnosis is reported to be 65%–86% and can reach 92% when normal endoscopic findings correspond to EUS findings. However, these diagnostic capabilities drop for depressed lesions, undifferentiated cancers, cases accompanied by ulcers, cases of minute submucosal invasion, type 0-I lesions, and lesions located in the upper-third of the stomach. Accordingly, when it is difficult to diagnose lesion depth even with the combined use of EUS, endoscopic therapy can be conducted if there are no findings suggesting deep submucosal invasion. Apart from the utility of EUS for diagnosing invasion depth, EUS can be used preoperatively to assess the submucosal vasculature in order to predict intraoperative bleeding during endoscopic therapy.

Management of Early Gastric Cancer

Endoscopic mucosal resection or surgery, are the standard treatment options for Tis, T1 early gastric cancer. No further treatment is necessary if there is no residual or nodal disease [13].

Endoscopic Therapy

The frequency of lymph node metastasis, which accompanies early gastric cancer, is 3% for intramucosal carcinoma and 20% for submucosal carcinoma. Hence, a favourable prognosis can be expected for early gastric cancer with the standard therapy of gastric resection with lymph node dissection. However, endoscopic therapy for these early cases has significant advantages over surgery, as it is minimally invasive and preserves post-operative gastric function. Given that endoscopic therapy involves local excision and is not accompanied by lymph node dissection, the indications for endoscopic therapy need to be strictly limited to lesions where lymph node metastasis can be negligible.

Various methods of endoscopic mucosal resection (EMR) have been developed, and are widely used. Lesions with an extremely low likelihood of lymph node metastasis have been identified and compiled by the Japan Gastric Cancer Association. Broadly, the tumour should be of a size and in a site that allows it to undergo en bloc resection and the likelihood of lymph node metastasis is extremely low. Specifically, the lesion must be (1) a differentiated, elevated intramucosal cancer less than 2 cm in size or (2) a differentiated, depressed intramucosal cancer less than 1 cm in size without ulceration (Table **8**). However, due to the nature of the excision technique, which uses a snare, EMR also has the disadvantage that only a small area can be excised at a time. By contrast, endoscopic submucosal dissection (ESD) enables en bloc resection of larger lesions, with accompanying ulcer scarring, and those recurring after EMR because it involves dissecting along the submucosal layer directly [14]. As such, additional indications for ESD have been stipulated (Table **9**).

Table 8. Criteria for endoscopic mucosal resection (EMR) for early gastric carcinoma [14].

1	Differentiated intramucosal cancers without ulcer findings, irrespective of tumour size.
2	Differentiated intramucosal cancers less than 3 cm in size with ulcer findings
3	Differentiated minute invasive submucosal (less than 500 μm below the muscularis mucosa) cancers less than 3 cm in size.
4	Undifferentiated intramucosal cancers less than 2 cm in size without ulcer findings.

Although ESD is said to cause more complications than EMR, most instances of perforation or bleeding complications can be treated with endoscopy, and the risk for life-threatening complications is very low. The continuing modifications of endoscopic therapy devices and techniques have encouraged the widespread adoption of this utility globally.

The incidence of lymph node metastasis is one of the most important factors in determining the prognosis of patients with EGC. Long-term results after EMR and ESD are favourable, with both the 5- and 10-year survival rates over 90% with a low risk of local recurrence provided that complete excision is achieved. Patients should be advised to have annual endoscopic monitoring to detect metachronous cancers (3-year cumulative incidence rate of 5.9%) and recurrence. In addition, patients should be advised to have half-yearly abdominal computed tomography (CT) or endoscopic ultrasonography, for at least 3 years in order to detect lymph node or distant metastasis. If the pathological examination indicates non-curative resection, additional surgery including lymph node dissection should be strongly recommended.

Table 9. Criteria and extended criteria for endoscopic resection therapy for early gastric cancer [15].

Criteria
1. High probability of en bloc resection
2. Tumour histology: a. Intestinal type adenocarcinoma   b. Tumour confined to the mucosa   c. Absence of venous or lymphatic invasion
3. Tumour size and morphology: a. Less than 20 mm in diameter, without ulceration   b. Less than 10 mm in diameter if Paris classification IIb or IIc
(Extended Criteria)
4. Mucosal tumours of any size without ulceration
5. Mucosal tumours less than 30 mm with ulceration
6. Submucosal tumours less than 30 mm confined to the upper 0.5 mm of the submucosa without lymphovascular invasion

Although the number of early gastric cancer lesions in the West is relatively small, increased public awareness and diagnostic facilities are likely to increase the numbers. Lesions in the gastric fundus or greater curvature of the gastric corpus or lesions with severe ulcer scarring can be technically difficult for ESD. These lesions can be managed by conventional radical surgery or laparoscopy-assisted full-thickness resection of the stomach.

Surgical Management of EGC

Subtotal or total gastrectomy with regional lymphadenectomy is the standard surgical treatment for early stage gastric cancer with lymph node metastases. Less invasive gastrectomy with limited lymphadenectomy, such as pylorus-preserving gastrectomy and proximal gastrectomy, has been proposed for more advanced stages of EGC that has a low possibility of nodal metastasis and a high probability of cure.

Laparoscopic-assisted gastrectomy (LAG) has been used to treat EGC, which requires less extensive lymph node dissection. The use of LAG for EGC confers the benefits of less invasive surgery including reduced blood loss, decreased pain, early recovery of bowel movements, and a short hospital stay. Oncologically, it is equivalent to open gastrectomy but the technique does involve a steep surgical learning curve.

Advanced Gastric Cancer

In the majority of patients (more than 90%) particularly in the West, gastric cancer is diagnosed at a later stage than the first stage of the disease, with classic symptoms of weight loss, consistent and dull pain in the epigastrium, loss of appetite, nausea, vomiting and chronic bleeding. There is heterogeneity in the definition of AGC in the literature. The term 'advanced' encompasses resectable advanced stage (beyond the defined EGC), unresectable M0 and M1 cancers. Another term, which is frequently used in the literature, is 'locally advanced' gastric cancer presumably as distinct from 'metastatic' gastric cancer. According to the anatomical definition, the term implies a tumour without distant metastases which exceeds the anatomical boundaries of the stomach, that is, with, at least, serosal or lymph node involvement. However, this term also lacks rigor in the sense that patients with serosal disease have a different prognosis and response to treatment in comparison with patients with positive lymph nodes.

When analysing the literature, it must be recognised that the term 'advanced gastric cancer' includes a number of stages of the disease. In order to standardise the results and survival outcome for different therapeutic modalities, there has to be clarity on the stage of gastric cancer used for each treatment and uniformity in the comparisons made. The classification determined by lesion depth remains extremely important as it has been shown to correlate with patient prognosis.

Gastric cancer can be classified histologically into various types. Signet ring cell carcinoma is a distinct histological type with cells containing abundant intracytoplasmic mucin. It has been reported that 3.4% to 29% of gastric cancers are signet ring cell carcinomas. Although some studies have reported on the clinicopathological features and prognosis of signet ring cell carcinoma of the stomach, results have been inconsistent, but patients with SRC tend to present with a more advanced stage and poorer prognosis than patients with other types of gastric carcinoma.

Management of Advanced Gastric Cancer

Radical resection of the stomach and presumed areas of lymphatic drainage has been advocated as the definitive surgical treatment of advanced and lymph node positive early gastric cancer. There is controversy over the extent of lymphadenectomy. Theoretically, the removal of a wider range of lymph nodes which "may" harbour micro metastases by an extended lymphadenectomy increases the chances for cure / survival. Japanese surgeons assert that the extended lymphadenectomy (D2) removes all tumour deposits in the regional lymph nodes before they manifest as metastases. In addition, they stress that an extended lymphadenectomy improves staging accuracy. Western surgeons on the other hand, have found that the perceived benefits of an extended lymphadenectomy were overshadowed by a high complication rate in Western patients. The pattern of recurrence after extended surgery is completely different from that after limited surgery and mainly involves loco regional recurrence in the majority of cases. An extended lymphadenectomy might reduce the loco regional recurrence rate. However, if patients have already developed distant micro metastases at one extreme or if the lymph nodes are not involved at the other extreme, such extended resection might be harmful without altering the patient's survival benefit. It is unlikely that this controversy would be resolved until advances in imaging modalities improve the accuracy of gastric cancer staging. In the interim, surgeons would have to evaluate each case individually for tolerance of an extended lymphadenectomy provided that they have the technical expertise of extended lymphadenectomy. Studies estimate that lymph nodes will be involved with tumours in 3–5% of cases of gastric adenocarcinoma limited to the mucosa; 11–25% of cases for those limited to the sub-mucosa; 50% for T2; and 83% for T3 tumours. Lymph node dissemination is in an orderly fashion through lymphatic channels in gastric cancer. The Union Internationale Contrale Cancer (UICC)/American Joint Committee on Cancer (AJCC) classification, which is most widely used for the staging of gastric cancer, suggests that at least 15 lymph nodes should be examined for a correct assessment of N staging.

For medically fit patients, the recommended treatment for operable gastric cancers beyond stage T1N0 is surgery with both preoperative and postoperative chemotherapy. Radical gastrectomy with D2 lymph node dissection is indicated for resectable stage IB–III disease, although subtotal gastrectomy may be performed if a macroscopic proximal margin of 5 cm can be achieved between the tumour and the oesophagogastric junction (8 cm for diffuse-type cancers).

Extent of Resection

Similar to other organs cancer surgery, R0 resection indicates a microscopically margin-negative resection, in which no gross or microscopic tumour remains in the primary tumour bed. R1 resection indicates the removal of all macroscopic disease but microscopic margins are positive for tumours. R2 indicates gross residual disease with gross residual tumour that was not resected (primary tumour, regional nodes and macroscopic margin involvement). For gastric cancer, all surgeons should aim for an R0 resection in every patient. However, given the pattern of spread of gastric cancer, and the debate surrounding the extent of lymphadenectomy, a minority of resections can turn out to be R1 resections. However, an R2 resection is inexcusable.

Lymphadenectomy

The Japanese Research Society for the study of gastric cancer published a manual in 1963 standardizing lymph node dissection and pathologic evaluations for GC. The revised classification recognized 23 different lymph node stations that surround the stomach (Fig. **5**) (Table **10**). These 16 nodal stations are grouped according to the location and extension of the primary tumour (N0-N4) and the extent of lymphadenectomy is classified according the level of lymph node dissection - LND (D1-D4). In D1 dissections, only the perigastric nodes directly attached along the lesser curvature and greater curvatures of the stomach are removed (stations 1-6, N1 level). An incomplete N1 dissection is labelled a D0 lymphadenectomy [16]. D2 dissections (N2 level) add the removal of nodes along the left gastric artery (station 7), common hepatic artery (station 8), celiac trunk (station 9), splenic hilum, and splenic artery (station 10 and 11). D3 dissections include the dissection of lymph nodes at stations 12 through 14, along the hepatoduodenal ligament and the root of the mesentery (N3 level). Finally, D4 resections add the stations 15 and 16 in the para-aortic and the para-colic region (N4 level). The incidence of metastasis to any perigastric station is highest when the tumour location is close to it. There is little variation in the metastatic pattern along the lesser curvature between tumours of different thirds. For tumours of the antrum, right para-cardiac lymph nodes are staged as second tier while left para-cardiac lymph nodes are N3. For tumours of cardia, the 5th and 6th lymph node stations are in the second tier.

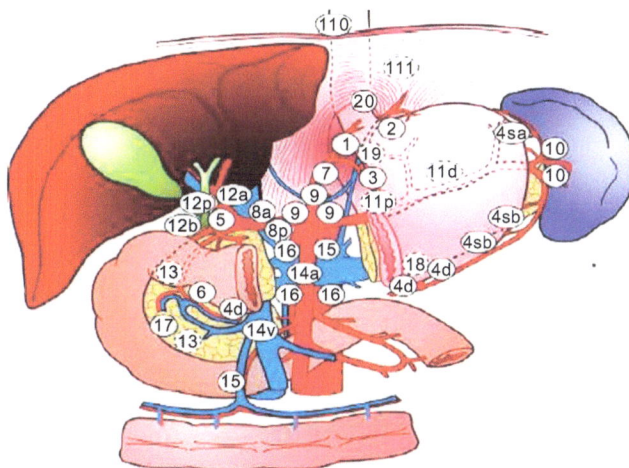

Fig. (5). Lymph node tiers around the stomach.

A number of investigators have observed a progressive decrease in survival with the increasing number of lymph nodes involved, with an apparent drop off in survival when 3 or more nodes are involved. Another drop off have been reported when more than 6 nodes are involved. Involvement beyond 15 or 16 nodes is thought to be largely incompatible with long-term survival. As a prognostic tool, the ratio between metastatic lymph nodes and the total number of lymph nodes examined was proposed. Several cut-offs were studied increasing in pentatonic or decimal scale starting from zero to mostly >30%; the survival decreases as the involved lymph node ratio increases. This scheme may also be useful for patients who had lower than 15 lymph nodes dissected [17].

Table 10. The regional lymph nodes of the stomach [16].

Station	Lymph Nodes	Station	Lymph Nodes
1	Right para-cardial	2	Left para-cardial
3	Along the lesser curvature	4sa	Along the short gastric vessels
4sb	Along the left gastroepiploic vessels	4d	Along the right gastroepiploic vessels
5	Supra-pyloric	6	Infra-pyloric
7	Along the left gastric artery	8a	Along the common hepatic artery (Anterosuperior group)
8p	Along the common hepatic artery (Posterior group)	9	Around the celiac artery
10	At the splenic hilum	11p	Along the proximal splenic artery
11d	Along the distal splenic artery	12a	In the hepatoduodenal ligament (along the hepatic artery)
12b	In the hepatoduodenal ligament (along the bile duct)	12p	In the hepatoduodenal ligament (behind the portal vein)
13	On the posterior surface of the pancreatic head	14v	Along the superior mesenteric vein
14a	Along the superior mesenteric artery	15	Along the middle colic vessels
16a1	In the aortic hiatus	16a2	Around the abdominal aorta (from the upper margin of the celiac trunk to the lower margin of the left renal vein)
16b1	Around the abdominal aorta (from the lower margin of the left renal vein to the upper margin of the inferior mesenteric artery)	16b2	Around the abdominal aorta (from the upper margin of the inferior mesenteric artery to the aortic bifurcation)
17	On the anterior surface of the pancreatic head	18	Along the inferior margin of the pancreas
19	Infra-diaphragmatic	20	In the oesophageal hiatus of the diaphragm
110	Para-oesophageal (in the lower thorax)	111	Supra-diaphragmatic
112	Posterior mediastinal		

D1 and D2 dissection have been defined by guidelines of the Japanese Research Society for the Study of Gastric Cancer, which have also been recommended by the American Joint Committee on Cancer. In these guidelines, 16 different lymph node stations are identified surrounding the stomach. Broadly, the perigastric lymph node stations along the lesser (stations 1, 3, and 5) and greater (stations 2, 4, and 6) curvature are grouped N1, whereas the nodes along the left gastric (station 7), common hepatic (station 8), celiac (station 9), and splenic (stations 10 and 11) arteries are grouped N2.

D1 dissection entails removal of the involved part of the stomach (distal or total), including the greater and lesser omentum. The spleen and pancreas tail are only resected when necessitated by tumour invasion. For a D2 dissection, the omental bursa is removed with the front leaf of the transverse mesocolon, and the vascular pedicles of the stomach are cleared completely. Standard resection of the spleen and pancreatic tail can be done only in proximal tumours to achieve adequate removal of D2 lymph node stations 10 and 11.

Reconstruction after Gastric Resection

Various reconstructive procedures have been proposed for patients undergoing distal gastrectomy for gastric cancer (Fig. **6**) [18]. In general, Billroth I (BI) reconstruction was the most common technique used clinically because it involves relatively simple reconstruction. However, bile reflux resulting in remnant gastritis and gastroesophageal reflux disease (GERD) has been noted as a problem associated with BI reconstruction after distal gastrectomy. Billroth II is also a simple reconstruction technique but like BI results in biliary gastritis. This could be improved by adding an entero-enterostomy creating an Omega loop reconstruction. Roux-en-Y (RY) reconstruction following distal gastrectomy is superior to BI reconstruction in preventing remnant gastritis and reflux esophagitis because it reduces duodeno-gastric and gastroesophageal reflux. The disadvantages of RY reconstruction include the possible development of stomal ulcers, increased probability of cholelithiasis, increased difficulty with an endoscopic approach to the papilla of Vater, and the possibility of Roux stasis syndrome. Furthermore, in the RY reconstruction all food passes through the jejunum and bypasses the duodenum, which causes one of the disadvantages of this procedure. J pouch reconstruction is popular after gastrectomy because it was found to improve early postoperative eating capacity, bodyweight and quality of life. Recently, double tract reconstruction (DT) after either total or subtotal gastrectomy has been introduced to remove the disadvantage of RY reconstruction. DT reconstruction is as simple as RY reconstruction and can be performed safely after distal gastrectomy with regional lymphadenectomy. The advantages of DT reconstruction following both total and distal gastrectomy include maintaining the physiological passage of food and allowing future diagnostic and therapeutic endoscopic interventions to be safely performed.

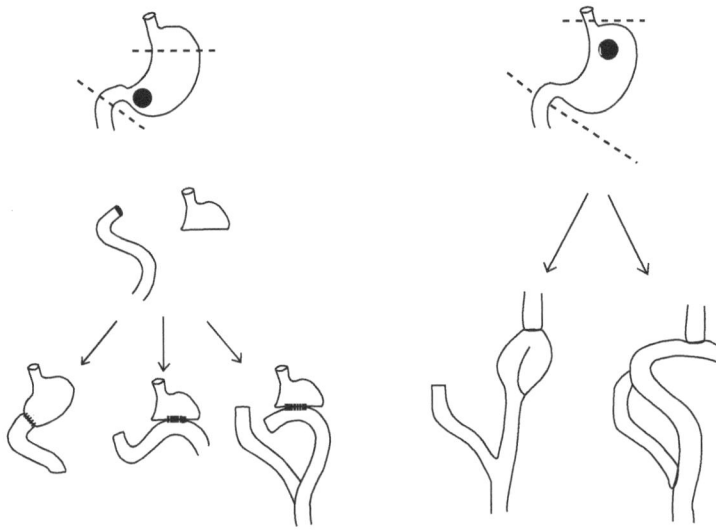

Fig. (6). Resection and reconstruction options for distal and proximal gastric cancers.

Gastrectomy

In Japan, D2 dissection was introduced in the 1960's and gastrectomy with D2 lymph node dissection has been regarded as a safe surgical procedure and performed regularly in most hospitals. However, whether D2 LN dissection in radical gastrectomy should be routinely performed is still unclear in the Western world. Most Western surgeons perform gastrectomy with only D1 dissection, because D1 was associated with less mortality and morbidity than D2 in prospective randomized trials preformed in the Netherland and the UK concluded that there was no survival benefit for D2 over D1 lymph node dissection [19]. With evolving experience in extensive lymphadenectomy, and better selection of patients, D2 gastrectomy is becoming accepted as a safe treatment for gastric cancer in high-volume centres, in western countries. Currently in the West, the choice of D1 *vs* D2 gastrectomy depends on the centre's experience, volume and the results of morbidity, mortality and survival.

According to Japanese Gastric Cancer Association (JAGA) classification, lymph nodes surrounding the stomach are divided into 20 stations and these are classified into three groups depending upon the location of the primary tumour. The grouping is based on the results of studies of lymphatic flow at various tumour sites, and observed survival associated with metastasis to each nodal station. (Recent publications from JAGA have matched these groups to the standard TNM classification of UICC). In this grouping system, the most perigastric LNs (stations nos. 1-6) are defined as group 1, whereas the nodes along the left gastric artery (station no. 7), common hepatic artery (station no. 8), celiac axis (station no. 9), splenic artery (station no. 11) and proper hepatic artery (station no. 12) are defined as group 2.

D1 gastrectomy is defined as dissection of all the Group 1 nodes, and D2 is defined as dissection of all the Group 1 and Group 2 nodes. The selection of D1 or D2 dissection is influenced by the type of gastrectomy, *i.e.*, total gastrectomy or distal gastrectomy, not by the location of the primary tumour. It should be emphasised that D1 gastrectomy includes the dissection of the nodes along the left gastric (station no. 7) as well as the perigastric lymph nodes (stations nos. 1–6), regardless of the location of tumour. D2 gastrectomy adds LN stations 8,9,11 and 12. LNs along the superior mesenteric vein (station no. 14v) are eliminated from D2 dissection for tumour in the lower third of the stomach. In other words, D1 distal gastrectomy consists of LN dissection of station nos. 1, 3, 4sb, 4d, 5, 6, and 7 and D1 total gastrectomy includes station nos. 1-6 and 7.

In order to improve the prognosis of patients with advanced gastric cancer, gastrectomy with more radical extended lymphadenectomy (D3 and D4) have been performed in Japan, since 1980's at many specialized centres. The more extensive lymph node dissection increased the complication rate with a very modest improvement in survival. For patients with oesophageal invasion from gastric cancer of more than 3 cm, the survival is poor and dissection of the lower oesophagus and mediastinal lymphadenectomy increase morbidity without improving survival.

In Japan, pancreaticosplenectomy for LN dissection around the splenic artery (station no. 11) and splenic hilus (station no. 10) were widely performed. However, Japanese retrospective analyses showed that there was no survival benefit of these procedures. Recently, pancreas-preserving splenectomy has been considered a safe and alternative procedure without decreasing surgical curability. Pancreaticosplenectomy in Western countries had a marked adverse effect on both mortality and morbidity and is considered beneficial only when the primary tumour or metastatic LN directly invades the pancreas.

The Surgical Procedure

The following section describes the basic steps in a D2 total gastrectomy. It is intended as a guide and not a technical manual. There are many valid variations on many of the steps, which suit patient anatomy, tumour location, available equipment, individual preferences and experience. A D1 total gastrectomy would have similar steps but the nodal dissection is limited to the perigastric lymph nodes (stations 1-6) and the left gastric lymph node (station 7). In a partial (subtotal) gastrectomy, the proximal portion of the stomach is left attached to the oesophagus but all lymph node stations are dissected according to D1 or D2 intent with the exception of lymph nodes along the superior mesenteric vein (station no. 14v) being eliminated from D2 dissection for tumour in the lower third of the stomach.

Key Steps:

Access

- For open surgery, a transverse upper abdominal incision is ideal. However, depending on surgeon's preference, a midline upper abdominal incision can provide adequate access.
- For laparoscopic surgery, an infra-umbilical port should be used for the endoscope/ camera. A midline sub-xiphistrenal port should be used for a Nathanson liver retractor. Two ports on each side of the abdomen should be used for dissection and retraction.
- Adequate retraction facilities should retract the liver to expose the stomach from OGJ to pylorus.

Exploration

- The procedure should commence with abdominal exploration to ensure the absence of metastatic disease and to assess the surgical stage of the primary tumour and lymph nodes.
- A mechanical retractor should be used to achieve adequate surgical exposure.

Dissection

- The dissection should commence at the gastro-colic ligament by separating the omentum from the transverse colon and mesentery ensuring to dissect the inferior omental bursa layer from the transverse colon mesentry.
- This dissection is extended upwards until the pancreatic capsule was completely dissected to reach the upper edge of the pancreas. At this stage, 14a and 14v nodal stations should be dissected from the superior Mesenteric vein and the aortocaval area respectively.
- The right gastro-epiploic artery and vein are ligated and divided. Nodal stations 4d and 6 should be included in this dissection.
- The short gastric vessels (station 4sa) are divided, and the left gastroepiploic vessels (station 4sb) is divided. Lymph nodes of stations 11 and 10 were then

dissected along the splenic artery, vein and their branches.

- The splenorenal, phrenicosplenic and splenocolic ligaments are then dissected. The spleen is flipped and raised, enabling the dorsal tissues of the pancreas to be separated, and the pancreatic tail and spleen can be lifted to the wound. Lymph nodes along the upper edge and dorsal side of the pancreas can be dissected along the splenic artery. After that, the spleen and the pancreas should be replaced back in position without the need for fixation.
- A Kocher incision is made around the duodenum. The duodenum and the head of the pancreas are mobilized. Nodal station 12b should be included in this dissection.
- A plane should be established around the duodenum and a 60 mm dividing stapler should be used to close and divide the duodenum.
- The hepato-duodenal ligament is then dissected. The lymph nodes to be dissected from right to left of the patient.
- The hepato-gastric ligament (pars flaccida) is then divided and lymph nodes around the proper hepatic artery (station 12a) should be dissected until the portal vein is reached.
- The right gastric artery is then ligated and divided (station 5), and lymph nodes to the left and posterior side of the portal vein should be dissected (station 12p).
- The dissection should continue to the celiac trunk (station 9) along the common hepatic artery (station 8).
- The left gastric artery (station 7) and coronary vein should be ligated and divided at their origins.
- The lesser omentum is then divided close to the liver, and stations 3 and 1 at the lesser curvature side should be dissected.
- The phreno-oesophageal membrane should be divided; both vagus nerves are then divided, and lymph nodes (station 2) to the left of the cardia should be dissected.
- The lower 5 - 7 cm portion of abdominal oesophagus should be dissected free and divided above the oesophago-gastric junction. A purse string suture should be applied to the end and ligated around the anvil of a circular stapler.
- The stomach with attached lymph nodes should be removed and submitted for histology.
- The duodenal stump should be consolidated with additional sutures.

Reconstruction (Rou-en-Y with a Pouch)

- A loop of small intestine based on a vascular arcade is selected and divided using a linear stapler approximately 20 cm from the ligament of Treitz.
- The distal part of this loop is delivered to the supra-colic compartment through the transverse colon mesentry. A J pouch is constructed using linear staplers. The circular stapler (25 mm) is inserted through an enterotomy in the pouch and

the dome of the pouch is approximated to the oesophagus by uniting the circular stapler and the previously inserted anvil. The circular stapler is triggered and then removed. Additional serosal anchoring sutures may be required.

- A naso-jejunal tube should be inserted with its distal end positioned just below the J pouch.
- An end-to-side anastomosis is made between proximal intestine and the small intestine 50 cm below the previous oesophageal anastomosis using sero-muscular sutures.
- All anastomoses can be consolidated with absorbable interrupted suture if necessary. Defects in the small bowel mesentery will need to be closed using interrupted or continuous sutures.
- A feeding jejunostomy tube should be inserted percutaneously for post-operative feeding.
- Abdominal lavage and drainage should be established.
- The abdomen should be closed.

Post-operative Course

- The patient should be nursed in a high dependency unit with appropriate monitoring of vital parameters.
- The patient should be nursed without oral intake and all fluids and medication should be administered intravenously.
- Feeding *via* the feeding jejunostomy tube should commence after 24 hours and stepped up slowly over days.
- A water-soluble contrast swallow test should be arranged on day 5 post-operatively to check the integrity of the oesophago-jejunal anastomosis.
- Provided that the contrast swallow test shows no leakage, the naso-jejunal tube could be removed and the patient is given fluids to drink. The volume of fluid intake is stepped up gradually over 48 hours. At the end of this period, small amounts of semi-solid food could be introduced and if tolerated, substituted with more solid food.
- The patient should be ready for discharge home when sufficiently mobile and independent.
- Feeding *via* feeding jejunostomy could be continued nocturnally for three months after discharge.

Anticipated Complications

- Primary or secondary haemorrhage should necessitate either re-operation if the haemorrhage is profuse or angiographic imaging to determine the source and attempt radiological embolization if less profuse.
- Respiratory infection or compromise should necessitate antibiotics and pulmonary toilet by physiotherapy. Depending on the level of respiratory

compromise, additional measures may be necessary such as positive airway pressure (CPAP) or ventilation.

- Leakage from the anastomosis should necessitate antibiotics and antifungal agents, cessation of oral intake, drainage and considerations for sealing the anastomosis. This could be done conservatively with a monitoring policy until the anastomosis is healed. Alternatively, a self-expanding covered stent could be placed across the leaking anastomosis to provide a scaffold for healing.
- Pancreatitis could occur as a result of pancreatic injury during the dissection. Supportive measures should be instituted for all affected body systems until resolution of the inflammation. Repeated cross sectional imaging is necessary to monitor recovery or untoward further deterioration in the pancreas.
- Abscess formation can occur due to a surgical site infection and manifest in septic deterioration. The site and size of the abscess could be delineated by cross sectional imaging. Drainage of the septic collection either surgically or radiologically should lead to noticeable improvement.
- Multi-system organ failure can occur as a result of sepsis. Broad-spectrum antibiotics should be commenced and the source of sepsis should be identified by cross sectional imaging and managed. All affected body systems should be supported until discernible improvements are achieved.

Laparoscopic Gastrectomy

The key technical issues of laparoscopic surgery, for gastric cancer, center on lymph node dissection and reconstruction. When laparoscopic gastrectomy was first introduced, D1 lymph node dissection was performed because of the technical difficulties involved in systemic lymph node dissection. However, advances in laparoscopic instrumentation, such as an ultrasonic coagulating shears to seal blood vessels, have made feasible extended lymph node dissection that includes supra-pancreatic lymph nodes. The frequency of D2 lymph node dissection has gradually increased because of these advances. Laparoscopy-assisted surgery has been widely performed in reconstruction in which the intestine is pulled out of the body through a small laparotomy wound. Reconstructive methods have included, Billroth-I reconstruction, and Roux-en-Y reconstruction. Recently, pure laparoscopic surgery has also been used in which a series of procedures of lymphadenectomy, resection, and reconstruction is completely performed intra-abdominally. In addition, recent improvement in anastomosis devices and modifications in various anastomotic techniques have enabled oesophago-jejunostomy and anastomosis between the esophagus and remnant stomach. Laparoscopy-assisted proximal gastrectomy (LAPG) and laparoscopy-assisted total gastrectomy (LATG) have begun to be performed. In particular, the introduction of circular stapler with trans orally inserted anvil has enabled oesophago jejunostomy and esophagus-remnant stomach anastomosis.

These procedures closely approach conventional anastomosis by laparotomy.

The short- and long-term outcomes are similar if not better than open surgery. The 5-year disease-free survival rate is around 99.8% for stage IA disease, 98.7% for stage IB disease, and 85.7% for stage II disease. These therapeutic outcomes are at least non-inferior to those of conventional open surgery.

Oncological Management of Gastric Cancer

The high mortality rate in gastric cancer reflects the prevalence of advanced disease at presentation. In population-based series of Western populations, the five-year survival rate for patients with completely resected stage I gastric cancer is approximately 70 to 75 per cent, while it drops to 35 per cent or less for stage II disease and beyond. These results have spawned efforts to improve the treatment results for this group of patients using adjuvant (postoperative) or neoadjuvant (preoperative) therapies [20, 21].

The positive impact of such therapies on survival in patients with resected gastric cancer is becoming clearer over time, although there is no consensus as to the best approach. In many parts of the world, chemotherapy (either following surgery or combined pre-operative and post-operative administration) is the preferred treatment strategy [22]. On the other hand, a significant survival benefit for chemoradiotherapy after complete resection resulted in the adoption of this strategy in the United States.

Another controversial issue is the management of cancers arising at the oesophagogastric junction (OGJ). Classification and management of these tumours has evolved over time. In the latest edition of the TNM staging manual, tumours arising at the OGJ or in the cardia of the stomach within 5 cm of the OGJ that extend into the OGJ or oesophagus (the so-called Siewert III EGJ tumours) are staged and treated as oesophageal rather than stomach cancers. However, tumours that arise beyond 5 cm of the OGJ or are within 5 cm of the OGJ but without extension to the oesophagus or OGJ are still classified and treated as gastric cancers.

Palliation of Advanced Gastric Cancer

Unfortunately, many cases of gastric cancer are not diagnosed until late stages of the disease, which underscores the importance of the palliative treatment of gastric cancer. Palliative care is best defined as the active total care of patients whose disease is not responsive to curative treatment. The main indication for the institution of palliative care is the presence of advanced gastric cancer for which curative treatment is deemed inappropriate either due to patient or disease stage factors. The primary goal of palliative therapy of gastric cancer patients is to improve quality, not necessarily length, of life. Every case must be considered individually taking into account the patient's and carer's views. Four main modalities of palliative therapy for advanced gastric cancer are appropriate: resection, bypass, stenting, and chemotherapy. The choice of modality depends on a variety of factors, including individual patient prognosis and goals, and should be made on case-by-case basis.

A number of clinical trials have produced evidence that chemotherapy improves survival in comparison to best supportive care in selected patients. However, the impact on quality of life remains unclear. Although, a wide range of chemotherapeutic regimens, have been tested in clinical trials, most are 5-flurouracil (5-FU) based. The combination of epirubicin, cisplatin and 5-FU (the ECF regimen) is widely used but has not been accepted worldwide because of concerns for systemic toxicity. A number of new and less toxic agents particularly in the immunotherapy group are emerging with good results. A number of patients may require nutritional supplementation from the outset or during chemotherapy. These patients may benefit from stenting and or the insertion of a feeding jejunostomy either surgically or radiologically. In a number of patients with advanced gastric cancer, diffuse bleeding from the tumour surface can be troublesome and necessitates repeated blood transfusions. Treatment with a PPI and tranexamic acid can help reduce the rate of bleeding. Endoscopic argon plasma coagulation is also useful. In refractory patients, single-fraction radiotherapy is useful for the management of diffuse bleeding from gastric cancer.

For inoperable or metastatic gastric cancer, treatment is with palliative chemotherapy, or best supportive care if the patient is unfit for treatment. In HER-2 negative disease, combination regimens based upon a platinum–fluoropyrimidine doublet are generally used; triplet regimens are controversial, but the addition of an anthracycline (*e.g*, epirubicin) has demonstrated benefit. In HER-2 positive disease, recommended chemotherapy is with trastuzumab plus cisplatin and either 5-fluorouracil or capecitabine. Second-line chemotherapy options include irinotecan and docetaxel or paclitaxel.

Surgical Palliation

There is some evidence that gastric resection in the palliative setting can lead to a small survival benefit, but only in a highly selected group of patients. Young patients with a high performance status, lower tumour burden and a favourable histology can derive a favourable but small survival benefit especially if they were able to receive post-operative chemotherapy. The effect of such resection on quality of life remains unclear. Patients with disseminated peritoneal disease, bilobar liver metastases, and metastases in more than one organ are less likely to derive a survival benefit. Emergency surgery for bleeding, obstruction or perforation is associated with a shorter survival than operations done electively. In the setting of a palliative resection, the goal is to reduce tumour burden without an extensive dissection. In this setting, minimal or no lymph node dissection is acceptable.

Palliative Surgical Bypass

Gastric outlet obstruction is a troublesome complication of advanced distal gastric cancer. It results in troublesome persistent vomiting, dehydration and emaciation due to reduced oral intake. Traditionally, this has been treated with open gastrojejunostomy and more recently by laparoscopic gastroenterostomy. Endoscopic stenting is another alternative that should be considered. The decision of operative bypass versus endoscopic stenting should be made on a case-by-case basis taking into account each patient's life expectancy. Gastrojejunostomy is associated with good symptomatic relief and less need for re-intervention but is also associated with significant morbidity. The laparoscopic approach is an option, which provides the same benefit as open surgery but with less pain, earlier recovery and shorter hospital stay for a selected group of patients.

Stenting of Distal Gastric Cancer

Endoscopic stenting has become an attractive alternative that avoids the need for an abdominal procedure. The majority of patients can resume oral intake with minimal morbidity. Early complication rates are minimal in experienced centres. Late stent failure due to tumour ingrowth or stent migration remains a problem in up to 40% of patients, which necessitates re-intervention in a substantial proportion of patients.

Palliative Gastro-enterostomy (GE)

The indications for this procedure include gastric out let obstruction of any cause or symptomatic persistent delayed gastric emptying. The obstructing lesion could be in the distal stomach, the duodenum or elsewhere but causing obstruction to the flow of gastric contents into the small bowel. Ideally, a retro colic, iso-peristaltic GE should be formed. However, an ante colic GE is equally effective particularly if it achieves limiting the incision wound and dissection. With an ante-colic GE, patients may suffer intermittent delayed gastric emptying and more bile reflux causing biliary vomiting and gastritis. The procedure can be done laparoscopically with early recovery and rapid discharge from hospital.

Access

- For open surgery, a limited transverse upper abdominal incision to the left of the midline is ideal. However, depending on preference, a small midline upper abdominal incision can provide adequate access.
- For laparoscopic surgery, an infra-umbilical port should be used for the endoscope/ camera. Two ports on each side of the abdomen should be used for dissection and retraction.

Exploration

- The procedure should commence with a limited abdominal exploration to assess the feasibility of gastroenterostomy in palliating obstruction and the feasibility of a retrocolic approach.
- The merits of a limited dissection with an antecolic approach should be weighed against a more extensive dissection for the retro-colic approach. The important factors to consider include the patient's condition and comorbidities, the site and size of the tumour as well as the presence of metastases.

Dissection

- In a retrocolic approach, a window is created in the transverse colon mesentry to the left of the middle colic vessels.
- A 5 cm length of the greater curvature of the stomach is withdrawn to the infra-colic compartment.
- A loop of proximal jejunum approximately 15 cm from the ligament of Treitz is identified and sited alongside the greater curvature of the stomach in the infra-colic compartment.

Reconstruction (Omega Loop)

- The jejunum is approximated to the greater curvature of the stomach using either sutures or a linear stapling device.
- The two sides of the jejunum on either side of the gastroenterostomy are approximated using either sutures or a linear stapling device. This is termed as a Braun entero-enterostomy or Omega loop.
- The abdomen should be closed.

Post-operative Course

- The patient should be nursed on an appropriate ward with appropriate monitoring of vital parameters.
- The patient should be nursed without oral intake and all fluids and medication should be administered intravenously for at least 24 hours.

- After 24 hours, the volume of fluid intake is stepped up gradually over 48 hours. At the end of this period, small amounts of semi-solid food could be introduced and if tolerated, substituted with more solid food.
- The patient should be ready for discharge home when sufficiently mobile and independent.

Anticipated Complications

- Primary or secondary haemorrhage from the edges of the gastroenterostomy should be managed by endoscopic haemostasis or surgery if necessary.
- Respiratory infection or compromise should necessitate antibiotics and pulmonary toilet by physiotherapy. Depending on the level of respiratory compromise, additional measures may be necessary such as positive airway pressure (CPAP) or ventilation.
- Intestinal obstruction due to tumour or metastatic progression remains a possibility.

Surgical Insertion of Feeding Jejunostomy

The procedure is indicated for complete or partial inability to progress oral food intake through the oesophagus, stomach or duodenum. This could be due to mechanical obstruction or functional abnormality. In addition, the procedure is commonly used to supplement oral intake in the post-operative period. Feeding could be continuous or intermittent [23]. The GE could also be used to administer all enteric medication.

Access

- For open surgery, a limited transverse abdominal incision to the left of the midline (above the level of the umbilicus) is ideal. However, depending on preference, a small midline upper abdominal incision can provide adequate access. If a laparotomy is carried out for another procedure, the same wound could be used.
- For laparoscopic surgery, an infra-umbilical port should be used for the endoscope/ camera. Two ports on each side of the abdomen should be used for dissection and retraction.

Exploration

- The procedure should commence with abdominal exploration to ensure that an adequate proximal jejunal loop is sufficiently free for the feeding jejunostomy.

Dissection

- The distal end of the jejunostomy tube is brought into the abdomen through a separate stab incision to the left of the transverse incision used for access.

Reconstruction

- A purse-string suture is placed at the potential site of insertion of the feeding tube into the jejunum.
- An enterotomy is created in the centre of the purse-string suture on the selected jejunum.
- The feeding tube is inserted through the enterotomy into the jejunum (to the required length).
- The purse-string suture is ligated to close the enterotomy around the feeding tube. (The balloon on the feeding jejunostomy is inflated).
- A running suture on the jejunum starting distal to the enterotomy inlays the enterotomy and tunnels a 5 cm length of the feeding tube.
- The jejunum at the proximal end of the tunnel is approximated to the anterior abdominal wall.
- Other anchoring sutures are placed between the jejunum and anterior abdominal wall will prevent twisting of the jejunum around the fulcrum of the tube entry site.
- The abdomen should be closed.

Post-operative Course

- The patient should be nursed on the ward with appropriate monitoring of vital parameters.
- The patient's oral intake should be resumed rapidly.
- Feeding *via* the feeding jejunostomy tube should commence after 24 hours and stepped up slowly over days.
- The feeding tube should be flushed with water after every feed and after administering medication.
- Partially dissolved enteric medication is likely to block small calibre feeding tubes. Maximal dilution of such medication is recommended.
- The patient should be ready for discharge home when sufficiently mobile and independent.
- Feeding *via* feeding jejunostomy, could be continued nocturnally or as required.

Anticipated Complications

- Small bowel obstruction due to a twisted small bowel requires revision surgery.

Prognosis of Gastric Cancer

The overall prognosis of AGCs is poor, with 5-year survival rate of 10% in the West. Median survival for metastatic or unresectable disease is approximately 8 to 10 months. The main poor prognostic factors include: advanced stage at presentation, type of gastric cancer (diffuse type tumours have a worse prognosis than the intestinal type), grade of the tumour, lymph node metastases (a higher N ratio describing the number of nodes involved divided by the number of nodes examined, have a worse prognosis) and tumour location (proximal tumours have a worse prognosis than distal tumours). Tumours with lymphatic and vascular invasion and those with positive peritoneal cytology tend to recur earlier.

Pattern of Relapse

Recurrence following surgical removal of gastric carcinoma can manifest in one or more sites: Local, including lymph nodes or remnant stomach, Regional within the peritoneal cavity and distant. Two thirds of gastric cancer patients succumb to recurrences within the first 2 years. Gastric cancer prefers to spread intra-abdominally, and hence loco regional control is very important issue in treatment strategy. Loco regional recurrence rates vary from 25% to 96% depending on different detection methods. Haematogenous or lymphatic spreads without intra-abdominal metastases occur rarely.

Supportive Care

A considerable number of patients with advanced gastric cancer are either unfit for any therapeutic modality or develop advanced disease with a limited expectation of survival. Equally, a number of patients will relapse after previous radical curative measures to a point beyond any treatment benefit. These patients should be offered best supportive care in liaison with the "palliative care team". Such teams offer expert support in terms of analgesia, anti-nausea agents, drying of secretions, hydration and nutritional supplementation and general palliation of all symptoms on an individual basis in a supportive environment. Eventually, these teams offer the necessary expertise in "end of life care" for the unfortunate patient while supporting their relatives.

GASTRO-INTESTINAL STROMAL TUMOURS

Gastro-intestinal stromal tumours (GISTs) are the most common type of mesenchymal tumours of the gastrointestinal tract and can occur anywhere along the GI tract, but over 60% are found in the stomach. The clinical presentation of patients with GIST varies depending on the anatomic location of the tumour and the tumour size and aggressiveness. The most common presentation of GIST is GI bleeding, which may be acute (melena or hematemesis) or chronic and results in anaemia. Patients with GIST can also present acutely due to tumour rupture or gastric outlet obstruction. Others present with dysphagia (proximal obstructing tumours), early satiety (large tumours), or fatigue due to chronic blood loss.

Smaller lesions may be incidental findings during surgery, radiologic studies, or endoscopy. The natural history of these incidental tumours and the frequency of progression to symptomatic disease are unknown. There may be a substantial reservoir of small GIST tumours that do not progress to symptomatic stages.

Presentation

GISTs are responsible for 2.2% of malignant gastric tumours without any gender preference (male: female 1.1:1). The predicted age groups are in the 6th to 8th decade. Small GISTs (<2 cm) are usually asymptomatic and detected incidentally during endoscopy, surgery or physical examination. The majority GISTs (69%) is diagnosed at the time of presentation with nonspecific symptoms such as nausea, vomiting, early satiety, melena and anaemia (due to bleeding caused by intraluminal erosion or intraperitoneal rupture), abdominal pain, distension, fever, or leukocytosis. A significant number of gastric GISTs present with acute bleeding and are diagnosed at endoscopy to investigate the cause of the bleeding.

Most GISTs present as a single endophytic or exophytic nodule with a well-defined border and a median size of 3–5 cm. They rarely invade adjacent structures, but penetration through the stomach wall, organ invasion, adenopathy, cystic degeneration, irregular margins, mesenteric fat infiltration, ulceration, haemorrhage, and necrosis are likely and indicate malignancy. GISTs are also highly vascular and friable. Thus, they are prone to rupture and dissemination, which greatly increase the risk of recurrence.

Pathology and Molecular Genetics

GISTs typically arise within the muscle wall of the stomach. They range in size from less than 1 cm to more than 40 cm, with an average size of approximately 5 cm when clinically diagnosed. Small GISTs may form solid subserosal, intramural, or, less frequently, polypoid intraluminal masses. Large tumours tend to form external masses attached to the outer aspect of the stomach involving the muscular layers. As they grow, they can become adherent to perigastric organs and tissues. GIST morphology is quite varied; the tumours are composed of spindle cells (70%), epithelioid cells (20%) and mixed spindle and epithelioid components (10%). GISTs encompass a broad continuum of histologic patterns, ranging from bland-appearing tumours with very low mitotic activity (previously designated leiomyomas) to very aggressive-appearing patterns (previously called leiomyosarcomas). They originate from the interstitial cells of Cajal (ICC).

The most commonly used marker for GIST is KIT (cKIT, CD117) antigen, a marker expressed by the ICC. Approximately 95% of GISTs are positive for the CD117 antigen, an epitope of the KIT receptor tyrosine kinase. However, CD117 immunohistochemistry is not specific for GIST, as weak reactivity occurs with other mesenchymal neoplasms. In doubtful cases, morphologic examination and the use of other immuno-stains (DOG1, CD34, and α-smooth muscle actin) help with the pathological diagnosis.

Approximately 85% of GISTs contain oncogenic mutations in one of two receptor tyrosine kinases: KIT or PDGFRA (platelet-derived growth factor receptor alpha). Constitutive activation of either of these receptor tyrosine kinases plays a central role in the pathogenesis of GIST. Wild-type tumours, with no detectable *KIT* or *PDGFRA* mutations, account for 12% to 15% of all GISTs. Fewer than 5% of GIST occur in the setting of syndromic diseases, such as neurofibromatosis type 1 (NF1), Carney triad syndrome, and other familial diseases. The correct characterisation of GIST is very important because of the availability of specific, molecular-targeted therapy with KIT/PDGFRA tyrosine kinase inhibitors (TKI) such as imatinib mesylate or, in the case of imatinib-resistant GIST, sunitinib malate. Four different regions of KIT and three different regions of PDGFRA have been found mutated in sporadic GISTs. The location of the mutations strongly impacts on the response to systemic therapy with tyrosine kinase inhibitors. Exon 9 KIT mutant GISTs are less sensitive to imatinib than exon 11 KIT mutant tumours, and tumours with exon 18 mutation in PDGFRA are resistant to imatinib. The analysis of the mutational status is therefore part of the routine work-up in GISTs requiring systemic therapy.

Evaluation and Staging

Imaging is used to characterize extent of disease, and assess response to therapy. Endoscopy and endoscopic ultrasound (EUS), computed tomography (CT) with contrast enhancement, magnetic resonance imaging (MRI), and positron emission tomography (PET) can be used to evaluate suspected GISTs. The endoscopic characteristics of GISTs include smooth shape, normal overlying mucosa, occasional mucosal ulceration, and firm consistency on compression. Superficial forceps biopsies are usually non-diagnostic due to the sub-epithelial position. However, deeper forceps biopsies obtained through repeat biopsies at the same location ('ink pod' biopsies) can provide diagnostic tissue. EUS can determine additional lesion features, including hypoechoic appearance, oval shape, and wall layer of origin, which may aid in diagnosing GIST and determining malignant features. EUS-guided fine needle aspiration, provides adequate tissue for histologic and mutational analyses.

Contrast-enhanced CT is the best radiological technique for the characterization of GISTs and for the evaluation of the extent of disease. GISTs typically appear as hyper dense, enhancing masses on CT. When present, calcification, ulceration, necrosis, cystic areas, fistula, metastases, ascites, and infiltration indicate malignancy. MRI provides higher sensitivity for small liver lesions and should be used to evaluate liver metastases or when CT is inconclusive or contraindicated. 18FDG-PET is highly sensitive (80%) and a valuable imaging tool for diagnosis and as a predictor of clinical outcome.

Management

Small (<2 Cm) GISTs discovered accidentally, without high-risk features may be followed up by endoscopic surveillance for signs of transformation or until they become symptomatic. For larger GISTs >2 cm, abdominal/pelvic CT recommended to identify potential metastases and determine surgical risk. Resection is the preferred primary treatment for localized GISTs >2 cm, with a goal of R0 margins, intact pseudo capsule, no tumour rupture, and minimal morbidity. Surgery is the primary treatment for resectable GIST, but this approach is not always curative. A complete (R0) resection can be achieved in up to 85% of patients with primary disease. However, approximately 50% of patients develop recurrences or metastases within 5 years of primary resection. With surgery alone, the 5-year recurrence-free survival (RFS) rate is around 45–65%. Surgical options for GISTs range from minimally invasive endoscopic techniques for small tumours to open surgery for large malignancies. Because lymph node metastases are uncommon, lymphadenectomy is not generally indicated. Gastric GISTs located away from the gastroesophageal junction may be adequately resected with a gastric wedge resection, rather than by gastrectomy with lymphadenectomy. The lack of need for lymphadenectomies, combined with advances in minimally invasive techniques, has resulted in wider acceptance of minimally invasive approaches for resecting larger GISTs. Endoscopic techniques of resection are not recommended, as this has been associated with high rates of margin positivity and perforation.

Adjuvant/ Neo-Adjuvant Therapy

The tyrosine kinase inhibitor (TKI), imatinib, which selectively inhibits the KIT receptor, has demonstrated clinical benefit for patients with GIST. In clinical trials, imatinib treatment resulted in response rates of 40–55%, improved progression-free survival (PFS) for patients with KIT-positive unresectable or metastatic GIST, and extended RFS and overall survival (OS) in the adjuvant setting. Currently, imatinib is approved as first-line treatment in both settings.

Treatment of GIST depends on several factors such as the presence of metastases, expected difficulty of surgery, size of the primary tumour, and overall health of the patient. The optimal duration of adjuvant imatinib is still unknown, however, current guidelines recommend at least 3 years of adjuvant imatinib treatment for patients with KIT-positive GIST who are at high risk of recurrence based on tumour size, MI, site, rupture, and completeness of surgery [24].

The risk of GIST recurrence can be predicted based on mitotic index (MI: mitoses per 50 high-power fields), tumour size and location, and tumour rupture. Various stratification strategies have been developed to quantify the risk of recurrence in patients with primary GISTs (Table **11**).

Neoadjuvant imatinib therapy may reduce the risk of surgical morbidity and improve the probability of achieving complete resection. Surgical resection of metastases may even allow prolonged or complete remission in patients who respond to neoadjuvant imatinib and continue imatinib therapy afterwards. Patients with advanced primary or metastatic/recurrent GIST may have improved outcomes with surgical resection if they respond to neoadjuvant/preoperative imatinib as compared to those patients who have progressive disease on therapy. Perioperative imatinib can also improve outcomes in metastasectomy patients who present with metastatic GIST.

Table 11. Risk Stratification of Primary gastric GISTs by Tumour Size and Mitotic Index [24].

Size (cm)	≤ 2		$>2 \leq 5$		$>5 \leq 10$		>10	
Mitotic index per 50 hpf.	≤ 5	>5	≤ 5	>5	≤ 5	>5	≤ 5	>5
Risk of progressive disease	None	None	Very low	Moderate	Low	High	Moderate	High
% Risk of progressive disease	0	0	2	15	5	55	10	85

Hpf: High Power Field.

Prognosis

The overall disease-specific survival is 35% at 5 years. After treatment, less than 10% manifest with isolated local recurrence and 50% with metastasis. The site of relapse for GISTs is usually intra-abdominal, involving the peritoneum, the liver, or both. True local recurrences are uncommon, and typically there is widespread intraperitoneal recurrence that may not be detectable by imaging techniques. The median disease-specific survival of patients with metastatic GISTs is around 2 years.

Follow-up and Monitoring

Follow-up recommendations are based upon the risk of tumour progression. Low-risk lesions do not need routine follow-up. Abdominal/pelvic CT may be performed regularly for higher risk GISTs. The intervals between scan are based on the percentage risk of disease progression and clinical judgment. Low risk lesions require repeat scan every 5 years. High risk GISTs may require scans annually. CT is also used to monitor therapeutic effects in patients receiving systemic therapy for unresectable, metastatic, or recurrent disease.

18FDG-PET may be helpful in detecting resistance to TKI. If 18FDG-PET is used to monitor therapy with a TKI, a baseline FDG-PET should be performed before kinase inhibitor administration. Because 18FDG-PET imaging may detect the activity of imatinib in GIST much earlier than CT imaging, imaging of GIST with 18FDG-PET may represent a useful diagnostic modality for the very early assessment of response to imatinib therapy; a decrease in tumour avidity for 18FDG may be detected as early as 24 hours after a single dose of imatinib.

Wedge Resection of GISTs

Surgical resection with free margin is the gold standard treatment for GIST lesions and complete surgical resection is the only curative treatment of GISTs. Laparoscopic wedge resection is considered as the procedure of choice and a valid alternative to the conventional open approach for the resection of gastric Gastro-intestinal stromal tumours (GISTs) smaller than 2 cm. However, there is still debate regarding the most appropriate operative approach for larger GISTs. The development of endoscopic stapling devices has facilitated both the laparoscopic and open approach.

GISTs on the anterior surface of the stomach could be resected using an extra gastric wedge resection. This may necessitate prior ligation of the short gastric vessels in a fundic GIST or the gastro-omental branches in a greater curvature corpus GIST. GISTs on the posterior surface of the stomach are best managed through an intra-gastric wedge resection. GISTs close to the oesophago-gastric junction should be approached through an intra-gastric approach with a bougie (52 FG) across the oesophago-gastric junction to prevent its narrowing with closure. Rarely, narrowing of the oesophago-gastric junction is estimated as inevitable. In these cases, a formal wedge resection / proximal gastrectomy with oesophago-gastric anastomosis should be carried out. A stay suture on the epithelium or serosa should be used to manipulate the GIST. Multi-fire staplers (when available) should be used to resect the GIST with adequate margin. For lesions close to the oesophago-gastric junction, multiple firing of short staplers should achieve a semi-circular wedge resection without compromising the patency of the oesophago-gastric junction. In laparoscopic cases, extraction of the resected GIST out of the abdomen should observe oncological principles by protecting the wound. A bag would serve such a purpose but also keep the tumour intact for pathological processing and evaluation of completeness of resection. Most surgeons advocate over-sewing the staple line, unless the staple line is protected by membrane (*e.g.* seam guard). Post-operatively, patients should be managed without oral intake for at least 24 hours to protect the stapled closure. Patients who have had a proximal gastrectomy and oesophago-gastric anastomosis may require a longer abstinence from oral intake due to the tenuous nature of these anastomoses. All other patients who had a wedge gastrectomy could have oral fluids and diet reintroduced gradually after the first 24 hours.

GASTRIC NEURONEDOCRINE TUMOURS

The incidence of neuroendocrine tumours (NETs) is constantly rising. Gastric NETs show an additional increase in proportional incidence compared to all NETs of the gastroenteropancreatic system, accounting now for about 6-23% of gastrointestinal NETs. It is not clear whether this is a consequence of rising numbers of esophagogastroduodenoscopies performed with increasing awareness of these lesions or a true incidence effect.

Although the majority of gastric NETs have a benign course and asymptomatic behaviour, a subgroup has the potential to become aggressive and mimic the clinical course of gastric adenocarcinoma. In general, all NETs have malignant potential. In the stomach, three distinct types of neuroendocrine neoplasms are distinguishable.

Type 1 gastric NETs constitute 70-80% of gastric NETs. They are often <2 cm, polypoid in the majority of cases and multiple in 65% of cases. They develop on the background of chronic atrophic gastritis, either due to autoimmune gastritis or as a consequence of *H. pylori* infection, and are predominantly found in the gastric corpus or fundus. Atrophy of the fundic glands leads to hypochlorhydria and hypergastrinaemia, resulting in hyperplasia of enterochromaffin-like cells. Female patients are more frequently affected than male patients. These gastric NETs are usually asymptomatic except for anaemia, well differentiated and show benign behaviour with excellent survival rates, although a small proportion of patients develop distant metastases.

Type 2 gastric NETs are associated with hypergastrinaemia as a consequence of Zollinger-Ellison syndrome, almost exclusively within the MEN-1 syndrome, and account for 5-6% of gastric NETs. Endoscopically, they present as small, frequently multiple and polypoid lesions located mainly in the gastric fundus. Distant metastases can be found in 10-30% of cases.

Type 3 gastric NETs are not related to any chronic gastric pathology and occur as sporadic tumours. Macroscopically they present as unique, large (>2 cm), polypoid and ulcerated lesions. The majority of them are poorly differentiated. Male patients >50 years are predominantly affected. These tumours frequently are symptomatic, causing pain and/or weight loss. More than half of the patients with these type 3 gastric NETs present with distant metastases, resulting in a rate of 25-30% of tumour-related deaths.

The WHO classification discriminates four subtypes of gastric NETs, with a distinct category for poorly differentiated high-grade malignant NETs.

Evaluation and Staging

In type 1 and 2 gastric NETs, upper gastrointestinal endoscopy is the only imaging procedure recommended for staging purposes. In polyps >1 cm in size, endoscopic ultrasound may be used to rule out invasion of the depth of the gastric wall. Additional staging by computed tomography and somatostatin receptor scintigraphy are recommended in patients with type 3 gastric NETs. Gallium PET CT has become the gold standard for assessing metastatic disease from NETs.

All patients with gastric NETs should have serum gastrin and chromogranin A levels measured. In addition, characterization of underlying chronic gastric disease should be made by endoscopy and biopsies. Genetic analysis is recommended in case of suspected MEN-1 syndrome.

Management

Endoscopic surveillance is mandatory for type 1 NETs as they usually recur and progress to neuroendocrine carcinoma in about 3% of cases. In case of submucosal involvement, incomplete endoscopic resection or metastases in lymph nodes or distant organs, a surgical approach is the treatment of choice. Type 2 gastric NETs should be treated by local excision with yearly endoscopic surveillance. Type 3 NETs should be treated by multi-modality therapy. The surgical approach in type 3 NETs should be similar to the treatment of gastric adenocarcinoma.

Patients with advanced and progressive disease should be treated with anti-proliferative therapy. Somatostatin analogues and peptide receptor nucleotide therapy are options in differentiated tumours, while patients with poorly differentiated neuroendocrine carcinoma should be treated with chemotherapy, applying a combination of cisplatin and etoposide.

GASTRIC LYMPHOMA

Primary lymphoma of the stomach is defined to either originate from the gastric wall or from the adjacent lymph nodes. More than 40% of non-Hodgkin lymphomas arise from extra-nodal locations, and the gastrointestinal tract is one of the most common extra-nodal sites. The prevalence of primary lymphoma of the gastrointestinal tract ranges from 4 to 18% in the Western world (25% in the Middle East). The stomach is the most frequent site of origin in the Western world, but the midgut is predominantly involved in the Middle East. The average age of onset is in the 5th decade without any gender differences. Acquired or congenital immunosuppressive conditions are risk factors for lymphoma.

H. pylori infection is the leading cause of gastric mucosa-associated lymphoid tissue (MALT) lymphoma, accounting for about 90% of cases. B-cell-associated antigens such as CD19, CD20, CD22 and sIg are frequently positive in immunohistochemical staining, whereas CD5, CD10, CD38 and IgD are negative. B-cell MALT lymphomas are the only low-grade lymphomas of the stomach, whereas the majority of gastric lymphomas belong to the high-grade B-cell lymphomas.

Presentation

Symptoms are frequently unspecific, with abdominal discomfort and nausea, vomiting or signs of bleeding. Large lesions may be palpable in the epigastrium in advanced situations. Endoscopic biopsies are not always diagnostic and additional biopsies obtained at laparoscopy are frequently essential.

Management

The therapeutic approach depends on histopathological classification and staging (Ann Arbor classification for lymphoma) (Table **12**) [25]. Early-stage MALT lymphoma regresses in most cases after *H. pylori* eradication therapy. This should constitute the first line of treatment following diagnosis. Infrequently, multi-resistant *H. pylori* may not respond to conventional eradication measures. Tests of eradication will ensure that these individuals are identified early for treatment with other antibiotics. Lymphomas with genetic alterations {t(11:18) (q21:q21)} are at risk for eradication failure and the development of diffuse large B-cell lymphoma. Advanced MALT lymphoma should be treated by radiotherapy with curative intent, and mantle cell lymphoma, diffuse large B-cell lymphoma or rare Burkitt lymphoma are treated by systemic chemotherapy in accordance with the stage of disease. Surgical therapy is indicated in case of complications such as bleeding or perforation. In addition, surgical therapy can be considered when other modalities of treatment have failed or when complications arise from other modalities of treatment (*e.g.* Radiotherapy induced stenosis).

Table 12. Ann Arbor classification for lymphoma [25].

Stage	Features
I	Disease in single lymph node or lymph node region.
II	Disease in two or more lymph node regions on same side of diaphragm.
III	Disease in lymph node regions on both sides of the diaphragm is affected.
IV	Disease is wide spread, including multiple involvement at one or more extra-nodal (beyond the lymph node) sites, such as the bone marrow (which is involved commonly), liver, pleura (thin lining of the lungs).
Extra-nodal lymphoma is denoted by the prefix E before the stage. Stage II *contiguous* means two or more lymph nodes in close proximity (side by side).	

CONSENT FOR PUBLICATION

Not applicable.

ACKNOWLEDGEMENT

Declare none.

CONFLICT OF INTEREST

The author declares no conflict of interest, financial or otherwise.

REFERENCES

[1]   Choi JI, Joo I, Lee JM. State-of-the-art preoperative staging of gastric cancer by MDCT and magnetic resonance imaging. World J Gastroenterol 2014; 20(16): 4546-57.
[http://dx.doi.org/10.3748/wjg.v20.i16.4546] [PMID: 24782607]

[2]   Ramos RF, Scalon FM, Scalon MM, Dias DI. Staging laparoscopy in gastric cancer to detect peritoneal metastases: A systematic review and meta-analysis. Eur J Surg Oncol 2016; 42(9): 1315-21.
[http://dx.doi.org/10.1016/j.ejso.2016.06.401] [PMID: 27432515]

[3]   Washington K. 7th edition of the AJCC cancer staging manual: stomach. Ann Surg Oncol 2010; 17(12): 3077-9.
[http://dx.doi.org/10.1245/s10434-010-1362-z] [PMID: 20882416]

[4]   Tsai MM, Wang CS, Tsai CY, Chi HC, Tseng YH, Lin KH. Potential prognostic, diagnostic and therapeutic markers for human gastric cancer. World J Gastroenterol 2014; 20(38): 13791-803.
[http://dx.doi.org/10.3748/wjg.v20.i38.13791] [PMID: 25320517]

[5]   Wittekind C. The development of the TNM classification of gastric cancer. Pathol Int 2015; 65(8): 399-403.
[http://dx.doi.org/10.1111/pin.12306] [PMID: 26036980]

[6]   Zhang J, Zhou Y, Jiang K, Shen Z, Ye Y, Wang S. Evaluation of the seventh AJCC TNM staging system for gastric cancer: a meta-analysis of cohort studies. Tumour Biol 2014; 35(9): 8525-32.

[http://dx.doi.org/10.1007/s13277-014-1848-6] [PMID: 24696259]

[7]   Siewert JR, Stein HJ. Classification of adenocarcinoma of the oesophagogastric junction. Br J Surg 1998; 85(11): 1457-9.
[http://dx.doi.org/10.1046/j.1365-2168.1998.00940.x] [PMID: 9823902]

[8]   Kleinberg L, Brock M, Gibson M. Management of locally advanced adenocarcinoma of the esophagus and gastroesophageal junction: finally a consensus. Curr Treat Options Oncol 2015; 16(7): 35.
[http://dx.doi.org/10.1007/s11864-015-0352-6] [PMID: 26112428]

[9]   Japanese A. Japanese classification of gastric carcinoma: 3rd English edition. Gastric Cancer 2011; 14(2): 101-12.
[http://dx.doi.org/10.1007/s10120-011-0041-5] [PMID: 21573743]

[10]   Lauren P. The two histological main types of gastric carcinoma: diffuse and so-called intestinal-type carcinoma. An attempt at a histo-clinical classification. Acta Pathol Microbiol Scand 1965; 64: 31-49.
[http://dx.doi.org/10.1111/apm.1965.64.1.31] [PMID: 14320675]

[11]   Ming SC. Gastric carcinoma. A pathobiological classification. Cancer 1977; 39(6): 2475-85.
[http://dx.doi.org/10.1002/1097-0142(197706)39:6<2475::AID-CNCR2820390626>3.0.CO;2-L]
[PMID: 872047]

[12]   Schulz C, Schütte K, Malfertheiner P. Rare Neoplasia of the Stomach. Gastrointest Tumors 2015; 2(2): 52-60.
[http://dx.doi.org/10.1159/000435899] [PMID: 26674659]

[13]   Espinel J, Pinedo E, Ojeda V, Del Rio MG. Treatment modalities for early gastric cancer. World J Gastrointest Endosc 2015; 7(12): 1062-9.
[http://dx.doi.org/10.4253/wjge.v7.i12.1062] [PMID: 26380052]

[14]   Maple JT, Abu Dayyeh BK, Chauhan SS, *et al.* Endoscopic submucosal dissection. Gastrointest Endosc 2015; 81(6): 1311-25.
[http://dx.doi.org/10.1016/j.gie.2014.12.010] [PMID: 25796422]

[15]   Chung JW, Jung HY, Choi KD, *et al.* Extended indication of endoscopic resection for mucosal early gastric cancer: analysis of a single center experience. J Gastroenterol Hepatol 2011; 26(5): 884-7.
[http://dx.doi.org/10.1111/j.1440-1746.2010.06611.x] [PMID: 21198830]

[16]   Degiuli M, De Manzoni G, Di Leo A, *et al.* Gastric cancer: Current status of lymph node dissection. World J Gastroenterol 2016; 22(10): 2875-93.
[http://dx.doi.org/10.3748/wjg.v22.i10.2875] [PMID: 26973384]

[17]   Chan BA, Jang RW, Wong RK, Swallow CJ, Darling GE, Elimova E. Improving Outcomes in Resectable Gastric Cancer: A Review of Current and Future Strategies. Oncology (Williston Park) 2016; 30(7): 635-45.
[PMID: 27422110]

[18]   Lehnert T, Buhl K. Techniques of reconstruction after total gastrectomy for cancer. Br J Surg 2004; 91(5): 528-39.
[http://dx.doi.org/10.1002/bjs.4512] [PMID: 15122602]

[19]   Ku GY, Ilson DH. Management of gastric cancer. Curr Opin Gastroenterol 2014; 30(6): 596-602.
[http://dx.doi.org/10.1097/MOG.0000000000000115] [PMID: 25197781]

[20]   Marrelli D, Polom K, de Manzoni G, Morgagni P, Baiocchi GL, Roviello F. Multimodal treatment of gastric cancer in the west: Where are we going? World J Gastroenterol 2015; 21(26): 7954-69.
[http://dx.doi.org/10.3748/wjg.v21.i26.7954] [PMID: 26185368]

[21]   Quiros R M, Bui C L. Multidisciplinary approach to esophageal and gastric cancer 2009.
[http://dx.doi.org/10.1016/j.suc.2008.09.019]

[22]   Biondi A, Lirosi MC, D'Ugo D, *et al.* Neo-adjuvant chemo(radio)therapy in gastric cancer: Current status and future perspectives. World J Gastrointest Oncol 2015; 7(12): 389-400.

[http://dx.doi.org/10.4251/wjgo.v7.i12.389] [PMID: 26690252]

[23]   Rosania R, Chiapponi C, Malfertheiner P, Venerito M. Nutrition in patients with gastric cancer: an update. Gastrointest Tumors 2016; 2(4): 178-87.
[http://dx.doi.org/10.1159/000445188] [PMID: 27403412]

[24]   Sicklick JK, Lopez NE. Optimizing surgical and imatinib therapy for the treatment of gastrointestinal stromal tumors. J Gastrointest Surg 2013; 17(11): 1997-2006.
[http://dx.doi.org/10.1007/s11605-013-2243-0] [PMID: 23775094]

[25]   Fischbach W. Gastric MALT lymphoma - update on diagnosis and treatment. Best Pract Res Clin Gastroenterol 2014; 28(6): 1069-77.
[http://dx.doi.org/10.1016/j.bpg.2014.09.006] [PMID: 25439072]

CHAPTER 5

Oncological Management of Oesophageal and Gastric Cancer

Russell Petty[*] and **Asa Dahle-Smith**

Department of Oncology, Ninewells Hospital and Medical School, Dundee, Scotland, UK

Abstract: In current clinical practice the majority of patients diagnosed with oesophageal or gastric cancer have metastatic disease at the time of diagnosis. In order to manage these patients successfully, effective systemic treatments are necessary and the impact of these systemic therapies in reducing tumour burden, improving symptoms, quality of life and extending survival in the palliative setting are all-important.

Given the early propensity of these cancers to progress and the potential for dissemination, even in patients with early cancers, local and systemic therapy must be considered along with surgery. The concept of multi-modal treatment is at a well-developed stage in oesophago-gastric cancer treatment and best exemplified by neoadjuvant chemo-radio therapy for oesophageal cancer. Adjuvant therapy remains an option in locally advanced cancers. Similar treatments can be used for recurrent disease.

Systemic treatments for oesophageal and gastric cancer have evolved from cytotoxic chemotherapies to the more recent emergence of rationally designed targeted therapies which act by inhibiting specific molecular drivers of oncogenesis. They are often used in combination with predictive biomarkers that identify those patients most likely to respond- the precision medicine strategy. Despite their cost, their benefits include reduced toxicity and increased efficacy

Keywords: Adjuvant therapy, Chemo/radio therapy, Chemotherapy, Gastric cancer, Multi-modality treatment, Neo-adjuvant therapy, Oesophageal cancer, Palliative treatment, Performance status, Radiotherapy.

RATIONALE AND ASSESSMENT

Rationale

It is well recognised that both gastric and oesophageal cancers disseminate

---

[*] **Corresponding author Russell Petty:** Department of Oncology, Ninewells Hospital and Medical School, Dundee DD1 9SY, Scotland, UK; Tel/Fax: +44 1382 660111; E-mail: r.petty@dundee.ac.uk

beyond their primary site at an early and commonly asymptomatic stage in their natural history. This means that in current clinical practice the majority of patients have metastatic disease either clinically or radiologically apparent or below the threshold of detection, that is micro-metastatic, disease at the time of diagnosis. This represents one of the most challenging aspects of these diseases in terms of developing effective clinical management strategies, especially those that will lead to long term disease control or cure. In short, to treat oesophageal and gastric cancer successfully effective systemic treatments are needed and the impact of systemic therapies as adjuvant treatments and in reducing tumour burden, improving symptoms, quality of life and extending survival in the palliative setting provide clinical evidence for this concept.

Systemic treatments for oesophageal and gastric cancer have evolved from cytotoxic chemotherapies which still remain useful in clinical practice to the more recent emergence of rationally designed targeted therapies which act by inhibiting specific molecular drivers of oncogenesis, and which are used in combination with predictive biomarker tests that identify those patients most likely to respond- the precision medicine strategy. Targeted therapies have benefits in terms of reduced toxicity and increased efficacy. Progress in the development of targeted therapies for oesophageal and gastric cancer has lagged behind other tumour types, but more recently targeted therapies together with predictive biomarkers have been established and this has led to the development of a new molecular sub-classification of the disease, where subgroups are defined by biomarkers that indicate which targeted agents should be used. The development of targeted therapies together with this molecular classification as part of a precision medicine strategy is the cutting edge of oncological management of the disease. However, anatomical and histopathological classification remain and are likely to remain important in oncological management as these features capture key aspects of disease biology which are relevant to systemic treatments. Anatomical considerations are also critical for use of radiotherapy and the development of concurrent chemoradiotherapy as a radical treatment for oesophageal cancer has been a key development in oncological management in recent years.

Assessment of Patients for Oncological Management

Performance status (PS), which captures the general condition of the patient represents a central clinical tool in assessment of patients for oncological management. In UK and European practice, the Eastern Co-operative Oncology Group (ECOG) scale is most commonly used (Table **1**).

PS is easy to assess, reproducible and is a powerful prognostic tool for patients with oesophageal and gastric cancer, especially in the palliative treatment setting.

While potentially readily reversible causes of poorer PS should be determined and addressed in general terms, individuals with ECOG PS 3 and 4, have an extremely poor prognosis regardless of disease stage, are likely to experience severe toxicity from cytotoxic chemotherapy and generally speaking are not candidates who will benefit from oncological management. In these individuals, supportive/ symptomatic care measures only are likely to be more appropriate. Individuals with ECOG PS 01 or 1 in general terms will be suitable and can potentially benefit from oncological interventions. ECOG PS2 patients represent an area of more uncertainty, because the PS 2 category captures a wider range of clinical condition and there is less clinical trial evidence regarding oncological interventions in PS 2 patients (trials predominately enrol PS 0 and 1 patients only). While this applies in all cases, especially for PS 2 individuals with oesophageal and gastric cancer clinical judgement of an experienced site specialised oncologist is critical in assessment for oncological interventions.

Table 1. The Eastern Co-operative Oncology (ECOG) Performance status (PS) grading.

Grade	ECOG Performance Status
0	Fully active, able to carry on all pre-disease performance without restriction
1	Restricted in physically strenuous activity but ambulatory and able to carry out work of a light or sedentary nature, e.g., light house work, office work
2	Ambulatory and capable of all self-care but unable to carry out any work activities; up and about more than 50% of waking hours
3	Capable of only limited self-care; confined to bed or chair more than 50% of waking hours
4	Completely disabled; cannot carry on any self-care; totally confined to bed or chair
5	Dead

Bone marrow, renal function and other medical co-morbidities must also be considered as there may be specifics contraindications to chemotherapy, or dose reductions and modifications may be required. Assessment of left ventricular function is important if the use of the anthracycline epirubicin is considered.

Age in itself is not considered a barrier to the use of oncological treatments, but there is evidence that older individuals even with similar PS, and co-morbidly experience more toxicity from chemotherapy and most clinical trials have a minority of individuals over 75 years of age. Accordingly, many oncologists will be cautious about treating older individuals and more clinical research is required regarding the assessment of fitness for oncological intervention and the benefits versus toxicity balance of oncological interventions in older people.

As will be discussed in more detail in subsequent sections, concurrent chemoradiotherapy provides a radical potentially curative treatment option for oesophageal squamous cell carcinoma and adenocarcinoma. In order to proceed with this, it must be possible to include all the patients' sites of disease in a radiotherapy treatment field, which will allow a curative dose to be delivered without exceeding the tolerance of normal tissues. Advances in computed tomography (CT) in radiotherapy planning have facilitated this greatly in recent years and often, it will not be possible to determine if curative dose radiotherapy is possible until detailed CT planning is undertaken on the patient. However broadly speaking for radical treatment the tumour and involved regional lymph nodes must not extend beyond 10 cm cranio-caudal distance. Endoscopic ultrasound is a critical test to determine the extent of the primary tumour and location of involved regional lymph nodes for radiotherapy planning and assessment.

EARLY STAGE OESOPHAGEAL CANCER

Pre-operative Treatment

Patients with local lymph node spread (T1-2, N1-3) or more advanced T stage primary tumours (T3-4, Nx) who are deemed fit to proceed with surgical resection are candidates for neo-adjuvant therapy with either chemotherapy or chemoradiotherapy (CRT) which improves survival outcomes by improving probability of R0 resection and eradicating micro-metastatic disease. The optimum neo-adjuvant treatment modality/modalities and regimen remains controversial with no globally agreed standard schedule. Randomised controlled trials (RCTs) indicate that both neoadjuvant chemotherapy and neoadjuvant concurrent chemoradiotherapy improve R0 resection rate and overall survival, but the comparative effectiveness of each approach remains uncertain. The results look similar when different trails are compared (taking into account case mix), and have not yet been evaluated in a RCT. Histopathological response rates and R0 resection rates appear to be higher with CRT, but delivering concurrent CRT limits the dose of systemic treatment delivered and this could have a negative impact on the treatment of micro-metastatic disease which may be the critical aspect in terms of improving survival and cure rates.

Neo-adjuvant Chemoradiotherapy (NA CRT)

The recent Dutch CROSS RCT has established a standard of care for NA CRT in oesophageal cancer [1]. In this trial, 368 patients with locally advanced oesophageal cancer (Adenocarcinoma, 75%, and squamous cell carcinoma, 23%) were randomised to receive either, five weeks of pre-operative CRT (weekly administration of carboplatin and paclitaxel for 5 weeks and concurrent radiotherapy, comprising 41.4 Gy in 23 fractions, 5 days per week, followed by surgery), or surgery alone. R0 resection was achieved in 92% of patients in the CRT plus surgery arm compared to 69% in the surgery alone arm. This translated into survival benefit with median overall survival 49.4 months versus 24.0 months in favour of the CRT plus surgery arm. While earlier reports identified and expressed concerns regarding increased operative morbidity following NA CRT, this was not seen in the CROSS RCT, and more recent larger cohort studies have also been reassuring in this regard. However surgical experience in operating on patients who have had NA CRT may be a key factor.

On-going early phase trials are evaluating the addition of targeted therapies to NA CRT. It is unclear yet whether this will offer increased effectiveness. To determine the benefit, RCTs comparing targeted therapies + CRT in the NA setting to the standard of using NA CRT such as the CROSS regimen will be required. Any increased toxicity from the addition of targeted therapies will also need to be considered.

Neoadjuvant Chemotherapy (NAC)

The UK OEO2 study established a standard of care for NAC. In this trial, 802 patients with oesophageal adenocarcinoma (69%) or squamous cell carcinoma (31%) were randomised to two cycles of combination cisplatin and 5-fluorouracil (5FU) before surgery or surgery alone. Long-term results with a median follow up of 6 years have now been reported and show a long term maintained survival benefit for NAC, with the hazard ratio (HR) of 0.84 (95% CI, 0.72 to 0.98; P = .03) favouring chemotherapy, which in absolute terms is a 5-year survival of 23.0% compared with 17.1% for Surgery alone. The treatment effect seen for NAC is consistent in both adenocarcinoma and squamous cell carcinoma [2].

More recently the OEO5 study randomised 897 patients with oesophageal cancer to 2 cycles of Cisplatin and 5FU or capecitabine (an oral 5FU pro-drug) as in the OEO2 trial, versus 4 cycles of Epirubicin, Cisplatin and 5FU or capecitabine. The triplet regimen had greater toxicity and while there was some evidence of improved histopathological response, R0 resection rate and progression free survival, there was no improvement in overall survival. Accordingly, 2 cycles of Cisplatin and 5FU or capecitabine remains the standard of care at present.

Neoadjuvant Chemoradiotherapy or Chemotherapy?

Several meta-analyses have suggested that NAC seems to be relatively more beneficial in oesophageal adenocarcinoma, while NA CRT may be relatively more beneficial in squamous cell carcinoma [3]. However, this remains controversial and a RCT is required to determine a definitive answer regarding the comparative effectiveness of NAC and NA CRT. At the present time, both NA

CRT and NAC remain valid treatment options. Patient selection for each approach is likely to be critical and there is a consensus that some patients will more optimally benefit from one or other approach. However, at the present time it is not possible to determine which clinicopathological characteristics determine which approach is optimal. A RCT will enable this to be evaluated and investigators are also evaluating other approaches to optimise patient selection, such as the use of MRI to determine the risk of circumferential resection margin (CRM) positivity prior to surgery. In patients at high risk for CRM positivity, NA CRT may be preferable to NAC. Another approach to optimise patient selection is the use of predictive biomarker tests, including molecular tests and imaging biomarkers such as FDG PET scans is being investigated to determine sensitivity and clinical usefulness of NAC and targeted therapies.

Peri-operative Chemotherapy

Adjuvant chemotherapy (AC) also has a role in oesophageal adenocarcinoma, as part of a perioperative chemotherapy regimen. The UK MAGIC study of 503 patients with resectable adenocarcinoma of oesophagus, junction or stomach randomised participants to receive perioperative chemotherapy with three cycles of epirubicin, cisplatin and 5-FU before and after surgery, or surgery alone. Perioperative chemotherapy conferred an improvement in overall survival (HR for death 0.75, p=0.009), resulting in an improvement in five-year survival from 23% to 36% when compared to surgery alone [4]. Only 10% of enrolled patients had oesophageal adenocarcinoma, and while the subgroup analysis demonstrated benefit across all anatomical sites – oesophageal, junctional and gastric – some oncologists believe that the small number of oesophageal adenocarcinoma patients in this study together with the recent results of the OEO5 RCT question the generalisability of the MAGIC trial data. The utility of this perioperative approach over NAC with 2 cycles of Cisplatin and 5FU or capecitabine, specifically for oesophageal cancer remains unclear. However similar results demonstrating benefit of perioperative chemotherapy have been demonstrated in a French RCT with resectable oesophageal, junctional and gastric adenocarcinomas and accordingly without a RCT comparing NAC with perioperative chemotherapy, both approaches remain valid at the present time in oesophageal adenocarcinoma. Very recently the German FLOT4 study randomised 716 patients with adenocarcinoma oesophagus, junction or stomach to MAGIC type per-operative chemotherapy or the FLOT regimen comprising 4 cycles of 5FU, Leucovorin, oxaliplatin and docetaxel before surgery and 4 cycles afterwards. FLOT 4 demonstrated superiority for the FLOT regimen, with mean survival of 50 months for FLOT versus 36 months for MAGIC, HR 0.77, p=0.012). While there are some concerns regarding additional toxicity of the FLOT regimen when applied to a non-trial population FLOT is likely to become a new standard of care for perioperative chemotherapy. Perioperative chemotherapy has not been evaluated in oesophageal squamous cell carcinoma.

Definitive Chemo-radiotherapy (dCRT)

In cases of locally advanced oesophageal cancer in which R0 resection is felt to be unachievable or in patients who are deemed medically unfit for surgery, radical concurrent chemo-radiotherapy (CRT) is a viable alternative. Current European recommendations are for at least 50.4 Gray (Gy) delivered in 1.8Gy fractions for definitive chemo-radiation, usually with the addition of low dose weekly cisplatin and continuous capecitabine as radiosensitisers. Several RCTs, predominantly involving squamous cell carcinoma patients have demonstrated equivalent overall survival for dCRT versus surgery. The control dCRT arm in a recent UK trial SCOPE, showed a 5-year survival of 26% which is similar to survival seen in surgical series after taking into account case mix. The lower treatment related morbidity, faster recovery and quality of life have led oncologists to suggest that dCRT should be considered as an alternative to surgical resection especially for squamous cell carcinoma [5]. However, it is clear that local recurrence rates are higher for dCRT compared to surgery and this is a key factor in clinical decision making. Nevertheless, for high proximal oesophageal squamous cell cancers where surgery would involve laryngectomy there is now a general consensus that dCRT rather than surgery is the preferred approach.

For adenocarcinoma there is a lack of sufficient evidence from RCTs regarding the comparative effectiveness of dCRT and surgery. However a number of large cohorts and data from the control arm of the SCOPE trial, which comprised adenocarcinomas and squamous cell carcinomas, suggest that the outcomes for dCRT and surgery are similar stage for stage [6]. Similar to squamous cell carcinoma, there is a higher incidence of local recurrence with dCRT.

Due to lack of therapeutic equipoise it is unlikely or possible to perform a further RCT of dCRT versus surgery and so indirect comparison will need to be made. The introduction of more effective targeted therapies into dCRT regimens and further optimisation of radiotherapy delivery due to technical advances may improve effectiveness of dCRT regimens in the future. This could lead to improved survival and better local control with dCRT compared to surgery however this remains to be determined. At present the optimal approach is for multi-disciplinary clinical teams to consider either surgery or dCRT for each patient whose tumour is radically treatable, depending on patient fitness, co-morbidities and the patient's own preferences for treatment. The comparative effectiveness of dCRT and surgery in oesophageal cancer has been the subject of a very helpful recent Cochrane review, which provides a detailed evaluation and commentary [7].

EARLY STAGE GASTRIC CANCER

Peri-operative Treatment

As already discussed the UK MAGIC trial established a standard of care for perioperative chemotherapy in junctional and gastric adenocarcinomas, and the recently reported FLOT4 trial has established a new standard of care that is currently being implemented. On-going studies are evaluating the addition of targeted agents to perioperative chemotherapy.

Adjuvant Treatment

Adjuvant treatment is delivered post operatively and includes adjuvant chemotherapy and chemoradiotherapy.

Adjuvant Chemotherapy

Eastern RCTs performed in japan and South Korea have demonstrated clearly that the addition of adjuvant chemotherapy after R0 resection involving D2 lymphadenectomy improves survival. This includes the oral 5FU prodrug S1 as a monotherapy, which is not licensed in this indication in Europe or North America, and the XELOX regimen combining capecitabine and oxaliplatin, which was evaluated in the CLASSIC trial. In the CLASSIC trial, 1035 patients were randomly assigned to adjuvant capecitabine and oxaliplatin, or observation after surgery. 5-year disease-free survival was significantly improved with adjuvant chemotherapy - 68% in the adjuvant capecitabine and oxaliplatin group versus 53% in the observation alone group. For overall survival HR was 0·66, 95% CI 0·51-0·85; p=0·0015, favouring adjuvant chemotherapy and the estimated 5-year overall survival was 78% versus 69% [8]. A definitive RCT comparing pre and postoperative chemotherapy has not yet been undertaken.

Adjuvant chemotherapy is considered the standard approach in eastern countries, but due to demographic and likely biological differences between gastric cancer in east and west there are some concerns regarding extrapolation of this data to western patients. Accordingly, in the west peri-operative chemotherapy is preferred, but post-operative adjuvant chemotherapy will also be considered for patients who for whatever reason proceed directly to resection without preoperative chemotherapy.

Adjuvant Chemoradiotherapy

The intergroup 0116 trial demonstrated a benefit from post-operative concurrent

CRT following gastrectomy. In this RCT, 559 patients with ≥ T3 and/or node-positive gastric cancer were randomly assigned to observation or CRT (45 Gy with 5FU) after R0 resection. There was a survival benefit for CRT, which has been sustained in a recent long term follow up report with a hazard ratio for overall survival of 1.32 (95% CI, 1.10 to 1.60; P = .0046). However, most of the patients in this trial underwent D0 (41%) or D1 (35%) lymphadenectomy [9]. This study has been criticised on this basis suggesting that the adjuvant CRT was compensating for 'inadequate' or 'sub-optimal' surgery.

A more recent Korean RCT, ARTIST1 compared adjuvant chemotherapy and adjuvant CRT and provides useful data to determine the utility of these different adjuvant therapy approaches in gastric cancer. In ARTIST1, 458 patients with gastric cancer all of whom received gastrectomy with D2 lymph node dissection were randomised to adjuvant chemotherapy with 6 cycles of capecitabine and cisplatin or to two cycles of the same chemotherapy followed by chemoradiotherapy and then two additional cycles of chemotherapy. With 7 years of follow-up, disease free and overall survival were not different between adjuvant chemotherapy and adjuvant CRT. A subgroup analyses showed that chemoradiotherapy significantly improved survival in patients with node-positive disease and in light of this the authors have initiated the ARTIST2 RCT evaluating adjuvant chemotherapy and chemoradiotherapy in patients with node-positive, D2-resected gastric cancer [10].

Perioperative Chemotherapy, Adjuvant Chemotherapy or Adjuvant CRT for Gastric Cancer?

Based on evidence from RCTs, peri-operative or adjuvant chemotherapy remain valid options at present for gastric cancer even if a D2 lymphadenectomy has been performed. The peri-operative approach may be preferred since post-operative morbidity means that as many as half of patients, especially in the western clinical practice, may not be fit within an appropriate time frame after surgery to start adjuvant chemotherapy and so without a pre-operative treatment, these patients will miss out on potential survival benefits.

The role of adjuvant CRT and any advantage over adjuvant chemotherapy is less clear from RCT evidence, and remains controversial. However, even in patients that have had a D2 lymphadenectomy based on the ARTIST1 RCT, adjuvant CRT with the regimen used in this trial seems similar in efficacy to adjuvant chemotherapy. Adjuvant CRT is not routinely used in the UK and Europe, but there is more agreement and consensus that is may have a role in patients who for whatever reason, for example due to emergency presentation, have had a D0 or limited lymphadenectomy. Adjuvant CRT may have a role following D2 lymphadenectomy in node positive patients but the results of the ARTIST 2 RCT to determine this are awaited. If this trial is positive for adjuvant CRT in this group of patients, this would establish a clear role for adjuvant CRT as opposed to adjuvant chemotherapy.

The comparative effectiveness of adjuvant CRT versus peri-operative chemotherapy remains unknown, but is currently under evaluation in several RCTs. Data from the ARTIST1 trial illustrates clearly the key point that different perioperative and adjuvant approaches are likely to be more or less optimal for different patient subgroups and it is likely to be very important to identify these subgroups in the setting of RCTs.

ONCOLOGICAL MANAGEMENT OF ADVANCED OESOPHAGEAL AND GASTRIC CANCER

The majority of patients, in the region of 60-70% with oesophageal or gastric cancer present with disease that is not amenable to radical (potentially curative) treatment approaches. In addition, approximately half of those treated with radical intent will develop recurrent disease. For these patients palliative treatment approaches, designed to control symptoms, improve health related quality of life (HRQL) and prolong survival are the available therapeutic options. Palliative chemotherapy has a clear role but is suitable for only 50-60% of patients. Supportive care measures which may include stent insertion for dysphagia or gastric outlet obstruction and palliative radiotherapy for local symptoms e.g. pain or bleeding related to a specific site of disease are of paramount importance alongside palliative chemotherapy, and improve tolerance of chemotherapy as well as reducing side effects, and ultimately improve effectiveness. For those patients unsuitable for palliative chemotherapy supportive care measures are the mainstay of treatment. Targeted therapies have an emerging role in palliative management and may offer equal or improved efficacy to chemotherapy with less toxicity. Increasingly, the paradigm of precision medicine is developing in the palliative treatment setting with predictive biomarkers being evaluated in clinical trials to select patients for particular targeted therapies and this is leading to the development of a molecular sub-classification of oesophageal and gastric cancer which is likely to change the way the disease is viewed clinically and treated by oncologists in the near future.

There is very little difference in the effectiveness or clinical use of cytotoxic chemotherapy in oesophageal squamous cell carcinoma, adenocarcinoma, junctional adenocarcinoma or gastric adenocarcinoma. Accordingly, the use of palliative chemotherapy is discussed in this section collectively for these tumours. Given that targeted treatments are rationally designed medicines against specific molecules that are pathological drivers for the continued growth of tumours (in contrast to chemotherapies which have a less specific cell killing mechanism of action) biological differences between the anatomical and histological subtypes are more relevant for targeted therapies. Accordingly, the established use of targeted therapies, and their investigation in clinical trials is discussed with reference to use in specific anatomical and histological disease sites.

With supportive care measures only, the median survival for patients with advanced gastric and oesophageal cancers, is in the range 3-4 months reflecting a rapid 'week on week' clinical and symptomatic progression. In patients with progressive disease, symptoms can develop rapidly and this is associated with rapid deconditioning. In this scenario, clinicians most commonly have to act in a reactive rather than pro-active manner to optimise symptom control and this can be very challenging.

With palliative chemotherapy median survival is extended to 11-12 months. In patients with gastric or junctional adenocarcinoma who are HER2 positive (approximately 15%), the addition of the HER-2 monoclonal antibody trastuzumab to chemotherapy extends median survival to 14-18 months' dependent upon the degree of HER 2 positivity (most strongly positive have greatest benefit). Second line therapies, both targeted and cytotoxic drugs have recently been established in practice and median survival following second line systemic therapy is in the range 6-9 months. Overall, approximately 2 out of 3 treated patients with advanced disease will gain disease control following first line palliative systemic treatment. This will translate into improved quality of life and symptom control and disease control for typically 1-2 years. The increasing use of second line therapy is resulting in greater numbers of 2 year survivors but overall only 1 in 3 patients treated at present would be expected to remain well at 2 years and 10-20% at 3 years. Survival beyond 3 years is uncommon with current palliative systemic treatments.

Systemic Palliative Therapy in Advanced Oesophageal and Gastric Cancer

As already mentioned, historically, all advanced gastric and oesophageal cancer subtypes were treated in the same way. Early trials of single cytotoxic agents including methotrexate (MTX), 5-FU and mitomycin C (MMC) demonstrated modest response rates in small case series. This has led to randomised trials of combination regimens versus supportive care only, which demonstrated unequivocal benefit over supportive care [11]. Subsequently, small stepwise improvements have been demonstrated in RCTs as the efficacy and toxicity of combination chemotherapy regimens have been optimised. These randomised clinical trials have provided a robust evidence base for the use of palliative systemic chemotherapy in advanced gastric and oesophageal cancer (Fig. **1**).

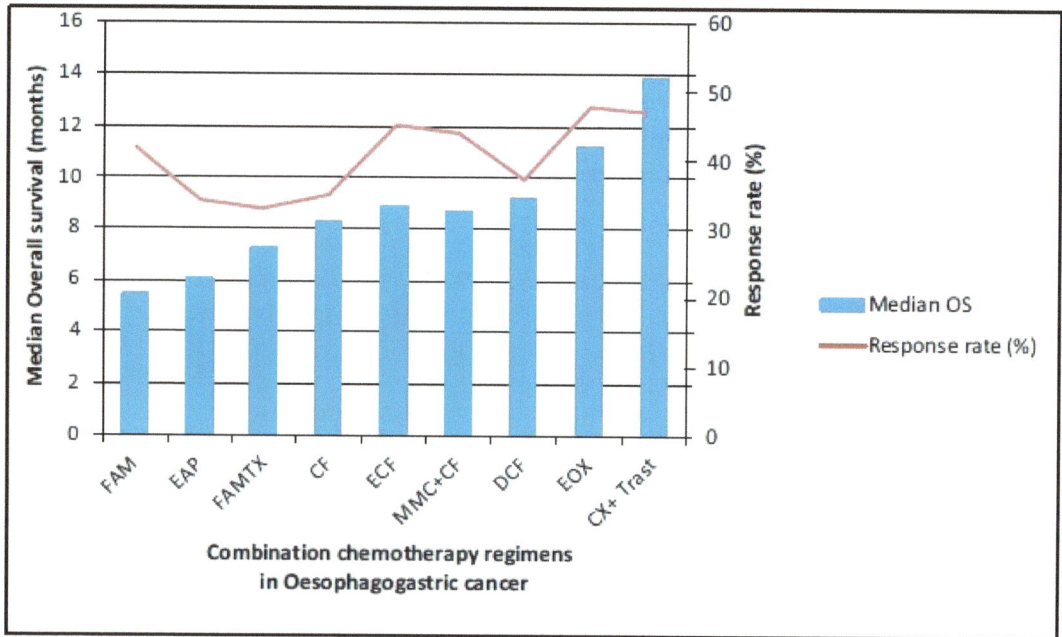

Fig. (1). Benefits of selected palliative systemic treatments from randomised controlled trials in advanced gastric and oesophageal cancer demonstrating stepwise incremental benefits achieved. Note that those patients with highest HER 2 protein expression, HER2 IHC score 3+, median survival is extended to 18 months. Median overall survival (OS) and Response rate comprising, partial and complete responses are shown. Patients without an objective response also benefit from achieving disease stabilisation. Median survival reported takes in to account those patients achieving disease control (partial or complete response plus disease stabilisation) who typically survive above the median and those not responding nor achieving disease control who survive much lower than the median, and similar to those receiving supportive care alone, typically 3 -4 months only. FAM (5-FU, doxorubicin and MMC), FAMTX (high dose 5-FU, doxorubicin and MMC), EAP (etoposide, doxorubicin and cisplatin), CF (cisplatin and 5FU), MMC +CF 9 mitomycin C, cisplatin and 5FU), DCF (docetaxel, cisplatin and 5FU), EOX (epirubicin, Oxaliplatin and Capecitabine), CX + Trast (cisplatin 5FU (or capecitabine) plus trastuzumab.

A pivotal phase III RCT, the REAL-2 study, has established the standard of care for palliative chemotherapy. A two by two design allowed patients with locally advanced or metastatic gastric and oesophageal cancer to be randomised to receive ECF (epirubicin, cisplatin, 5-FU), EOF (epirubicin, oxaliplatin, 5-FU), ECX (epirubicin, cisplatin, capecitabine) or EOX (epirubicin, oxaliplatin, capecitabine) with the primary end point of demonstrating non-inferiority of capecitabine over 5-FU and non-inferiority of oxaliplatin over cisplatin. Approximately 90% of cases enrolled were adenocarcinoma; squamous and undifferentiated tumours accounted for the rest of cases. Oesophageal, junctional and gastric tumours were included. The hazard ratio for overall survival was 0.86, non-significantly favouring capecitabine, in the capecitabine versus 5-FU comparison and 0.92 non-significantly favouring oxaliplatin in the oxaliplatin versus cisplatin comparison. Although no statistically significant difference was detected in progression free survival or disease control rate, overall survival was significantly longer in the EOX group, 11.2 *vs* 9.2 months (HR 0.8, p=0.02) compared with ECF. This study established equivalence of capecitabine as an oral alternative to infusional 5FU and of oxaliplatin to cisplatin [12]. There are small differences in the toxicity profiles, but this study led to the recognition of platinum based triplets, ECF, ECX, EOX, with EOF being considered as a standard of care. Notably the incidence of both venous and arterial thromboembolic events is significantly lower with oxaliplatin compared to cisplatin, and given the high risk of thromboembolism in advanced oesophageal and gastric cancer this is a significant observation for clinical practice [13].

Some oncologists have questioned the incremental benefit from addition of epirubicin to a platinum drug (Oxaliplatin or cisplatin) and a fluoropyrimidine (5FU or capecitabine) suggesting that epirubicin increases toxicity with only minimal if any additional efficacy in terms of symptom control and quality life or survival. There have been no definitive RCTs to determine this, but indirect comparisons and small underpowered randomised studies provide some support for this, especially in older and frailer patients. In addition, problems with increased and unacceptably high levels of toxicity have been encountered when some targeted agents have been combined with chemotherapy triplets resulting in the need to reduce the dose of the cytotoxics and reduce efficacy, for example when combining the anti-EGFR monoclonal antibody Panitumumab with EOX chemotherapy [14]. Combining targeted agents with platinum fluoropyrimidine doublets has not lead to excessive toxicity. In light of this many oncologists consider doublets rather than triplets as the standard of care for cytotoxic chemotherapy in advanced gastric and oesophageal cancer although this remains controversial and best practice suggests that an individual patient by patient approach should be undertaken where the balance of efficacy and toxicity are considered in each case.

The V325 trial group compared docetaxel, cisplatin and 5-FU (DCF) to CF as first line treatment in a phase III setting in patients with advanced gastric cancer. DCF demonstrated superior response rate compared to CF (37% v 25%, p=0.01), which translated to a statistically significant improvement in overall survival (9.2 months in DCF group *vs* 8.6 months in the CF group). The improvement in survival was at the expense of excess toxicity in the DCF group, and the observed survival in the study was less than expected in both arms [15]. While this triplet regimen is an option for first line treatment for advanced gastric cancer, many clinicians remain wary of this regimen due to the significant haematological toxicity. In practice, it is an option for selected patients only.

There has been a recent paradigm shift following the results of the TOGA study in which 594 patients with advanced junctional or gastric adenocarcinoma with tumour over expression of the HER-2 protein (determined by immuno-histochemistry, IHC) or HER2 gene amplification (determined by fluorescent in situ hybridisation, FISH) were randomised to receive, either capecitabine/ 5FU and cisplatin with or without the HER2 monoclonal antibody (mAb) trastuzumab. The median overall survival was superior in the trastuzumab arm compared to the chemotherapy alone arm, 13.8 versus 11.1 months, p=0.046. In a pre-planned subgroup analysis, patients who gained most benefit from the addition of trastuzumab were those with high levels of HER-2 expression (IHC2+ and FISH positive tumours or IHC 3+ tumours). The median overall survival was 16 months in the population who received capecitabine/ 5FU with cisplatin and trastuzumab compared to 11.8 months in the chemotherapy alone group. Further, patients with the highest levels of HER2 protein expression, HER2 - score IHC 3+, had a median overall survival of 18 months. Trastuzumab is now considered the standard of care for patients with HER-2 positive gastric or junctional adenocarcinomas [16].

Typically, 40-50% patients may be eligible for further treatment following progression after first line systemic therapy. Both single agent and combination chemotherapy regimens have been investigated in the second line. Recent RCTs have demonstrated survival and quality of life benefits for single agent chemotherapy with docetaxel, paclitaxel, or irinotecan in oesophageal adenocarcinoma, junctional and gastric cancers. RCTs comparing each of these regimens and a recent meta-analysis have suggested that each has similar efficacy and different but broadly similar toxicity with a median overall survival is in the range 4-6 months. In summary, about 1 in 3 patients gain disease control, which results in a disease control period of 9-10 months. Combinations of the cytotoxic agents have been evaluated but only in smaller randomised or cohort studies and from these it is clear that the combinations are significantly more toxic, with uncertain additional efficacy. Accordingly, particularly in the palliative treatment setting where life expectancy is very limited (especially if, as is the case for the majority of patients, that treatment is ineffective and does not achieve disease control), it is difficult on the basis of present evidence to justify the clinical use of combination chemotherapies as a second line treatment. For Squamous cell carcinoma there is no randomised evidence for second line treatment, only cohort studies which suggest similar efficacy for single agent docetaxel, irinotecan and paclitaxel as seen in adenocarcinomas. This has led to the extrapolation of the use of single agent chemotherapy in the second line setting here.

Two recent RCTs have established the effectiveness of the anti- VEGFR2 monoclonal antibody Ramucurimab, in gastric and junctional cancers either as a single agent on the basis of the REGARD trial [17], which demonstrated efficacy over supportive care alone, or in combination with paclitaxel on the basis of the RAINBOW trial which demonstrated efficacy of the Ramucurimab paclitaxel combination over paclitaxel alone [18]. Ramucurimab monotherapy offers efficacy which is similar to single agent chemotherapy, but with considerably less toxicity. A median overall survival of 9 months was reported for the Ramucurimab paclitaxel combination and the targeted agent added little to the toxicity of paclitaxel. Accordingly, in patients fit for second line cytotoxic chemotherapy the combination of Ramucurimab and paclitaxel is considered as a standard of care.

Emerging Targeted Therapies and Molecular Sub-Classification

The TOGA trial and the demonstration of the effectiveness of Trastuzumab in HER2 positive gastric and junction adenocarcinomas established the utility of a targeted agent for the first time in this disease area and also established molecular sub-classification [16]. In clinical practice, gastric and junctional cancers are referred to as HER2 positive, (approximately 15%) are defined as HER 2 IHC score 3+ (strongly positive) or HER2 IHC score 2+ (moderately positive) plus HER2 gene increased copy number (by FISH). By contrast, HER2 negative is defined as HER2 IHC score 0 (negative) or score 1+ (weakly positive only). This helps to identify those cancers for the different palliative treatment approaches with chemotherapy plus Trastuzumab or chemotherapy alone. HER2 status is also taken into account in on-going clinical trials reflecting the different treatment approaches.

While the TOGA trial did not include any patients with oesophageal adenocarcinoma, many oncologists consider with some biological justification, that similar efficacy would have been observed in HER2 positive oesophageal adenocarcinomas and use of Trastuzumab in oesophageal adenocarcinomas is becoming increasingly prevalent in clinical practice.

There have been no targeted therapies of proven benefit, and accordingly no molecular sub-classification yet used in clinical practice for Squamous cell carcinoma of the oesophagus.

Many RCTs of targeted therapies are on-going and it is likely that practice and standard of care will change in the coming years based on this emerging evidence. It is widely accepted now that targeted therapies must be used in practice guided by predictive biomarker tests to select patients who will benefit. Positive RCT results investigating this precision medicine strategy will expand and develop the molecular classification of the disease. These include recently developed checkpoint inhibitors, which as immunotherapies have demonstrated considerable efficacy in other tumour types. Recently the immune checkpoint inhibitor nivolumab has established efficacy as a 3rd line palliative treatment in advanced gastric or gastroesophageal junction adenocarcinoma. In the ATTRACTION-02 trial 493 patients were randomized to nivolumumab or placebo after at least 2 lines of previous systemic treatment. While there was only a modest improvment in median overall survival 5.26 months in the nivolumab group and 4.14 months in the placebo group (HR = 0.63, p<0·0001), the 12-month overall survival rates for nivolumab was 26.2% in thsi heavily pre-treated group of patients with high disease burdens, and with most responses maintained at 18 months indicating the occurrence of durable 'immune type' responses similar to those seen in other cancers with this class of therapies. Ideally a predictive biomarker to identify the minority subgroup of patients that have these durable responses will be identified in subsequent studies. Immune checkpoint inhibitors are being investigated in clinical trials in first and second line palliative as well as neo-adjuvant and adjuvant settings. It is important to emphasise that in order to change practice, large adequately powered randomised controlled phase III trials are required, which demonstrate superiority of novel targeted therapies over other standards of care. In addition, for widespread use in most healthcare systems, cost effectiveness as well as clinical effectiveness of new, targeted therapies need to be demonstrated. A detailed discussion of this aspect is out width the scope of this chapter, but a comprehensive review of the current state of the art of targeted therapy development in gastric and oesophageal cancer is included in the key reference list [19].

Most targeted therapies are evaluated initially in the second line setting, compared to single agent cytotoxics or even third line setting (where there is very little evidence to support any systemic therapy). Positive results have and will lead to evaluation in the first line setting and subsequently in neo-adjuvant, adjuvant, perioperative, and definitive chemoradiotherapy settings, where impact would be anticipated to be greater. For example, HER2 therapies are being evaluated in the neoadjuvant setting at present in HER2 positive gastric cancers, and following on from the demonstrated efficacy in the second line setting Ramucurimab is currently being evaluated as a first line treatment in combination with platinum fluoropyrimidine doublet chemotherapy in a large Phase III RCT, RAINFALL.

RARE OESOPHAGEAL AND GASTRIC TUMOURS

Gastrointestinal Stromal Tumours (GISTs) deserve specific mention due to recent significant advances in their systemic treatment. The majority of GISTs occur in the stomach and more than 90% have activating mutations in the KIT oncogene, which provides the sole oncogenic driver. Imatinib is a tyrosine kinase inhibitor initially developed for treatment of Chronic Myeloid leukaemia, targeting the

BCR-ABL oncogene but also found to inhibit KIT. In advanced GISTs, imatinib, which is an oral medication with a few significant toxicities, has proven very effective. In the pre Imatinib era, almost all patients with advanced or inoperable GISTs died within 2 years of presentation. Recent data has shown that Imatinib provides a median survival of more than 5 years for these patients and 20-30% will survive 10 years. In addition, second and third line, targeted therapies have been proven of benefit in RCTs and provide additional periods of disease control following the development of Imatinib resistance. Accordingly, the survival outcomes are expected to improve. Overall, the life expectancy of patients with advanced GISTs is now measured in years [20].

Imatinib is also used as an adjuvant treatment in resected GISTs that have on the basis of histopathological criteria, a high risk of recurrence. An initial RCT demonstrated the effectiveness of 1-year adjuvant treatment with Imatinib over surgery alone, and subsequently 3 years of treatment has been demonstrated to be superior to 1 year. This has now become the standard of care. On-going studies are evaluating the incremental benefit of longer periods of adjuvant imatinib.

Small cell carcinomas can rarely occur in the oesophagus or stomach and are worthy of mention since they are very sensitive to cytotoxic chemotherapy. Combination regimens involving cisplatin and etoposide can provide rapid responses, but unfortunately development of chemo resistance and disease relapse occurs rapidly. Extrapolating positive results from the treatment of small cell lung cancer, combination chemo and radiotherapy regimes are being evaluated in small cell cancers at other sites including oesophagus and stomach with some cohort studies reporting longer periods of disease control in patients with localised disease although these reports are preliminary at present.

Gastric Lymphoma can be effectively treated with chemotherapy and of the other rare tumour types melanoma is also worthy of mention. While most melanomas that are found in the oesophagus or stomach will be metastases, in some cases no primary tumour is evident. Recent success has been achieved with checkpoint inhibitors as an immunotherapy approach for cutaneous melanoma with approximately 1 in 5 patients gaining long-term disease control comprising several years. It is uncertain whether such approaches may be as beneficial for melanomas at other sites. At the very least, consideration should be given to these treatments in such patients.

CONSENT FOR PUBLICATION

Not applicable.

ACKNOWLEDGEMENT

Declare none.

CONFLICT OF INTEREST

The authors declare no conflict of interest, financial or otherwise.

REFERENCES

[1] van Hagen P, Hulshof MC, van Lanschot JJ, *et al.* Preoperative chemoradiotherapy for esophageal or junctional cancer. N Engl J Med 2012; 366(22): 2074-84.
[http://dx.doi.org/10.1056/NEJMoa1112088] [PMID: 22646630]

[2] Allum WH, Stenning SP, Bancewicz J, Clark PI, Langley RE. Long-term results of a randomized trial of surgery with or without preoperative chemotherapy in esophageal cancer. J Clin Oncol 2009; 27(30): 5062-7.
[http://dx.doi.org/10.1200/JCO.2009.22.2083] [PMID: 19770374]

[3] Sjoquist KM, Burmeister BH, Smithers BM, *et al.* Survival after neoadjuvant chemotherapy or chemoradiotherapy for resectable oesophageal carcinoma: an updated meta-analysis. Lancet Oncol 2011; 12(7): 681-92.
[http://dx.doi.org/10.1016/S1470-2045(11)70142-5] [PMID: 21684205]

[4] Cunningham D, Allum WH, Stenning SP, *et al.* Perioperative chemotherapy versus surgery alone for resectable gastroesophageal cancer. N Engl J Med 2006; 355(1): 11-20.
[http://dx.doi.org/10.1056/NEJMoa055531] [PMID: 16822992]

[5] Ilson DH. Surgery after primary chemoradiotherapy in squamous cancer of the esophagus: is the photon mightier than the sword? J Clin Oncol 2007; 25(10): 1155-6.
[http://dx.doi.org/10.1200/JCO.2006.09.4631] [PMID: 17401002]

[6] Crosby T, Hurt CN, Falk S, *et al.* Chemoradiotherapy with or without cetuximab in patients with oesophageal cancer (SCOPE1): a multicentre, phase 2/3 randomised trial. Lancet Oncol 2013; 14(7): 627-37.
[http://dx.doi.org/10.1016/S1470-2045(13)70136-0] [PMID: 23623280]

[7] Best LM, Mughal M, Gurusamy KS. Non-surgical versus surgical treatment for oesophageal cancer. Cochrane Database Syst Rev 2016; 3: CD011498.
[PMID: 27021481]

[8] Noh SH, Park SR, Yang HK, *et al.* Adjuvant capecitabine plus oxaliplatin for gastric cancer after D2 gastrectomy (CLASSIC): 5-year follow-up of an open-label, randomised phase 3 trial. Lancet Oncol 2014; 15(12): 1389-96.
[http://dx.doi.org/10.1016/S1470-2045(14)70473-5] [PMID: 25439693]

[9] Smalley SR, Benedetti JK, Haller DG, *et al.* Updated analysis of SWOG-directed intergroup study 0116: a phase III trial of adjuvant radiochemotherapy versus observation after curative gastric cancer resection. J Clin Oncol 2012; 30(19): 2327-33.
[http://dx.doi.org/10.1200/JCO.2011.36.7136] [PMID: 22585691]

[10] Park SH, Sohn TS, Lee J, *et al.* Phase III trial to compare adjuvant chemotherapy with capecitabine and cisplatin versus concurrent chemoradiotherapy in gastric cancer: final report of the adjuvant chemoradiotherapy in stomach tumors trial, including survival and subset analyses. J Clin Oncol 2015; 33(28): 3130-6.
[http://dx.doi.org/10.1200/JCO.2014.58.3930] [PMID: 25559811]

[11] Janowitz T, Thuss-Patience P, Marshall A, *et al.* Chemotherapy *vs* supportive care alone for relapsed gastric, gastroesophageal junction, and oesophageal adenocarcinoma: a meta-analysis of patient-level

data. Br J Cancer 2016; 114(4): 381-7.
[http://dx.doi.org/10.1038/bjc.2015.452] [PMID: 26882063]

[12]   Cunningham D, Starling N, Rao S, *et al.* Capecitabine and oxaliplatin for advanced esophagogastric cancer. N Engl J Med 2008; 358(1): 36-46.
[http://dx.doi.org/10.1056/NEJMoa073149] [PMID: 18172173]

[13]   Starling N, Rao S, Cunningham D, *et al.* Thromboembolism in patients with advanced gastroesophageal cancer treated with anthracycline, platinum, and fluoropyrimidine combination chemotherapy: a report from the UK National Cancer Research Institute Upper Gastrointestinal Clinical Studies Group. J Clin Oncol 2009; 27(23): 3786-93.
[http://dx.doi.org/10.1200/JCO.2008.19.4274] [PMID: 19398575]

[14]   Waddell T, Chau I, Cunningham D, *et al.* Epirubicin, oxaliplatin, and capecitabine with or without panitumumab for patients with previously untreated advanced oesophagogastric cancer (REAL3): a randomised, open-label phase 3 trial. Lancet Oncol 2013; 14(6): 481-9.
[http://dx.doi.org/10.1016/S1470-2045(13)70096-2] [PMID: 23594787]

[15]   Ajani JA, Moiseyenko VM, Tjulandin S, *et al.* Clinical benefit with docetaxel plus fluorouracil and cisplatin compared with cisplatin and fluorouracil in a phase III trial of advanced gastric or gastroesophageal cancer adenocarcinoma: the V-325 Study Group. J Clin Oncol 2007; 25(22): 3205-9.
[http://dx.doi.org/10.1200/JCO.2006.10.4968] [PMID: 17664467]

[16]   Bang YJ, Van Cutsem E, Feyereislova A, *et al.* Trastuzumab in combination with chemotherapy versus chemotherapy alone for treatment of HER2-positive advanced gastric or gastro-oesophageal junction cancer (ToGA): a phase 3, open-label, randomised controlled trial. Lancet 2010; 376(9742): 687-97.
[http://dx.doi.org/10.1016/S0140-6736(10)61121-X] [PMID: 20728210]

[17]   Fuchs CS, Tomasek J, Yong CJ, *et al.* Ramucirumab monotherapy for previously treated advanced gastric or gastro-oesophageal junction adenocarcinoma (REGARD): an international, randomised, multicentre, placebo-controlled, phase 3 trial. Lancet 2014; 383(9911): 31-9.
[http://dx.doi.org/10.1016/S0140-6736(13)61719-5] [PMID: 24094768]

[18]   Wilke H, Muro K, Van Cutsem E, *et al.* Ramucirumab plus paclitaxel versus placebo plus paclitaxel in patients with previously treated advanced gastric or gastro-oesophageal junction adenocarcinoma (RAINBOW): a double-blind, randomised phase 3 trial. Lancet Oncol 2014; 15(11): 1224-35.
[http://dx.doi.org/10.1016/S1470-2045(14)70420-6] [PMID: 25240821]

[19]   Dahle-Smith A, Petty RD. Biomarkers and novel agents in esophago-gastric cancer: are we making progress? Expert Rev Anticancer Ther 2015; 15(9): 1103-19.
[http://dx.doi.org/10.1586/14737140.2015.1071669] [PMID: 26313419]

[20]   Barrios CH, Blackstein ME, Blay JY, *et al.* The GOLD registry: a global, prospective, observational registry collecting longitudinal data on patients with advanced and localised gastrointestinal stromal tumours. Eur J Cancer 2015; 51(16): 2423-33.
[http://dx.doi.org/10.1016/j.ejca.2015.07.010] [PMID: 26248685]

CHAPTER 6

Endoscopic Therapeutic Procedures

Hugh Dalziel[1] and **Sami M. Shimi**[2,*]

[1] *Department of Gastroenterology and Surgery, Ninewells Hospital and Medical School, Dundee, Scotland, UK*

[2] *Department of Surgery, Ninewells Hospital and Medical School, Dundee, Scotland, UK*

Abstract: The application of endoscopic resection (ER) and endoscopic submucosal dissection (ESD) to gastrointestinal (GI) early neoplasms is limited to lesions with limited depth of invasion with no risk of nodal metastasis. Endoscopic electrosurgical knives are used in combination with high frequency electrosurgical current. Radio-frequency ablation (RFA) is the modality of choice for dysplastic lesions due to its efficacy and low side effect profile. ER and RFA could be used together in combination with encouraging results.

Acute upper gastrointestinal bleeding (UGBI) is a common medical emergency and has an average 10% in-hospital mortality rate. A risk stratification score should be calculated and used to guide subsequent management. Endoscopic therapy can be categorized into injection therapy, thermal coagulation, and mechanical haemostasis. The optimal choice of the endoscopic technique depends on the bleeding source, the endoscopists' skills, the available equipment, the patient's clinical condition and costs.

Endoscopic stenting has become the palliative treatment of choice for many patients with malignant oesophageal obstruction. However, the procedure is associated with a high incidence of complications. Stenting is widely used as a first line treatment option in patients that are not suitable for surgery and those with limited survival. Stents consist of a flexible framework of wire mesh, and are either uncovered or covered. Some have anti-reflux valves as an option.

Keywords: Dysplasia, Endoscopic treatment, Gastric cancer, Injection therapy, Oesophageal cancer, Oesophageal stenting, Pyloric stenting, Radio-frequency ablation, Rebleeding risk, Thermal coagulation, Topical therapy.

---

* **Corresponding author Sami M. Shimi:** Department of Surgery, Ninewells Hospital and Medical School, Dundee DD1 9SY, Scotland; Tel/Fax: +44 1382 660111; E-mail: s.m.shimi@dundee.ac.uk

ENDOSCOPIC DISSECTION AND RESECTION

Historical Background

Endoscopic mucosal resection (EMR) was initially developed in the Far East for the treatment of oesophageal superficial squamous cell carcinoma and early gastric cancer. Endoscopic resection (ER) of early neoplasms of the gastrointesti-

nal (GI) tract is subject to two main criteria: the index lesion should have a limited depth of invasion and the risk of nodal metastasis is negligible. The main benefits of endoscopic polypectomy or mucosal resection (EMR) are their low level of technical invasiveness and lower impact on the physiology of patients. These two factors will also confer additional advantages. In order to ascertain the curative potential of therapeutic endoscopic resection, accurate histopathological assessment of the resected tissue by experienced pathologists is an essential prerequisite. The depth of invasion and lymphovascular infiltration of a malignant lesion determine the risk of potential recurrence. These factors in turn determine the risk for lymph node metastasis. Every attempt should be made to obtain an en-bloc resection, which provides an accurate assessment of the depth of invasion. In recent years, a more refined technique of endoscopic resection has been developed; endoscopic submucosal dissection (ESD). This technique is more demanding but provides a reliable en-bloc resection to enable an accurate pathological assessment.

The technique of ESD evolved from EMR techniques. It was facilitated by local submucosal injection of a solution of hypertonic saline with noradrenaline. A variety of newly developed electrosurgical knives are used for this technique. A high frequency electrosurgical current generator powers the majority of the electrosurgical knives. The intensity of the high frequency current is automatically controlled. Further developments in the field saw new types of endoscopes or with a variety of additions to facilitate ESD procedures *e.g.* Water-jet system or multi-bending system (Fig. **1**).

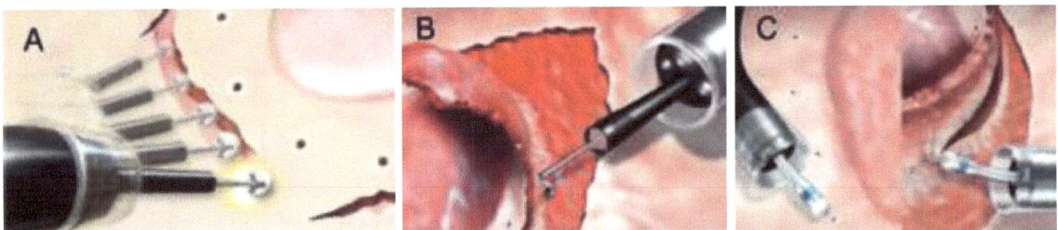

Fig. (1). Schematic drawing showing examples of ESD knives including the IT knife (**A**), the hook knife (**B**) and the Dualknife (**C**). Reproduced with permission.

In terms of the injectable solution to raise the lesion, a hyaluronic acid solution is reported to make a better and more durable submucosal space without damaging the surrounding tissue. Other reported improvements of hyaluronic acid solution include mixing it with glycerine or sugar. Regardless of which fluid is used, it is important for the endoscopist and the team to be familiar with the fluid, its injection technique and absorption time.

Endoscopic Mucosal Resection (EMR)

The technique of endoscopic mucosal resection for superficial oesophageal lesions, involves the formation of a suction pseudo-polyp, which includes the target lesion (either in its entirety if small, or, resected piecemeal) and subsequent electro-cautery snaring of this pseudo-polyp. Lesions up to 2 cm can be resected safely. Lifting of the lesion with saline prior to polyp formation can also be employed to reduce the risk of perforation. A cap device is attached to the end of the endoscope which, depending on which system is used, may place an elastic ligature band to maintain the pseudo-polyp prior to snaring. There are 3 main commercially available systems; the 'cap-and-band' systems, Duette (Cook Medical) and Captivator (Boston Scientific). The 'cap-and-snare' EMR-kit (Olympus) is an alternative, which omits the band ligature stage and simply snares the mucosa that is suctioned into the cap, the open diathermy snare being held in a groove just inside the distal rim of the cap until it is required to be closed.

The Duette system is the preferred instrument in our institution (Fig. **2**) below. Its operation is very similar to variceal banding but in this case it is the oesophageal mucosa (including the lesion) that is suctioned into the cap and a band (preloaded onto the cap) is deployed to maintain a mucosal pseudo-polyp. This method effectively lifts the mucosa, muscularis mucosa and a large proportion of the submucosa into the pseudo polyp, but leaves the muscularis propria and deeper structures *in situ*. This pseudo-polyp is then resected by electrocautery snare (Fig. **3**). Larger lesions can be removed in a piecemeal fashion by repeating the process. No more than 50% of the circumference of the oesophageal mucosa should be resected as this greatly increases the chance of stricture formation. Before resection is undertaken, the lesion is carefully inspected using a high-resolution white-light endoscope. Once the extent of the nodule/area of suspected dysplasia has been defined, the barely protruded tip of the electrocautery snare is used to carefully place dots of cautery on the normal mucosa, encircling the lesion to be excised. If none of these marks remain after either a single en-bloc resection or a piecemeal resection, then this provides confidence that the macroscopic extent of the lesion has been completely excised. If it is thought that a piecemeal resection is required, then the proximal edge of the lesion is targeted first. The next resection takes place by placing the suction cap at the distal or lateral resected edge so that there is a clean defect down to the muscularis propria for the second resection. This is repeated until the lesion, and marker dots, are removed and there is a clean defect in the mucosa. Any bleeding is usually easily controlled by cautery with haemostatic grasper forceps if arteriolar, and topical or submucosal adrenaline if mild ooze.

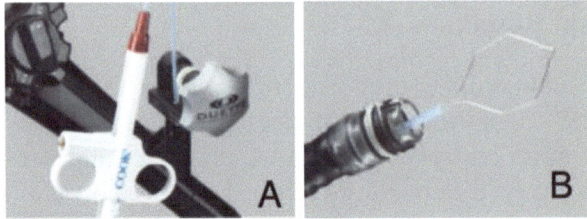

Fig. (2). (A) Operator end of the Cook Duette EMR system. Rotary handle deploys bands from the cap on the end of the scope *via* a string mechanism travelling through the working channel. The electrocautery snare can be simultaneously passed down the channel. **(B)**: cap with pre-loaded bands on the endoscope with open snare. Reproduced with permission.

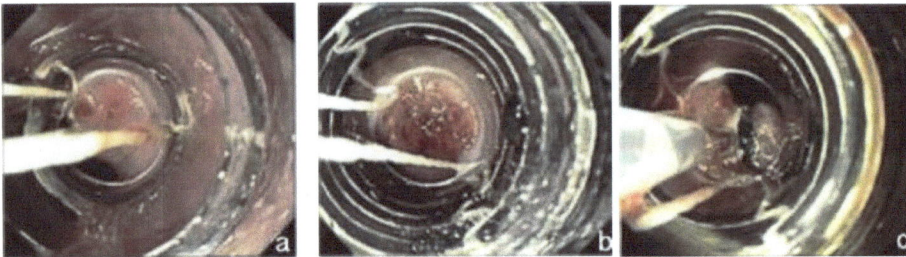

Fig. (3). (a) cap is brought into proximity to the nodule. **(b)** Suction is applied and a band deployed. **(c)** Electrocautery snare of the pseudopolyp on the mural side of the band. Reproduced with permission.

Specimen Preparation

The resected specimen is pinned out on a corkboard as quickly as possible. During the pinning process the specimen is gently stretched to avoid it curling into a pellet, and then immersed in a formalin specimen pot. Pinning allows the pathologist to ascertain depth of involvement and clarity of margins more accurately. When a lesion has been resected piecemeal, the endoscopist should endeavor to pin out each resected piece on the corkboard, as it was *in vivo* to effectively reconstruct the lesion. The accuracy of this reconstruction is crucial to ascertain margins are clear and allow certainty about a R0 resection.

Methodology of ESD

ESD consists of three steps: The first step involves elevation of the mucosa surrounding the lesion from the underlying muscle layer by injecting one of the preferred fluids into the submucosa. Around 10 -15 mls of fluid achieves the task. The second step involves circumferential division of the surrounding mucosa of the identified and marked lesion. The third step involves dissection of the areolar connective tissue in the submucosa. This technique has many advantages. 1. A more controllable resection size and shape, 2. The possibility of en-bloc resection, and 3. The ability to resect neoplasms with submucosal fibrosis. As such, this technique can potentially be used for en-bloc resection of large, complex, ulcerative lesions and some recurrent neoplasms. This technique has some disadvantages including the need for additional assistants, longer procedural time, and a higher risk of bleeding and perforation than EMR. Most centres, have adopted the emerging techniques and developments of ESD as a standard for early stage gastric tumours, particularly large or ulcerative ones. With increasing familiarity, ESD techniques are increasingly applied to oesophageal neoplasms in some centres.

The desired goal of ESD is to achieve an R0 *en-bloc* resection, which has a sufficient deep margin to ensure accurate histopathological assessment. At the same time, every attempt is made to avoid the described potential hazardous complications including perforation and bleeding. Various developments in endoscopes, knives and other accessories have all contributed to facilitate the technique and continue to do so.

In general, the devices used for ESD are one of two types: The needle-knife type and the cross action tips (grasping/scissors) type. The frequently used needle-knife devices are the Dual knife and the insulated knife. Many interventional endoscopists favour these since they perform a dual function minimising instrument changes. The grasping/scissors is less frequently used but are helpful when the submucosal plane could not be adequately elevated of to perform a safe submucosal dissection. Many endoscopists use a lifting technique where an additional external grasping forceps (EndoLifter) is used to provide counter-traction and make the submucosal plane wider. This is particularly useful in ESD for gastric lesions [1].

ESD has a long technical procedure time. In order to reduce operating time, the need for frequent instrument changes could be reduced by multi-tasking instruments. A new hybrid knife is such an instrument and combines the functions of both submucosal injection and dissection in one instrument. A pre-determined amount of fluid can be injected through the instrument into the submucosal. In addition, the endoscopist can mark, divide and dissect the tissue, with just one instrument. This and similar devices have reduced procedure time. Additional safety features in-built into these devices have contributed to a reduction in the perforation rate and an increase in the rate of en-bloc resection.

Indications for ESD

Early Gastric Cancer

Endoscopic resection is indicated for early gastric cancer with no 'known' risk of nodal metastasis, which can be resected *en-bloc*. Early gastric cancer is invasive gastric cancer (adenocarcinoma) limited to the mucosa, sub mucosa, or both, (T1) regardless of lymph node status. The term "early" describes the primary lesion features only. The essential criteria for node-negative gastric cancer have previously been defined [2]. Lesions with a preoperative endoscopic diagnosis of differentiated type intramucosal cancer without ulceration, differentiated type intramucosal cancer less than 3 cm in diameter with ulceration, differentiated type cancer invasive to the submucosa (less than 500 micrometres below muscularis mucosa) which is less than 3 cm in diameter are all considered as reasonable indication for endoscopic resection. Undifferentiated type cancers, and ulcerated lesions are more difficult to dissect with curative intent but some can be resected in experienced hands. For these lesions, ER should be carefully considered bearing in mind the available experience and equipment.

Early Oesophageal Cancer

Early oesophageal cancer (EOC) involving the epithelium (m1: carcinoma *in situ*) or the lamina propria (m2) are possible candidates for ER. These early cancers are much less likely to have lymph node metastasis. For early oesophageal cancer invading the muscularis mucosa (m3), the lymph node metastasis rate is around 9%. The rate is around 19% for cancer with submucosal invasion <200 micrometres below the muscularis mucosa (sm1). The rate for m3 or sm1 cancer without lymphovascular infiltration is around 4.7%. In these circumstances, ESD is reserved for patients either unwilling or unsuitable to have an oesophagectomy. Unsuitability for surgery may be due to the presence of comorbid diseases. Because of the relatively high risk of post-operative stricture formation, lesions spanning more than two thirds of the circumference of the oesophagus are unsuitable for ER.

Nodular HGD

EMR is now considered the gold standard treatment for oesophageal nodular HGD. It also provides the material for a histopathological diagnosis for evaluating the presence of adenocarcinoma invading the submucosa in HGD nodules and for the diagnosis of dysplasia in mucosal nodules. EMR can also be useful in accurate staging of early oesophageal cancer (EOC). Both EMR and ESD can be applied as formal dissection techniques or as a mucosectomy (multi-band mucosectomy MBM). This technique makes use of an endoscopic resection cap (ER-cap), together with a multi-band ligator. In both techniques, a diathermy snare can be used for the resection. In order to lift the submucosa, saline or a more viscous solution if preferred, can facilitate this technique. It can also be used prior to resection when using the ER-cap method and is sometimes with MBM.

After EMR, the reported short-term remission rates from HGD range from 87%-96% after a median follow-up of 22-28 months. The long-term remission rate of EMR as a single modality for treatment is not reliably reported. To establish the long term remission rate, all treated HGD patients should remain on a surveillance endoscopy program. The commonly reported complications of EMR include bleeding, perforation, and stricture formation. The rate of stricture development varies between studies, between 12.5% and 88%. The circumferential extent of EMR and number of sessions are important factors in the rate of stricture formation. Generally, the larger the area of circumferential resection, the higher is the rate of stricture formation.

The use of ESD techniques facilitates removing larger lesions with more precision in removing the area of dysplastic tissue than EMR. However, ESD technically differs from EMR. In ESD, a specialized knife is used to dissect the superficial lesion lifting it away from the submucosa. Similar to EMR, a fluid cushion is injected to lift the lesion to separate it from the underlying oesophageal musculature. This minimises inadvertent deep penetration of the ESD knife or electrosurgical current. Various viscous fluids are used to keep the mucosa lifted and some endoscopists add a dye to the fluid. This helps to identify tissue planes, which facilitates a precision in the dissection. ESD can also be used in the management of BE with HGD and early oesophageal adenocarcinoma. In the latter, satisfactory curative resection rates have been reported with a recurrence rate of 5.9% after two years' follow-up. The reported complication rate was 27%. ESD has also been used to resect early gastric cancers safely and effectively.

Endoscopic Full-Thickness Resection (EFTR)

This technique is relatively new. It involves a full thickness resection of the tumour and underlying serosa (en-bloc). After resection, the full-thickness defect requires closure using conventional clipping, endoloops, over-the-scope-clip or T-tags. The theoretical disadvantage of this technique is the potential peritoneal contamination from luminal contents or seeding of tumour cells into the surrounding body cavity. To overcome this, pre-resection closure using grasp-and-snare techniques have been advocated. The clip is applied at the base of the proposed resection before the resection is attempted above the clips or snares.

Preoperative Evaluation for Candidates of ER

In order to define and delineate the target lesion, high-resolution white light endoscopy preferably with chromoendoscopy if available, should be used. An experienced endoscopist should be able to assess the depth of the lesion, redness, size, presence or absence of ulceration, superficial morphology, and deformity of the wall of the organ. Magnification endoscopy with narrow band imaging technique (NBI) is a promising relatively new modality, which can help to evaluate the depth of cancer and delineate the border. Endoscopic ultrasonography is the gold standard modality to evaluate the depth of invasion. CT should be used evaluate lymph node status and EUS with fine needle aspiration cytology can be used for suspicious lymph nodes. More recently, CPET has been used to evaluate lymph node status.

Pathological Evaluation of the Removed Specimen

In order to achieve an accurate and reliable pathological assessment of the resected area, an *en-bloc* resection of the lesion is helpful. The removed tissue should be pinned with the correct orientation on a pre-prepared corkboard immediately after retrieval and before applying a preservative (formalin). The deep submucosal side of the tissue should be pinned facing the corkboard. At the pathology department, an imaginary line should be drawn across the tissue the tissue containing the lesion of interest. The tissue should be sectioned serially at 2 mm intervals parallel to this line. This enables the pathologist to assess both the longitudinal and horizontal margins. This should be followed by assessment of the circumferential margin (depth), the degree of differentiation and lymphovascular infiltration.

A curative resection should have an en-bloc resected lesion with negative margins where the deep margin is clear of invasion with no lymphovascular infiltration. Node negativity should be assessed separately by other tests. If all the preceding criteria are not met, interval endoscopic follow-up is recommended. At each repeat endoscopy, local recurrence (residual neoplasm) should be explored. In the absence of node-negativity, referral for surgery with lymphadenectomy is recommended.

Outcome Results and Complications of ESD

For gastric neoplasms, en-bloc resection rates exceeded 90% and local recurrence rates have become negligible. Early gastric cancer (EGC) treated by ESD has a 3-year disease-free survival of 90% with a local recurrence rate of 1%. Cancers, which satisfy the criterion of node negativity, are unlikely to represent with metastasis. However, metachronous cancers may be picked up during follow-up in 10. % of cases. After EMR, the long-term outcomes for small (less than 20 mm in diameter) differentiated mucosal gastric cancers are not too dissimilar to the outcomes after gastrectomy. Adjusted 5- and 10-year survival rates were above 90%. For early oesophageal cancers treated by ESD, the 3-year survival rate for m1-2 cancer and m3-sm1 cancer were 95.1% and 86.7%, respectively [3].

The common complications of ESD include bleeding, perforation, stricture formation and pain. Post-ESD, bleeding is more frequent in the stomach, and perforation is more frequent in the oesophagus. To prevent bleeding after ESD, adequate haemostasis should be attempted during the procedure. All vessels found on the resulting crater after removing the overlying tissue should be controlled using haemostatic forceps, hot biopsy forceps, endoclips or argon plasma coagulation depending on availability of the devices and familiarity with the technology. Any small perforation recognized at the time of the procedure should be sealed with endoclips and the patient managed conservatively by nasogastric aspiration, fasting and antibiotics for at least 48 hours. Perforations presenting late after the procedure (delayed perforations), will require emergency surgery as soon as they are detected. The reasons for the delayed perforations are unknown. Uncontrolled diabetes mellitus, chronic kidney disease and multiple comorbidities are patient related risk factors. The use of excessive coagulation and deep dissection and a previous anastomosis are procedure related risk factors.

Stricture formation may occur after ESD in the oesophagus when the residual ulcer crater is more than two-third of the circumference of the oesophagus, or in the stomach when the residual ulcer crater is more than three quarter of the pre-pyloric region. In such cases, stricture formation should be anticipated and pre-emptive intervention is preferable before evident obstruction. Pneumatic balloon dilation should be carried out two weeks after ESD and repeated dilatation should be carried out until complete healing of the residual ulcer has occurred. After ESD pain is not a common complaint. It is usually mild and can lasts up to 48 hours after the procedure. It is more frequent after oesophageal ESD than after gastric ESD.

Management after ESD

Provided there are no perceived complications after ESD, patients can commence eating the following day, and may be discharged home 2 - 3 days later. Acid suppression therapy in the form of PPIs should be prescribed to all patients after ESD to reduce the incidence of post-operative bleeding, create a more favourable environment for residual ulcer healing and reduce pain. After ESD, the majority of residual ulcers in the oesophagus and stomach heal within 6 to 8 weeks. After ESD endoscopic follow-up is recommended to detect local recurrence and metachronous cancers at an early stage. An annual surveillance endoscopic examination is safe and practical.

Future Perspectives

The technique of ESD requires specific training and mentoring and should be restricted to high volume centres. The practice of ESD requires experienced interventional endoscopists who have completed an advanced training program and a period of mentoring in a number of cases. Trainees contemplating a practice in ESD require a minimum, previous skills of diagnostic endoscopy, target biopsy, endoscopic haemostasis and should have mastered EMR techniques should be before embarking on ESD. It is estimated that a trainee would reach the plateau of the learning curve after 30 resections. The trainee should be mentored during these early cases. The technique of ESD continues to go through refinements with improvement in instrumentation and technology. In the fullness of time, it is proving to be a less invasive, safe and reliable treatment for patients with accessible GI neoplasms [4]. Given the pace of development in the technique and instrumentation, this is likely to happen in the short term.

ENDOSCOPIC MUCOSAL ABLATION

The initial modalities adopted in ablative endoscopic treatment were techniques such as multi-polar electrocoagulation, photodynamic therapy (PDT), argon plasma coagulation (APC) and cryotherapy.

Photo-dynamic Therapy (PDT)

This is an endoscopic technique for superficial mucosal ablation using a systemic photo-sensitiser and light of a specific wave-length applied endoscopically. The available photosensitisers are either 5-aminolevulinic acid or porfimer sodium. The photosensitiser is activated in the light exposed tissue and a photochemical reaction takes place, damaging mainly the mucosa (the level of light reach). Although high initial eradication has been reported, recurrence has been reported in over 50% of cases with progression to adenocarcinoma in proportion of these cases.

Nd:YAG and KTP Laser-Derived Thermal Therapies

This has historically been used as a treatment option for HGD in Barrett's oesophagus. However, despite initial enthusiasm, the technique has not proven to be a worthwhile method of mucosal ablation for a variety of reasons.

Cryotherapy

Cryotherapy using low-pressure liquid nitrogen or carbon dioxide delivered *via* an endoscopic spray catheter has also been historically tried for HGD ablation in BE. The sub-zero liquid gas freezes the tissue. Rapid freeze-slow thaw cycles are used for ablating the target tissue. Although high initial eradication rates have been reported, recurrence has been reported in up to 30% of cases. The technique is hardly used nowadays.

Argon Plasma Coagulation (APC)

APC applied endoscopically uses electro-thermal energy *via* the medium of argon gas to conduct the electrical current generated by the conventional electro-thermal devices to ablate tissue. The argon gas is administered *via* a catheter introduced through the endoscope's instrument channel.

There is limited evidence for safety and efficacy of PDT, Laser therapies, cryotherapy and electrocoagulation therapies for the treatment of HGD and BE. Currently, these treatments have largely been abandoned from mainstream use due to complexity of use, suboptimal efficacy, side effects and complications particularly that other therapies have become more popular with a more solid evidence base. APC however, continues to be used as an adjunct to treat small residual areas.

Radio-Frequency Ablation (RFA)

RFA is becoming the ablative modality of choice due to its efficacy (90% and 80% neo-squamous re-epithelialisation in LGD and HGD, respectively) and low side effect profile. RFA utilises various balloon or endoscope mounted probes to deliver microwave electromagnetic radiation to a carefully controlled depth of the mucosa (500μ to 1000μ). The result is a controlled thermal injury resulting in a sheet of dead cells, which sloughs away. Medtronic manufacture the generator units and delivery devices for this system (Fig. **4**).

Recently, RFA has emerged as the preferred ablative technique for BE with HGD because of evidence to support the ease of its administration, its efficacy (90% and 80% neo-squamous re-epithelialisation in LGD and HGD, respectively), and safety [5]. The basic principle involves the direct application of microwave radiofrequency energy to a carefully controlled depth of the mucosa (500μ to 1000μ) for molecular agitation and heat production. The resulting controlled thermal injury (Fig. **5**) destroys (ablates) a sheet of superficial mucosal cell, which eventually slough away.

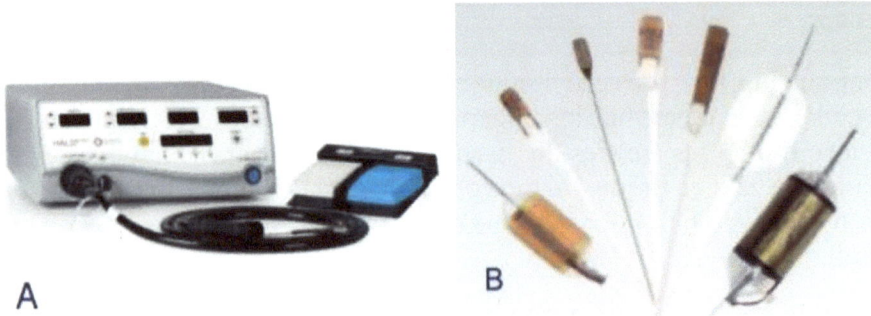

Fig. (4). (A) The HALO generator unit. **(B)** (from left to right) HALO 360 balloon, HALO 60 'on the scope', HALO 'through the scope', HALO 90 'on the scope', HALO Ultra long 'on the scope', HALO 360 sizing balloon and finally the HALO 360 Express combined sizing and therapeutic balloon. Reproduced with Permission.

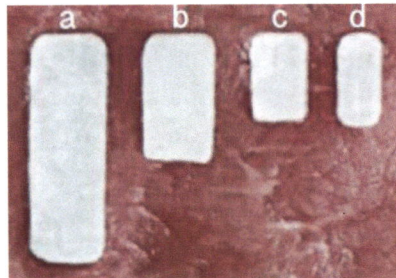

Fig. (5). Examples of the thermal injury caused by the various focal RFA probes (balloons) (seen here exemplified on beef steak) **(a)** Ultra long balloon, **(b)** Halo 90 on the scope, **(c)** Halo 60 on the scope, **(d)** Halo 60 through the scope. Reproduced with Permission.

RFA uses either a purpose-designed balloon for circumferential treatment or an attachment to the end of the endoscope or through a small catheter, which can pass through the working channel for more focal treatment (Fig. **6**).

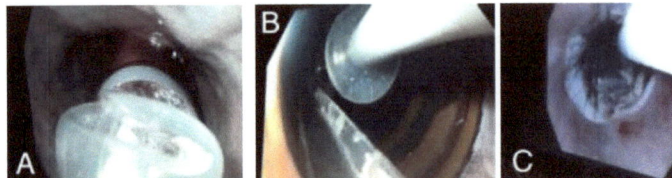

Fig. (6). (A) Balloon inserted into oesophagus over endoscopically placed wire. The gastroscope is re-introduced to allow targeting the Barrett's using direct vision. Balloon aligned with section to be ablated. **(B)** Balloon inflated, with automatic sizing by the generator unit's pneumatic sensors and radio-frequency ablation energy cycles applied. **(C)** Balloon catheter deflated to reveal thermo-coagulated mucosa. Reproduced with Permission.

Using one of the available devices, RFA can be applied to the oesophageal mucosa circumferentially or focally as required. There are two types of balloon catheter (ablation of large areas), three variations of 'on the scope' catheters (more focal targeted ablation of small or residual areas) and a 'through the scope' catheter (flexibility and ease of use) for different clinical situations (Fig. **7**).

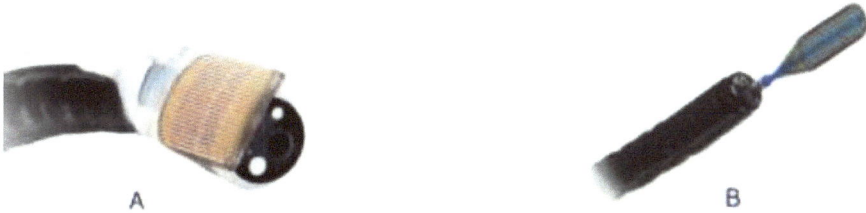

A   B

Fig. (7). (**A**) HALO 60 'on the scope' transducer mounted on a gastroscope. Power supply wire lies external and parallel to the scope and follows the transducer on intubation. (**B**) HALO 'through the scope' RFA catheter inserted into the working channel of a gastroscope. The transducer is now highly maneuverable using the endoscopes directional controls and the ability to rotate on its own axis. Reproduced with Permission.

The older balloon catheter (HALO 360) requires a sizing balloon to be used in the patient to measure oesophageal diameter before closing the appropriate ablation catheter from a range of sizes. The more recent HALO 360 Express balloon catheter has the sizing ability built into the treatment catheter and greatly speeds up the process and comfort for the patient as it involves far fewer instrument re-intubations (Fig. **8**).

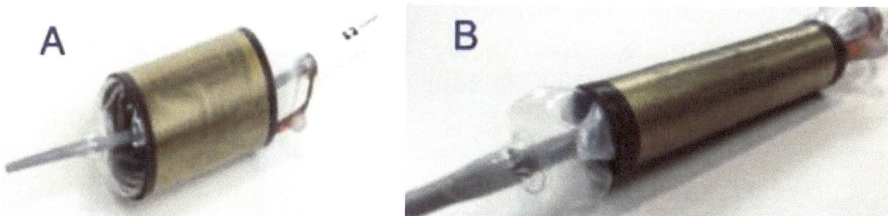

A   B

Fig. (8). (**A**) HALO 360 Express balloon catheter inflated. (**B**) Catheter deflated.

Patients with short segment Barrett's may only require treatment with a focal catheter. RFA is an out-patient procedure carried out under sedation with analgesia and the patient is discharged the same day with oral analgesia and high dose proton pump inhibitor therapy. The most common side effect is chest pain, which is short-lived and responds to analgesia. Post-RFA stricturing is reported in up to 8% of cases but responds to standard balloon dilatation. Peri-RFA perforation is extremely rare.

HG dysplastic lesions can be eradicated using RFA in 80% of patients. This modality is also thought to decrease the progression rate of the metaplasia - dysplasia – cancer sequence. The reported complications after RFA are rare and include a 10% rate of stricture formation after 12 months follow-up [6].

For patients with more extensive BE, circumferential treatment using a balloon at multiple endoscopic sessions are necessary. RFA is effective on smooth BE mucosa, and is not efficacious for the treatment of nodular dysplasia. When nodules are encountered, it is best to combine RFA with EMR or ESD. It is best to commence the treatment with EMR or ESD to remove nodular dysplasia, and after the EMR site has healed, any residual dysplasia or metaplasia can then be widely ablated with RFA. The combined modality therapy achieves a relatively high rate of complete eradication for HGD and early cancer and significantly high rate of complete eradication of intestinal metaplasia with very low recurrence rates. The main complications are those of ESD with the added complications due to RFA. The rate of oesophageal stenosis rate was reported around 6%.

The evidence for using RFA for the treatment of low-grade dysplasia or non-dysplastic BE is less abundant but major trials are underway. After RFA, lower rates of progression of LGD to either HGD or adenocarcinoma have been reported after three years follow-up [7].

ER and Mucosal Ablation

Historically, the accepted treatment for proven HGD in the oesophagus was oesophagectomy. This operation has well-recognised perioperative morbidity and mortality. More recently, the surgical community has used minimal access approaches and techniques such as the trans hiatal and minimally invasive oesophagectomy increasingly. These adjustments to the procedure have reduced the perioperative morbidity and mortality than the traditional oesophagectomy, including a reduced hospital length of stay, with fewer complications. Surgery is still indicated for patients in whom there is evidence or suspicion of invasive cancer to the level of the submucosa or lymph node metastases. In patients with early oesophageal cancer involving the submucosa, up to 20% will have lymph node metastases, with the risk increasing further as the depth of invasion increase. By comparison, the risk of lymph node metastases in patients with intra-mucosal adenocarcinoma, not invading the submucosa is less than 2%.

Endoscopic treatment has become the preferred treatment choice for HGD. Meanwhile, oesophagectomy of one type or another remains an option for some patients. This includes patients with large lesions, multiple lesions and where suspicion or confirmation of deeper invasion than the mucosa or in the presence of suspicious lymph nodes on CT.

The range of endoscopic treatments has also become more diverse. These include both mechanical resection of target lesions and ablative techniques for wider tissue changes. Methods that involve mechanical tissue resection include EMR and ESD. Ablative techniques include several older and largely abandoned techniques such as laser therapy, photodynamic therapy (PDT), argon plasma coagulation (APC), multipolar electrocoagulation (MPEC), and more recently introduced techniques such as cryotherapy and radiofrequency ablation (RFA). These endoscopic therapies can be tailored to the type of HGD present, specifically whether the dysplasia is visible, discoloured, raised or nodular. These features are more likely found in association with higher rates of malignancy compared to the flat mucosa. In order to allow healing of the mucosa after mechanical or ablative therapies, it is important that adjuvant acid suppression therapy is used after all these endoscopic ablative procedures.

Recurrence of metaplasia and dysplasia after endoscopic therapy of up to 30% remains a concern. Risk factors for recurrence include older age patients, higher scores of dysplasia on pre-treatment biopsies, and longer metaplastic segments. A systematic review and meta-analysis of prospective and retrospective studies of RFA found that recurrence of metaplasia or dysplasia was much lower after RFA, with a 0.9% pooled recurrence rate for dysplasia and a 13% rate for recurrence of metaplasia after an average follow-up of 1.5 years [8]. There is currently insufficient high quality evidence to support ablation of non-dysplastic Barrett's oesophagus (NDBE).

ENDOSCOPIC HAEMOSTASIS

Introduction

Globally, acute upper gastrointestinal bleeding (UGBI) is a common presentation as a medical emergency and has an average 10% in-hospital mortality rate. Despite evolution in the management of UGBI patients, the mortality rate has remained relatively high. Risk factors for mortality include advanced age and chronic comorbidities. These patients are less able to withstand the insult of acute upper gastrointestinal bleeding and have a higher risk of dying in the same hospital admission. The majority of patients who develop acute upper gastrointestinal bleeding are admitted to hospital. Peptic ulcer disease and oesophago-gastric varices are the commonest causes of acute upper GI bleeding.

The index investigation for all patients with acute upper gastrointestinal haemorrhage is diagnostic endoscopy. It is controversial whether urgent endoscopy is actually cost effective or merely useful. There is no doubting that endoscopy usually finds the bleeding lesion and can provide additional clinical information, which aids outcome prediction and importantly enables haemostasis and significantly reduce the risk of re-bleeding. In this setting, diagnostic endoscopy should be carried out by experienced endoscopists skilled in therapeutic upper GI endoscopic procedures and familiar with the range of haemostatic techniques carry out the initial endoscopy.

Over the last few years, endoscopic haemostasis has become so efficacious that surgery is reserved for very few patients where endoscopic treatment has failed. Most surgeons have encountered the familiar scenario of patients who presented massive UGIB, which could not be controlled endoscopically, with recurrent bleeding after several attempts of endoscopic haemostasis. There is no universally agreed number of attempts at endoscopic haemostasis before referral for surgery. However, it is important that surgical assessment and intervention is carried out expeditiously and before the patient decompensates markedly. Resuscitation is paramount to increasing the chances of a positive outcome. This should include restoration of circulating blood volume, coagulation parameters, in liaison with cardiology and respiratory services. The majority of patients will require intensive care monitoring in the post-operative period.

Recent guidelines on the management of acute UGIB recommend that an initial risk stratification score be calculated before endoscopy for all patients presenting with acute UGIB. The scoring systems can predict low risk patients who can be safely discharged from hospital with or without additional outpatient treatment. In addition, they are used to predict high-risk patients for early intervention and closer monitoring. There are several scoring systems that determine the need for hospital admission and intervention. It is recommended that each unit adopts such a scoring system and be familiar with its application. All the scoring systems have advantages and some drawbacks and staff familiarity with the system in use and nuances of its interpretation are essential.

Risk Stratification Scores

Various risk-scoring models for upper gastro-intestinal bleeding are widely available. The validated Glasgow Blatchford score (range 0-23) uses pre-endoscopic clinical parameters to predict the need for subsequent interventions (blood transfusion, endoscopy or surgery), rebleeding and death [9]. A Blatchford score of 0 selects patients who do not require urgent intervention. A score of 0 to 3 is used to identify patients who may be managed safely as outpatients.

The Rockall scoring system is another risk stratification system based on multivariate analysis of health informatics including history, examination, blood tests, and endoscopic investigation. This scoring system can be used to subdivide patients presenting with UGIB, into different risk groups (Table **1**). Originally, the system was developed to predict mortality. However, it has also been used for the prediction of the risk of rebleeding [10]. The Rockall score (range 0–11) incorporates both clinical and endoscopic findings to predict mortality. Scores of 2 or less indicate a low risk.

The Blatchford score is better than the Rockall score in estimating mortality and the need for interventions. Ideally, the Blatchford score may be used in the initial assessment of a patient with UGIB by primary care practitioners, whereas the Rockall score is suited to hospital clinicians especially gastroenterologists and surgeons, who are usually involved after admission and may find the score more relevant and informative. The Rockall system includes three clinical variables (age, shock, and comorbidity) and two endoscopic variables (diagnosis and major stigmata of recent haemorrhage - SRH), each categorised and scored with 0–3 points, to give a maximum score of 11 points. For patients with an initial Rockall score >0, endoscopy is recommended for a full assessment of bleeding risk. The score is also used to predict the risk of recurrent bleeding and mortality. Patients with higher scores may benefit from enhanced monitoring and a lower threshold for repeat endoscopy or reintervention. Whether the use of such scoring systems will increase cost efficiency or save lives remains to be seen.

Table 1. Rockall Scoring system [11].

Variable	Score			
	0	**1**	**2**	**3**
Age (years)	< 60	60 - 79	≥ 80	
Shock	No Shock SBP ≥ 100 mm Hg HR < 100/min	Tachycardia SBP ≥ 100 mm Hg HR > 100/min	Hypotension SBP < 100 mm Hg	
Comorbidity	No major comorbidity		CCF, IHD, any major comorbidity	Renal failure, liver failure, disseminated malignancy
Endoscopic diagnosis	Mallory-Weiss tear, No lesion identified.	All other diagnosis	Malignancy of Upper GI Tract	
Endoscopic signs of recurrent haemorrhage	None or dark spot only		Blood in upper GI tract, adherent clot, visible vessel, or squirting vessel	
Score ≤ 5: recurrent bleeding risk < 14.1%, risk of death 5.3%,				
Score > 5: Recurrent bleeding risk > 24.1%, risk of death 10.8%,				

Endoscopic Therapy

For the past thirty years, endoscopic haemostasis has been accepted within the first-line management strategies for upper-gastrointestinal bleeding (UGIB). The efficacy of endoscopic haemostasis has been established by several clinical trials and meta-analyses. There is now sufficient evidence that endoscopic haemostasis can reduce the rate of recurrent bleeding and the need for surgery to rescue bleeding patients.

Despite the established efficacy of endoscopic haemostasis, rebleeding still reported in up to 25% of cases, regardless of the haemostatic therapy used. A "second look endoscopy has been proposed to proactively assess the risk of rebleeding and counter this with appropriate therapy. However, the benefits of a 'second-look' endoscopy after the initial haemostasis in all patients remain controversial. A selective approach for second-look endoscopy is more likely to be beneficial. The selection should be based on endoscopic findings including the features of the ulcer, the bleeding vessel, adequacy of primary haemostasis and pre-existing comorbidities of the patients. If recurrent bleeding ensues, ulcers which are large or chronic should be treated by urgent surgery. Patients who are unlikely to survive surgery may benefit from repeat endoscopic haemostasis using the same or different modality from the one used previously. However, it is essential that repeat endoscopic assessment and treatment is undertaken by experienced skilled endoscopists familiar with the available endoscopic haemostasis therapies together with adequately trained nursing assistance.

The combined benefits of pharmacologic agents and endoscopic haemostasis for non-bleeding peptic ulcers with adherent clots are not established. In these cases, endoscopic manipulation can provoke bleeding by displacing the adherent clot. If the ulcer is bleeding, combined therapy using proton pump inhibitors (PPIs) and endoscopic haemostasis is better than either modality alone in controlling the bleeding.

If *Helicobacter pylori* infection is found in the stomach of a patient with of a bleeding ulcer, eradication of the infection with a course of antibiotics significantly reduces the risk of ulcer recurrence and recurrent rebleeding. Repeat endoscopy is advisable to check on ulcer healing and repeat testing is essential to ensure *H. pylori* eradication. The timing of the check endoscopy and repeat *H. pylori* testing should be between 6 and 12 weeks depending on availability of appointments, staff and equipment.

Endoscopic Risk Stratification

Forrest and colleagues devised an endoscopic risk stratification system. This is based on the characterization of stigmata of recent haemorrhage (SRH) found at endoscopy and aims to predict the risk of rebleeding, requirement for surgery and mortality. In addition, it can serve as a guide for additional endoscopic and medical therapy. Endoscopic management has been based on the Forrest classification of the bleeding lesion [12]. In patients with bleeding ulcers or those exhibiting high-risk features (Forrest Ia, Ib, or IIa), the use of endoscopic haemostasis with two different methods (Table **2**), including an injection of noradrenaline, is effective in reducing the risks.

The identification and features of the bleeding ulcer, endoscopic skill of the endoscopist, available endoscopic tools, familiarity and experience of the team all influence the choice between mechanical or thermal haemostasis methods to be used together with an injection of noradrenaline in and around the bleeding lesion. If a peptic ulcer with an adherent clot (not bleeding) is found, the endoscopist needs to carefully evaluate the decision to use haemostatic methods. If an endoscopic procedure is considered appropriate, an injection of adrenaline must precede removal of the clot. Subsequently, thermal therapy or clipping should be used.

Table 2. Forrest Classification of bleeding ulcers and indicative prognosis [12].

Class	Endoscopic Picture	Rebleeding Risk (%)	Requirement for Surgery (%)	Death Incidence (%)
I	Active haemorrhage	55 - 100	35	11
I a	Spurting	80 - 90		
I b	Oozing	10 - 30		
II	Signs of recent haemorrhage		34	11
II a	Visible vessel	40 - 50		
II b	Adherent clot	20 - 30	10	
II c	Haematin covered flat spot (black spot sign)	10	6	3

Types of Endoscopic Therapy

Endoscopic haemostasis can be classified into local injection methods, thermal coagulation, and mechanical methods of haemostasis.

The choice of the endoscopic method used for haemostasis depends to a large extent on the bleeding lesion, the experience and skills of the endoscopists, the available equipment and haemostatic tools, the patient's clinical condition and to a smaller extent on a cost benefit evaluation.

Injection Therapy

Diluted noradrenaline (1:10,000) injection is used widely because of its availability and simplicity. A sclerotherapy injecting needle should be available in all endoscopy departments where therapeutic endoscopy is practiced. The mechanism of action of diluted noradrenaline injection is mainly by a pressure effect due to the amount of vasoactive solution injected around the bleeding vessel. It is questionable whether the vasoactive nature of the solution exerts a profound effect in this setting. It is essential that a large volume (35-45 ml) of noradrenaline solution be used. The solution should be injected into and around the base of the ulcer in small amounts. Other agents in solutions such as polidocanol, or dextrose, can have a similar result using a similar volume. All solutions used for endoscopic injection haemostasis are similar in achieving haemostasis. The use of sclerosants solutions in injection therapy to control peptic ulcer bleeding is not recommended. These can cause extensive and uncontrolled tissue necrosis. This in turn can result in localised perforation of the ulcer base and other untoward complications in surrounding tissues.

Thermal Devices

These can be classified into contact devices (heater probe, monopolar and bipolar electrocoagulation) or non-contact devices (laser treatment, argon plasma coagulation - APC). They are very useful for more difficult to reach lesions such as tangential ulcers. Generally, the contact devices have a higher perforation risk due to tissue thermal destruction and subsequent necrosis. The popular Injection Gold Probe is a multi-task device, which enables thermal therapy and injection using the same instrument. This minimises instrument changes when the combined approach is used in an actively bleeding ulcer. Haemostatic forceps have traditionally been used for prophylactic or definitive haemostasis during after EMR or ESD of mucosal lesions. The forceps jaws can be approximated over the visible bleeding vessel or the base of the ulcer.

Coagulation Forceps

The use of haemostatic forceps for soft coagulation to control bleeding occurring during EMR or ESD has proven to be safe and efficacious. Effectively this is a monopolar electrocoagulation system that works by raising the temperature of the tissue between the jaws to just below boiling point. This in turn causes vascular protein denaturation and tissue dehydration without carbonisation. The denatured protein within the grasped vessel effectively seals it. Actively bleeding ulcers can be controlled by this method successfully.

Mechanical Devices (Clips)

Mechanical haemostasis aims to permanent occlusion of bleeding vessels. Every attempt should be made to apply Clips on the vessel and for them to remain *in situ* until natural clotting and tissue healing have occurred. Due to the lower perforation rate associated with clips mechanical haemostasis is preferable to other modalities of endoscopic haemostasis. Clearly, the bleeding source should be in an accessible location and the endoscopist must be familiar with the technique for this to be successful. Various clips are available for endoscopic haemostasis. They differ in their reopening capacity, rotation, jaw width, and cost. The technique of clipping is simple when the endoscope is axially straight and can be pushed axially into the bleeding ulcer. The ease or difficulty of successful application determines the efficacy of clipping to achieve haemostasis. Deployment and anchoring of the clip on rigid fibrotic ulcer bases can be challenging in ulcers, which can only be reached tangentially. Those ulcers requiring haemostasis in retro-flexion are particularly difficult since this can jam the release mechanism of the clips. To remedy this, the clip can be partly pushed in the straight position before retro-flexion. Final deployment can then be achieved without jamming the release mechanism. Recent developments in design of clips and their release mechanisms will obviate many of the technical problems. An example is the "Resolution clips", which are easier to apply when the target vessel necessitates torquing or retro-flexion of the scope.

Through the Scope Clips

The main difference between different "through the scope" clips (TTS) is the lengths of the occlusive arms, which strangulate the tissue between them. The more recently available clips 'Instinct Clip' have rotatable occlusive arms with a wide angle in the open position. These clips can be re-opened and closed repeatedly to achieve a desirable position in the process of haemostasis. This means that the same clip can be redeployed if it was initially misplaced or placed at a suboptimal position. Usually, multiple clips are required to achieve haemostasis. Multi-clip applicators can be used to fire several clips without the need to renew the applicator after firing each individual clip. MRI scans can be performed safely with all available clips due to the innate material of the clips.

Over the Scope Clips

Originally, over the scope clips (OTSC) were used to approximate the edges of defects and repair fistulae. Subsequently they have been used for endoscopic haemostasis. The mechanism of action consists of two sharp claws advancing around tissue and vessels to close tightly to mechanically compress intervening tissue and seal the bleeding vessel (Fig. **9**).

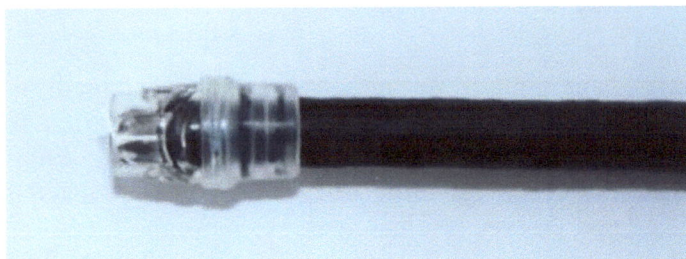

Fig. (9). Over the scope cap containing the clip applicator attached to the endoscope end.

The applicator houses the metal clips preloaded on a cap, which is attached to the end of the endoscope. The target tissue is sucked into the cap (using the intrinsic scope suction) or pulled into the cap using forceps down the instrument channel. A hand wheel attached to the instrument channel is rotated to pull a thread, previously passed through the scope's instrument channel. This releases and deploys the clip. The varix band ligation device is similar to this arrangement. (Fig. **10**).

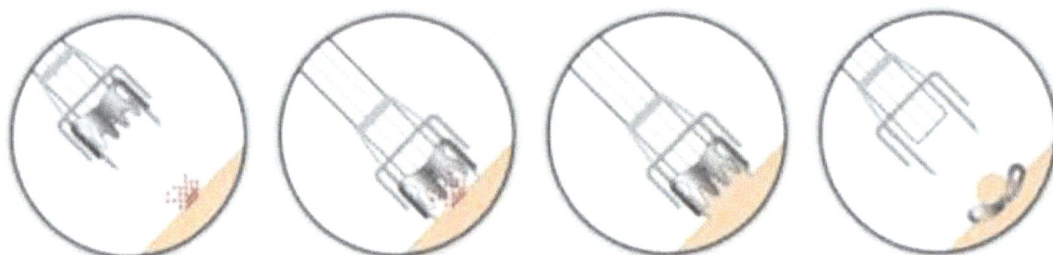

Fig. (10). Schematic diagram showing the steps in clipping a bleeding lesion using the over the scope clip applicator.

Due to the lesser constraint on clip size, the amount of tissue grasped by the claws in OTS clips is larger than with the TTS clips. Similar to the TTS clips, OTS clips are also made from biocompatible non-reactive nitinol. Normally, the clips remain permanently but rarely, can be removed if necessary. Tissue trauma can result from this removal.

Several clips and applicators are available for endoscopic haemostasis (Table **3**). Experienced endoscopists tend to have a wide knowledge of available clips, their features and optimal use. However, they tend to preferentially use and be familiar with a limited range of clips.

Table 3. Different clip models available.

Clip	Company	Opening Diameter (mm)	Characteristics
Through the scope clips (TTS)			
Resolution	Boston Scientific	11	Long retention
Quick Clip 2	Olympus	9	Rotatable
Clipmaster 2	Medwork	12	3 clips in a row
Instinct	Cook Medical	16	Rotatable, strong closing
Over the scope clips (OTSC)			
OTSC	Ovesco	11,12,14	Release mechanism through working channel
Padlock	Diagmed	11	Deployment cable parallel to scope, free working channel

Mechanical Ligation

Detachable Snares

These are used for mucosal lesions projecting into the lumen of the organ like polyps. They are usually used for post-polypectomy bleeding and ligation of oesophageal varices. However, they are unsuitable for flat or excavated tissue as in ulcers. For difficult non-variceal bleeding or rebleeding, a combination therapy using clips followed by detachable snare application can be effective to stop the bleeding. Mechanistically, the clips are positioned adjacent to but around the bleeding vessel. The tightened snare is used as a purse-string mechanism to approximate the clips over the tissue in-between.

Band Ligation

Interventional endoscopists in most units around the world use endoscopic band ligation for the acute management of oesophageal variceal bleeding and prophylactic band ligation in susceptible individuals. Band ligation has a better record of safety and efficacy in controlling variceal bleeding with lower re-bleeding rates than sclerotherapy. However, band ligation is less effective in non-variceal bleeding.

Combined Therapy

Combined therapy is the gold standard for actively bleeding lesions. This consists of injection of diluted noradrenaline solution, followed by thermal coagulation. The initial injection can diminish or even stop bleeding. This provides a clearer view of the field and enables the identification of the pathology and the source of bleeding. Subsequently, thermal coagulation can be applied precisely to the bleeding vessel with little collateral damage. This reduces the risk of subsequent tissue necrosis and perforation at the site of thermal coagulation.

The established benefits of combination therapy include reduction rebleeding episodes, the need for emergency surgical intervention and the mortality rate particularly in high-risk bleeding peptic ulcers. The risks include gastric-wall necrosis and perforation. The commonest combined therapy used is diluted noradrenaline solution injection, before thermo coagulation using the heater probe. The combined action of the injection gold probe is ideal for this purpose as it allows for both injection and followed by thermo-coagulation without the need to change the instrument.

Topical Haemostatic Agents

It is very difficult to treat diffuse multi-focal bleeding from either a large lesion or from a severely inflamed organ using conventional endoscopic methods. Dilute solutions of noradrenaline injections can stem the bleeding for short periods. Argon-plasma-coagulation can be used but it is often challenging and time consuming to apply over large areas. New topical haemostatic agents have emerged on the market. These substances include, Hemospray, Ankaferd Blood Stopper and Endoclot. They are all useful for the endoscopic treatment of bleeding from the upper GI tract with the exception of variceal bleeding. Haemostatic powders can be useful for haemostasis in various awkward scenarios including difficult locations such as posterior duodenal wall or lesser curvature of the stomach, and diffuse bleeding. However, the evidence on their efficacy is limited, these topical agents, including. The safety profile and potential side effects are acceptable. Usage of these powders seems uncomplicated and does not require above average endoscopic skills. Consequently, these powders can be helpful in out of hours' emergency situations when expertise may be limited. While these new endoscopic haemostatic agents are potentially useful, they lack scientific rigor in evaluating their efficacy, safety and role in the bleeding patient.

Hemospray is a synthetic inert powder, which was used in military trauma to control bleeding from skin wounds in addition to standard gauze tamponade. The powder is sprayed through a 10- or 7-French catheter advanced through the endoscope's instrument channel onto the bleeding source using a firing device powered by a carbon dioxide cartridge housed in the firing device to pressurise the powder through the catheter (Fig. **11**).

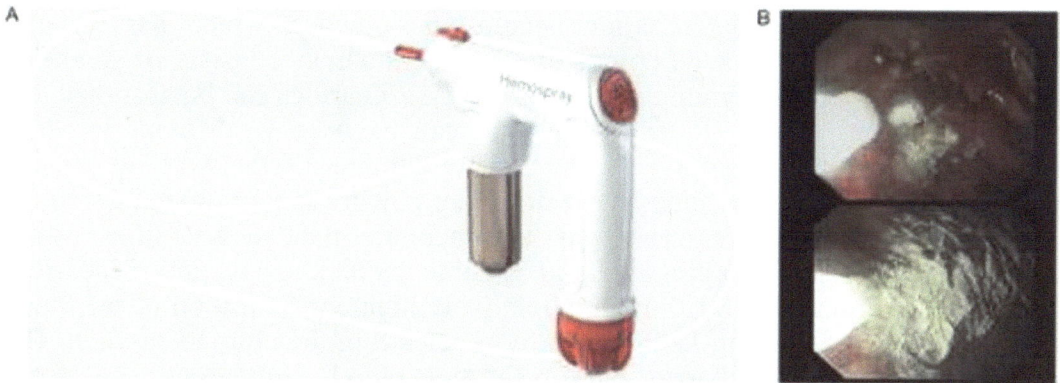

Fig. (11). (A) The endoscopic Hemospray system. **(B)** Endoscopic pictures of sprayed Hemospray on a bleeding lesion in the stomach. With permission.

The substance is haemostatic when in contact with blood products. For the powder to exert its haemostatic effect active bleeding is a requisite. The powder has three main mechanisms of action. (a) The sprayed powder forms a thin layer over the bleeding source acting physically as a barrier. (b) The powder absorbs the serum, thus increasing the concentration of clotting factors within. (c) The negatively charged foreign body powder activates the intrinsic clotting cascade. The use of Hemospray alone or in combination with other modalities achieved successful haemostasis in more than 90% of patients. The advantages of using hemospray include its ease of use, the ability to spray it in difficult to reach locations, and its efficacy irrespective of the cause of bleeding. The disadvantages include its high cost and the difficulty to flush the powder to use another haemostatic therapy if haemostasis was unsuccessful. In these cases, the powder would camouflage the area making visibility of the bleeding lesion difficult. In such cases, repeated forceful flushing using saline solution together with mechanical dislodgement can uncover the bleeding source before a different haemostatic therapy can be used.

Ankaferd Blood Stopper (ABS) is a biological mixture of traditional herbs, which was used to control bleeding from difficult superficial sources. This powder is made in Turkey. It is a mixture of several dried herbs (liquorice, thymia vulgaris, galgant brennnessel). The presumed mechanism of action of the powder is through initiation of the clotting cascade and activation of coagulation. However, the precise mechanism of action is not clear. Ankaferd has been used endoscopically to stop bleeding in cases of Mallory Weiss lesions, GAVE syndrome, variceal bleeding and anastomotic ulcers. The powder of Ankaferd is delivered through a spray catheter, which is advanced through the instrument channel of the endoscope. Until this powder has gone through scientific validation by randomised controlled trials, it is unlikely to be available for general use.

The *EndoClot* is a polysaccharide haemostatic powder, which has recently become available. It is a biocompatible powder, which consists of modified polysaccharides derived from starch. These polysaccharides can be absorbed and readily degraded in the GI tract. Endoclot can be used in difficult to reach locations. The powder is sprayed *via* a catheter fed through the working channel of the endoscope onto the bleeding lesion. The powder is pressurised down the catheter using available pressurised gas. This facilitates the delivery of the powder down the catheter without clogging and possible occlusion. The polysaccharides absorb fluid from the blood, leaving a relatively high concentration of red blood cells, platelets and clotting factors thereby accelerating the clotting cascade. The powder forms a gel-like barrier on contact with blood. This gel adheres to the mucosa and seals the bleeding site as well as accelerating the clotting cascade. The application device consists of a powder/gas mixing chamber, which is attached to a delivery catheter. A gas source pressurises the powder down the catheter.

Removable Covered Stents

Fully covered self-expandable metal stents (SEMS) can be placed in the oesophagus in patients with refractory bleeding from oesophageal varices. It is regarded as an alternative method for haemostasis in patients in whom first line medical and endoscopic methods have failed to control the bleeding. Once fully expanded, the radial forces of the covered stent compress the bleeding varices, to an extent, which stops the bleeding. The mechanism of action is *via* tamponade. This temporary effect can tide a patient over to realise resuscitation efforts and stabilise a perilous situation. Subsequently, a resuscitated and stable patient could be transported into an interventional centre for more definitive management including TIPS.

The stent is constructed with radiopaque markers in the middle and at both ends. This facilitates endoscopic placement with the aid of fluoroscopy. Most stents have hooks at one or both ends to aid the endoscopic atraumatic stent retrieval. This is usually carried out after a few weeks using specialised forceps. Reported complications include oesophageal ulcerations, stent migration and bronchial compression.

Bleeding Lesions in the Oesophagus and Stomach

Peptic Ulcer Upper GI Bleeding

Peptic ulcers are focal lesions, which are usually excavated and depressed from surrounding tissue. In addition, the ulcerated area can be fragile. Bleeding can be slow ooze or a more sustained arterial haemorrhage. Each year, a significant number of patients are admitted to hospital with acute upper GI bleeding. The largest proportion of these is due to peptic ulcer bleeding. The majority of these patients are managed endoscopically with over 90% overall bleeding control. Although the associated costs are high and continue to rise, they are justified on the basis of clinical efficacy and safety. Prediction of adverse outcomes for patients presenting with acute upper GI bleeding can potentially reduce hospital admissions but at the same time flag patients who would benefit from enhanced monitoring. Over the past decades, different scoring systems have been developed and used in the initial assessment of patients presenting with acute upper GI bleeding. These scoring systems have prioritised the prediction of rebleeding as an important predictor of mortality and/or the need for reintervention to either identify the risk of rebleeding or to control a rebleeding episode. These scoring systems differ significantly, with suboptimal formal methodological development, and little external validation.Currently, the standard management for patients with peptic ulcer bleeding is endoscopic haemostasis followed by intravenous proton pump inhibitor (PPI) infusion. The components of a successful outcome in these patients are urgent risk scoring, resuscitation of the patient, urgent endoscopic haemostasis followed by a PPI infusion. Appropriate selection of the patients who require repeat (second look) endoscopy comes with experience. Combined modality endoscopic haemostasis should be considered in every case. Noradrenaline injection followed by thermal coagulation or clipping can control the bleeding in the vast majority of patients.

Mallory–Weiss Syndrome

This is usually a focal lesion but often in a difficult place to reach (OG junction). The lesion is best seen on retro-flexion of the scope. In patients presenting with bleeding from this entity, all haemostatic therapies (injections, thermal coagulation, and clipping) are effective equally. However, bleeding tends to be limited and short lasting.

Dieulafoy's Lesions

This is a focal lesion in an otherwise normal stomach tissue. Potentially, any endoscopic haemostatic method can be used. Mechanical haemostasis (clipping, band ligation) tends to have a lower rebleeding rate than noradrenaline injections for these lesions. If multiple Dieulafoy's lesions are found, these are best managed with topical and spray agents such as Hemospray or APC.

Tumours

Although tumours tend to be focal, they can extend over relatively large areas. Bleeding occurs from fragile neo-vessels exposed to the GI milieu. Neoplastic tissue is cheese soft and cannot sustain mechanical endoscopic haemostatic methods. Endoscopy is a holding therapy for tumour bleeding in the GI tract before more definitive treatments. Tumour bleeding is often a challenge to manage endoscopically because of their size, slow bleeding from ectatic blood vessels. Clips are of limited value in neoplastic tissue due to their poor anchoring capacity and the fragility of the tissue. Noradrenaline injections or conventional thermal coagulation are also less likely to stop bleeding from GI tumours. Topical therapy such as APC or sprays can be used to treat bleeding GI tumours. These can be applied to manage the whole large oozing area of the tumour and the treatment repeated over successive days if necessary. However, the control of bleeding is likely to be short-term with recurrent bleeding a feature of neoplastic tissue. Hemospray can also potentially be used for GI tumour bleeding. More definitive surgery or radiotherapy will be needed for more durable control of bleeding GI tumours.

Gastric Antral Vascular Ectasia

With such lesions being relatively widespread within the distal stomach, topical methods of haemostasis are more appropriate. Thermal electro-coagulation, using APC, is the gold standard treatment for GAVE (watermelon stomach). Repeated treatments are often necessary to achieve haemostasis. Recently, there has been increased use of endoscopic band ligation. This has been shown in studies to significantly reduce bleeding episodes, reduce hospital bed days and blood transfusions. More recently, radiofrequency ablation has been used for GAVE with satisfactory results.

Angiectasia

Ectasia of gastric vessels can be widespread and topical therapy is recommended. In particular, APC coagulation has been recommended as the treatment of choice for this condition. However, this therapy can be cumbersome and the APC devices are not universally available.

Bleeding related to ESD

Intra-procedural or post procedural bleeding is one of the recognised complications of Endoscopic submucosal dissection. The bleeding emanates from the submucosal plexus of vessels exposed during the procedure. Meticulous dissection with inspection of the field is pivotal to recognise and control potential bleeding. Pre-procedural patient preparation such as stopping all anti-platelet agents *e.g.* aspirin is essential. During ESD, prophylactic coagulation is equally important. Diffuse bleeding can be controlled with electrocoagulation. Direct arterial bleeding is best controlled by electrocoagulation. Mechanical clipping can is not suitable during ESD procedures since these can be inadvertently displaced during the dissection. Hence, they are mainly used for arterial bleeding or after the ESD procedure is completed. A noradrenaline injection coupled with tamponade pressure by the end of the scope can control the bleeding in the short term. However, it clarifies the dissection field to recognise vessels, which require more formal haemostasis by one or other methods.

After gastric ESD, Infusion of proton-pump inhibitors is important in preventing post-procedural bleeding. After gastric ESD, a prophylactic second-look endoscopy can serve to recognise or prevent post-procedural bleeds. At repeat endoscopy, noradrenaline injection and thermo-coagulation of visible vessels is recommended. Mechanical endoscopic haemostasis can also be used.

Bleeding related to Endoscopic Mucosal Resection (EMR)

There is a considerable bleeding risk associated with EMR. Bleeding can be encountered during the procedure (intra-procedural) or discovered after the procedure (post-procedural). Intra-procedural bleeding is more likely with EMR of larger lesions, deeper lesions (Paris classification of 0–IIa + Is), and tubovillous or villous adenomas. Post procedural bleeding is more likely with lesions in the duodenum; those resected using electrosurgical devices without a microprocessor; and where intra-procedural bleeding was encountered.

Like ESD, a meticulous dissection is the key to recognise potential bleeding vessels. These can be controlled before bleeding ensues during the procedure and also ensures that these vessels do not bleed after the procedure. Closing the residual ulcer after EMR with clips can also prevent delayed bleeding. If bleeding is encountered during the procedure, noradrenaline injections should be used to stem the bleeding and this should be followed by thermo-coagulation with haemostatic forceps. Clips are not suitable during the resection and can be accidentally knocked or displaced during the procedure.

There are different electrosurgical units available on the market. For EMR resection, it is important to select one with microprocessor control. This limits the applied current intensity to the local tissue resistivity. The settings on the electrosurgical unit are of equal significance in delivering the appropriate coagulation, cutting or a blend of both. Intra-procedural bleeding is more likely with a pure cutting setting whereas a pure coagulating setting is more likely to cause post-procedural bleeding. Microprocessor controlled units which respond instantaneously to tissue parameters are more expensive in the short term but cost effective in the long term.

Bleeding Lesions related to Portal Hypertension

Varices

In patients with portal hypertension, bleeding from oesophageal varices is common. The gold standard management of bleeding oesophageal varices is with pharmacotherapy and Band ligation. As a haemostatic therapy, the latter is preferred to injections using sclerosing agents for in terms of mortality, complications and rebleeding. Ideally, band ligation should start at the GOJ and gradually proceed upwards covering the circumference of the oesophagus or GOJ.

The historical management of bleeding oesophageal varices commenced with balloon tamponade (Blakemore and Linton tubes) particularly in the emergency setting. However, significant complications were attributed to the use of balloon tamponade including oesophageal rupture and transmural necrosis. Subsequently, patients were managed by injection of sclerosants. A decade later, with advances in pharmacology and endoscopic haemostasis, these have become the main tenets of management of acutely bleeding varices. In particular, band mechanical ligation became the gold standard of endoscopic therapy. Recently, dedicated covered, self-expandable metallic stents have been used for the acute management of bleeding from oesophageal varices with proven efficacy [13]. Stenting (using covered stents) has been acknowledged as rescue therapy for patients with bleeding oesophageal varices where band ligation has not been successful in controlling the bleeding episode and as a bridge to transjugular intrahepatic porto-systemic shunt (TIPS) therapy by interventional radiologists.

Gastro-oesophageal Varices

In patients with type 2 gastro-oesophageal varices and in those with isolated gastric varices, Injection of cyanoacrylate or tissue adhesive (Histoacryl) is the recommended therapy. This is on the basis of good results for haemostasis, rebleeding, subsequent scarring, and mortality rates.

The injection is carried out endoscopically. The glue should be mixed with Lipiodol and injected down a larger catheter (20-FG) passed down the working channel of the endoscope. The working channel should be pre-lubricated to enable the large catheter to pass down easily. Once the glue has been injected, no suction should be applied to protect the scope. After injecting the glue, it is advisable to keep the needle within the varix for 10-15 seconds before carefully withdrawing the needle. After completing the injections, the scope must be quickly withdrawn to clean the working channel before any glue residue have set. The patient and all personnel in attendance should don protective eyewear to avoid ocular.

In EUS-guided angiotherapy endoscopic ultrasonography (EUS) can be used to guide haemostasis. EUS images can aid precise localisation and visualisation of bleeding varices and direct haemostatic injection. Radiological coils can also be delivered through fine needles advanced through the working channel of the EUS endoscope. These are used for embolisation of bleeding vessels. The improved haemostatic efficacy of EUS angiotherapy using combined coil–glue, especially for cases of refractory gastric variceal bleeding is advantageous. However, the procedure requires additional expertise in guiding the EUS scope and interpreting the ultrasonographic images.

Radiological Methods of Haemostasis

Trans-arterial embolisation (TAE) of bleeding vessels in the lower GI tract has long been used in place of surgery in high-risk patients. TAE for UGIB took longer to become established [14]. It provides a percutaneous minimal access embolisation of bleeding vessels especially for high-risk patients who are refractory to endoscopic haemostasis. The typical scenario is that of a patient presenting with massive blood loss and high transfusion requirements with possible haemodynamic instability with continued bleeding that has failed to respond to conservative medical therapy and endoscopic haemostasis. Percutaneous embolisation therapy can be life saving for these critical high-risk patients. In addition, this procedure can be used after surgical intervention if rebleeding occurs [15]. Radiological haemostasis is a demanding interventional radiology procedure, which requires specific expertise to negotiate tortuous and often difficult vessels. The bleeding vessel may have inflow from more than on feeding artery and all will need to be controlled to stop the bleeding. After the procedure, the patient will need continuous monitoring to evaluate the risk of focal ischaemia and tissue necrosis in the area served by the feeding vessels subsequent to embolisation.

Types of Procedure

Typically, the source of UGI haemorrhage will have been identified by diagnostic endoscopy with possible attempts at endoscopic haemostasis. Angiography is usually performed as a precursor to trans catheter embolisation therapy to identify the bleeding source and vascular supply. The bleeding source is identified angiographically by extravasation of radiological contrast or abnormal mucosal blush. Approximately one third of patients do not show these features on angiography limiting the sensitivity of angiography in identifying the source of the bleeding. In such cases, empirical embolisation of a targeted vascular bed guided by endoscopic findings can achieve haemostasis in the majority of such patients. This is effective in achieving bleeding control in the majority of cases.

The endoscopist can also mark the bleeding sites with clips placed at endoscopy around the periphery of the bleeding source. This can help guide super selective angiography and embolisation. Endoscopy at the time of angiography can also guide the radiologist in more complex cases with multiple or large bleeding lesions.

Radiological intervention to control UGIB is broadly divided into two types: trans-catheter infusion of a vasoconstriction medication (*e.g.* vasopressin), and mechanical occlusion (TAE) of the arterial supply responsible for the bleeding. Recently, there has been less enthusiasm for using vasoactive infusions. This is mainly because the techniques and results of trans-arterial embolisation have advanced rapidly.

TAE is now an established method of haemostasis in most internal organs and in a variety of scenarios. The risk of bowel ischaemia and/or infarction of areas supplied by the same vascular arcade have always been appreciated. However, selective and super-selective embolisation has enabled precise embolisation of one or more feeding vessels without compromising the arterial input to the rest of the organ. This has reduced the rate of these untoward complications.

The technical and clinical success rates of TAE have been reported to be above 69 and 63% respectively [16]. These results are promising and encouraging and various centres are increasingly adopting these techniques. TAE is currently indicated in high-risk patients, with previous failed endoscopic therapy and those with recurrent bleeding after surgery. Rebleeding can also occur after successful embolisation. Patients in whom TAE has failed to achieve haemostasis or who experienced rebleeding after embolisation should be managed by repeat embolisation or rarely surgery. If surgery is contemplated, this should be done urgently and expeditiously on an adequately resuscitated patient. Surgical resection should be anticipated and a planned recovery in intensive care should be expected. Rebleeding can occur after TAE for patients with duodenal ulcers. The duodenum has an abundant collateral circulation and the collaterals can open up and start bleeding. Successful embolisation must include the proximal and possibly the distal end of the vessel with exclusion of its side branches. After TAE, selective angiography should be carried out to rule out the contribution of a collateral blood supply to the bleeding source.

After TAE, complications occur in around 10% of patients. These include access-site complications (wound infection, pseudo aneurysm formation), vessel dissection, and organ infarction. Acute ischaemia requiring surgery after TAE is rarely encountered. This is presumably due to rich collateral blood supply and use of super-selective angiographic techniques. Rarely, embolisation of the gastroduodenal artery (GDA) can cause ischaemia with subsequent duodenal stenosis.

There are a variety of embolic agents available for TAE. The use of particular agent is at the discretion of the interventional radiologist and usually based on personal experience, availability, angiographic findings, and capability to perform super selective catheterization of the bleeding vessel. Gelfoam® used alone, has a high rate of rebleeding. By contrast, glue used alone has a higher rate of clinical success with fewer complications. *N*-butyl cyanoacrylate glue can reflux into other vessels and cause unintended ischaemia. Coils used alone have a higher rebleeding rate. They should be combined with Gelfoam® or glue using the 'sandwich technique' in areas with rich collaterals.

Predictors of Outcome

After TAE for UGIB, the mortality rate varies between 5 and 40%. Several factors have been associated with a poor outcome after TAE. These include coagulation disorders, delayed treatment, multiple blood transfusions before TAE, and multiple co-morbidities. TAE should be considered and used early before multiple organ failure occurs Coagulation disorders should be corrected before, during and after the embolisation. During the procedure, medical personnel should be available to manage monitoring and resuscitation.

ENDOSCOPIC STENTING OF OBSTRUCTING LESIONS

The insertion of hollow tubes in the narrowed oesophagus to provide immediate relief of dysphagia symptoms started over 4 decades ago. Previous stents were large and with procedure related complications. Some stents were inserted endoscopically while others required surgical insertion. These stents provided some but incomplete relief from dysphagia. The larger stents were not popular with physicians and patient outcomes were not ideal. Stenting using self-expanding metallic stents is now established as the optimal treatment for many patients with wide adoption by clinicians due to their superior outcomes. A variety of self-expanding metallic stents have evolved with different features. However, stents have continued to have a high incidence (23-50%) of untoward complications.

Stenting is now used globally as the treatment of choice for patients who are unsuitable for surgery and those with limited survival. Self-expanding metallic stents consist of a framework of flexible wire mesh made of a biocompatible metal alloy nitinol (nickel and titanium), which are either uncovered or covered by a polyurethane, polytetrafluoroethylene, or silicone membrane. Some have anti-reflux valves as an option.

Indications and Contraindications

Oesophageal stenting is currently used mainly in the palliation of dysphagia in patients with inoperable oesophageal cancer. However, some patients who are potential candidates for surgery who have dysphagia can have retrievable or biodegradable stent placement to improve their nutritional intake while waiting for surgery especially during the period of neoadjuvant chemo or chemoradiotherapy. More recently, covered stents have been used for spontaneous perforation of the oesophagus [17]. The indications and contraindications for oesophageal stenting are listed in Table **4**.

Table 4. Indications and contra-indications to stenting

Indications	Contra-indications
Malignant oesophageal obstruction	Uncorrectable bleeding diathesis
Extrinsic oesophageal compression by mediastinal malignancy	High malignant strictures (within 2 cm of cricopharyngeus.
Tracheo-oesophageal Fistula	Risk of airway compression
Oesophageal perforation including anastomotic leaks	
Malignant pyloric obstruction	

Pre-stenting Patient Preparation

All patients with oesophago-gastric cancer should be reviewed by a multidisciplinary team, which entails a decision on treatment intent and may include a recommendation of a particular treatment option. For patients with advanced disease, the goal of management is to improve the quality of remaining life and palliate symptoms using less invasive therapies. From the patient's perspective, they need a clear understanding of the stage of the disease, treatment options, goals of therapy, benefits and risks of any intended procedure and a relative prognosis. All diagnostic and staging investigations are necessary to facilitate such discussion. Informed consent can be obtained after such discussion. The review of investigations also helps the clinician to have the ability for pre-procedure planning including the type and length of stent required.

It is often preferable to pre-plan oesophageal stenting in all patients who require stenting. However, infrequently, the procedure has to be undertaken urgently due to risks of aspiration, leak from a ruptured oesophagus, an anastomosis or a fistula. The option of placement of a removable stent or a biodegradable one, as a temporary measure, may be appropriate. Patients who may potentially require radiotherapy are probably better stented using covered removable stents rather than permanent ones due to better outcomes.

Techniques of Oesophageal Stenting

Self-expanding metallic stents mounted on an introducer are inserted into the oesophagus *via* the mouth and positioned across the stricture using fluoroscopy, endoscopy or both. The approach using fluoroscopy may require interventional radiology expertise depending on the length and tortuosity of the obstructing lesion. However, some endoscopists routinely combine the use of endoscopy and fluoroscopic guidance when the latter is readily available. This helps in accurate positioning of the stent prior to deployment. Pyloric stents are typically inserted using endoscopy for guide wire insertion and fluoroscopy to position the stent prior to deployment. However, some centres prefer the fluoroscopic approach without endoscopy. Endoscopic stenting is usually done under sedation using a sedative (*e.g.* midazolam) with or without an opiate (*e.g.* fentanyl). Naso-pharyngeal anaesthesia using xylocaine reduces the discomfort of the procedure. However, some patients may require general anaesthesia depending on their tolerance, the position of the tumour and the degree of narrowing of the lumen.

The left lateral decubitus position is ideal since all gastric secretions gravitate towards the gastric antrum and reduce the risk of aspiration. Some patients cannot tolerate this position and stenting may be carried out with the patient supine. The supine position is the position selected when the patient is under general anaesthesia. An anti-Trendelenberg tilting of the endoscopy couch or operating table places the head in a higher position. This decreases the risk of aspiration during stenting. Adequate monitoring of the patient should be carried out throughout the procedure and pharyngeal suction may be necessary intermittently.

Endoscopic Insertion of Stent

An endoscope is inserted per orally and the distance from the incisors to landmarks identified and recorded during endoscopy. These should include the upper oesophageal sphincter (particularly for high lesions), the proximal and distal ends of the tumour and the length of the tumour. If the endoscope is not able to negotiate the oesophageal obstruction, gentle dilation usually with a through the scope10-14 mm balloon will suffice. The endoscope should be negotiated to the duodenum and a guide wire inserted through the scope. The scope can then be withdrawn. The stent with its deployment device can then be passed over the guide wire and positioned to traverse the tumour guided by graduated measurement on the deployment device against the recorded proximal and distal ends of the tumour from the incisors measured during endoscopy. After deployment of the stent, a repeat endoscopy can be carried out to confirm accurate positioning of the stent. If the stent requires proximal or distal displacement, this could be achieved to a limited degree. For displacement, the stent could be pulled or pushed using a rat-toothed grasper. This is not ideal and with experience should be minimal.

Radiological Insertion of Stent

Although this is performed typically in the radiology department, adequate monitoring and intermittent pharyngeal suction is mandatory. A wide catheter may be inserted into the oropharynx for all subsequent manoeuvres. A biliary manipulation catheter (BMC) (6FG) and a standard guide wire are inserted per orally (*via* the wide catheter) and used carefully to negotiate the oesophageal stricture under fluoroscopic control. If this proves challenging, the guide wire can be replaced with an angled hydrophilic guide wire. After repeated manipulations, both the wire and catheter should be negotiated through the stricture into the stomach or for better security into the duodenum.

The guide wire is then withdrawn and replaced with a stiff, 260 cm long Amplatz guide wire which can support the oesophageal stent on an introducer system. In order to assess the length of the oesophageal obstruction and the degree of luminal narrowing, a long sheath can be passed over the Amplatz guide wire, beyond the stricture. Radiological contrast can be injected through the sheath whilst it is withdrawn across the stricture. Using a combination of radiological contrast and air, double-contrast images can be obtained if required. This will enable a more accurate assessment of the position, and length of the malignant stricture as well as the degree of luminal narrowing.

At this stage, an informed selection of the stent can be made. Ideally, the stent should be at least 4 cm longer than the stricture to ensure satisfactory stent coverage across the entire neoplasm with at least 2 cm coverage beyond the lesion at both ends. If there is an abundance of stent length with a short lesion, it is preferable that 2/3 of the stent is placed above the obstructing lesion. In the event of partial stent migration, the obstructing lesion should still be stented. Due to the potential risk of perforation, oesophageal stricture pre-dilation is unnecessary. However, dilatation can be carried out in very narrow lesions to enable the passage of the stent on the deployment device. In these cases, gentle dilation using a pneumatic balloon dilator inflated to a diameter of 12 mm is sufficient. The dilator balloon can be advanced over the guide wire, positioned across the stricture and inflated to achieve the required dilatation. If the stent does not expand sufficiently after deployment, dilatation can be done post stenting. After deployment of the stent, water-soluble contrast can be Injected through a fresh catheter to confirm stent position, patency and exclude a perforation. However, this is not essential.

For pyloric stenting, the initial steps are similar but the guide wire needs to reach at least the distal duodenum and this can be time consuming. Subsequent steps are similar but the proximal end of the stent is positioned 2-3 cm proximal to the obstructing lesion.

Combined Method of Stent Insertion

This is the most commonly used method and requires endoscopic experience and fluoroscopic guidance. This method achieves accurate positioning of the stent aided by fluoroscopy and the facility to examine accurate placement by repeat endoscopy.

After endoscopic intubation, relevant land-marks such as the upper oesophageal sphincter, the proximal and distal ends of the tumour can be identified fluoroscopically by either injecting water soluble contrast (1 -2 mls of gastromiro) into the mucosa or by means of radio-opaque markers taped to the patient's skin. A guide wire can then be inserted through the endoscope which traverses the tumour with its end in the stomach. The endoscope is then withdrawn. The stent on the deployment device is passed over the guide wire and positioned accurately across the tumour guided by radio-opaque markers indicating the positions of the proximal and distal ends of the tumour and the markers on the stent indicating the proximal and distal ends of the stent. After deployment of the stent a repeat endoscopic examination is carried out to ensure accurate positioning of the stent and the absence of complications. This method is suitable for oesophageal, oesohago-gastric junctional and pyloric channel tumours.

After stent placement, dilation is usually unnecessary. Over the following 24-48 hours the stent expands gradually to its stated diameter. Some centres perform a water-soluble contrast study 24 or 72 h. after the procedure to confirm accurate stent placement, expansion, patency and the absence of potential complications.

Stenting of obstructing lesions in the cervical oesophagus or upper thoracic oesophagus can be challenging due to patient intolerance, repeated coughing, throat discomfort and foreign body sensation. However, provided that the stent does not cross over crycopharyngeus (upper oesophageal sphincter), the proportion of patients with these symptoms is minimal. If, however these symptoms persist despite all measures of symptom control, then stent removal becomes a preferred option. This has to be balanced carefully with return of obstructive symptoms, other treatment options available and most importantly, the patient's wishes.

Stent Options

Due to a number of reported unsatisfactory clinical outcomes great interest and attention has been devoted into stent design. In general, stents consist of nitinol, stainless steel or plastic constructed as a mesh, coil or spring and can be either covered or uncovered with or without anti-reflux valves. The old plastic stents (*e.g.* Celestin or Atkinson tubes) have now become obsolete. They have been superseded by self-expanding metal stents (SEMS). These have now become the standard for the management of dysphagia caused by malignant obstruction. They provide effective relief of symptoms, rapidly and safely. The metallic mesh of the stents provides internal support to keep the lumen patent by exerting a radial force against the narrowing neoplasm. The cover of the stents guards against tumour ingrowth. The widening of the ends of the stents impedes stent migration. More recently stents are made from nitinol which is biocompatible, inert and follows the physical principles of shape memory to conform to a predetermined shape and diameter after insertion.

Several types of self-expanding metallic stents are available on the market (Table **5**). Biodegradable stents are the most recent stent innovation (ELLA-BD stent by ELLA-CS) [18]. In these biodegradable stents, degradation of the mesh takes place gradually over 12 weeks' after placement. The degradation is facilitated by acid reflux from the stomach. Stent, which migrate, can be left to disintegrate in the new position or can be overlapped by additional stents. However, this stent is not easily visible radiologically and disintegration time can be variable.

Table 5. Available stents for oesophageal malignant strictures.

Stent	Manufacturer
Wallstent	Boston Scientific, MA
Ultraflex stent	Boston Scientific, MA
Gianturco-Rosch stent (with or without anti-reflux valve)	Cook, Denmark
Flamingo stent	Boston Scientific
FlerX- Ella stent (covered and uncovered with or without anti-reflux valve)	Radiologic
ELLA-CS stent	Hradec Kralove
Choo stent	Stentech, South Korea
Single or double NiTi-S stent	Taewoong Medical, South Korea
ComVi stent	Taewoong Medical, South Korea

Uncovered *vs* Covered Stents

In general, stents can be covered, partially covered or uncovered (Fig. **12**).

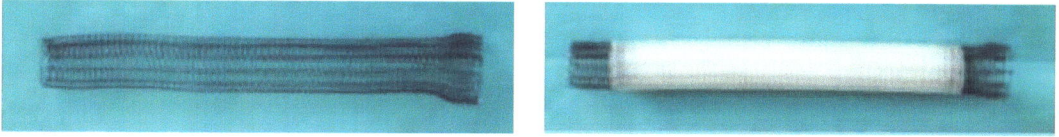

Fig. (12). Uncovered and partially covered oesophageal stents.

Self-expanding metal stents provide better palliation for malignant dysphagia with fewer complications compared to the old prosthetic plastic stents (Atkinson and Celestin tubes). They are also easier and safer to insert. Swallowing is also better with the newer SEMS. When they were first introduced to the market, only uncovered self-expanding metallic stents were available. There was wide adoption of these stents due to their ease of insertion. Epithelisation of the stent took place in the first 3-6 weeks after insertion and this epithelialisation reduced the risk of migration. However, tumour in- growth through the spaces of the mesh was common and resulted in luminal narrowing with recurrent dysphagia. Covered metallic stents were designed to prevent tumour ingrowth and subsequent obstruction. However, the smoother outer surface made these stents more prone to migration. This is more frequently encountered in the lower oesophagus. Another disadvantage of covered stents is the requirement of larger delivery systems than that for uncovered stents. The tumour may require mild dilatation to enable the passage of the covered stent on the larger delivery system. Covered stents have a migration rate of up to 32% whereas uncovered stents have a significantly lower migration rate of 3%.

Uncovered metallic stents are usually selected in patients with extrinsic oesophageal compression, the presence of a markedly dilated oesophagus above a tumour and in cases of recurrence following oesophagectomy. In a dilated oesophagus, food residue can be trapped between the proximal end of the stent and the oesophageal wall. An epithelialized uncovered stent would militate against this occurrence. In cases of local tumour recurrence after oesophagectomy, uncovered stents would be held in place by the external compression and stent migration is minimised. Metallic stents are marketed with a variety of lengths and diameters. It is important to select a stent length to straddle across the whole tumour. Standard stents have a diameter of 18 mm expanding to 23 mm at either end. These can be used for the majority of cases. For a dilated oesophagus and to seal a fistula, a larger diameter stent (up to 25 mm) can be selected.

Covered stents are useful for the management of fistulas such as tracheo-oesophageal or broncho-oesophageal fistulas. These stents can provide rapid relief of respiratory symptoms and repeated coughing episodes in these patients. Stenting of the trachea and oesophagus can also be carried out at the same time using metal stents for the management of malignant trachea-oesophageal fistulae. In this way, the symptoms of both dysphagia and airway compromise are treated simultaneously. However, the overall procedure is challenging for the patient and physician. The use of temporary retrievable covered stents is particularly useful for the management of oesophageal perforation from any cause.

Recently two new types of stents have become available which capitalise on the benefits of both covered (low tumour ingrowth) and uncovered (low migration) stent designs. In the Niti-S covered oesophageal stent a braided nitinol (braided nickel titanium alloy) mesh is covered with a polyurethane membrane over the whole length of the stent. The covering prevents tumour ingrowth. The stent flares to 26 mm at both ends in a "dog-bone end design" reducing the possibility of migration. The other type is the oesophageal double-layered Niti-S stent (Fig. **13**). T basic design of this stent is similar to the covered stent but has an additional, nitinol mesh on the outer surface of the body of the stent. These stents are less amenable to migration or tumour ingrowth while maintaining the intended function of keeping the oesophagus patent.

Both the wholly covered and the double layer stents are available in various lengths (6 to 15.5 cm) and are mounted on an 18 Fr delivery catheter. The stent is held, compressed and elongated on the delivery catheter by a cylindrical outer sheath. The delivery catheter has two markers at the proximal end of the stent, two in the middle of the stent and two at the distal end of the stent. Deployment of the stent is accomplished by withdrawing the outer retaining sheath while the inner catheter holding the stent is fixed relative to the position across the tumour. As the stent is deployed, it shortens by 35% from the distal side, whereas the proximal end does not foreshorten.

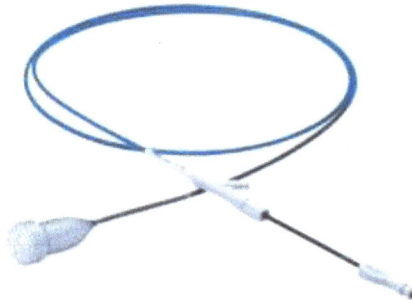

Fig. (13). Niti-S Stent which can be deployed over a guide wire.

After Care and Nutrition

Although stent insertion is described as a day-case procedure, in practice this is rarely achieved. Before stenting, patients should be informed of the 20% risk of developing transient chest pain in the 24-48 hours following stent insertion. This chest pain is caused by the gradual expansion of the stent, which continues after insertion for up to a week. Opioid analgesia maybe required during this period and patients should be given opioids at the earliest opportunity if they complain of chest pain. Patients should also be informed of the potential risks of early or late bleeding and fistulation. These tend to occur much less frequently but are alarming when they do.

Although the stent should restore oesophageal patency, full swallowing may still be impaired and this may impact on nutrition and quality of life [19]. Ideally, patients should be provided with a pamphlet providing clear information on nutritional intake and useful contacts details for further questions. After normal oesophageal stenting, patients should remain abstinent from fluids and food for four hours. If no complications are encountered, patients can then commence taking free fluids and by the following day progress to a soft, low fibre diet with encouragement to drink adequate amounts of fluids and carbonated drinks, which encourages food, remnants wash out. These patients should be advised to sleep with head of the bed elevation at a 30° angle and should eat in the upright position. Proton pump inhibitors should be prescribed to all patients to reduce acid reflux following stenting across the GOJ. Stents with anti-reflux valves may preferentially be selected for stenting across the OG junction.

Stenting Across OG Junction

The need to stent the lower oesophagus and across the GOJ is increasing due to the increasing incidence of lower oesophageal and junctional tumours. Stent placement across the GOJ is technically similar to oesophageal stenting. However, specific problems care attributed to this anatomic location. These include stent migration, angulation and gastro-oesophageal reflux.

Migration rates for covered oesophageal stents vary from 5% to 50%. The reason behind the increased migration rate in the lower oesophagus is due to the distal part of the stent projecting into the stomach lumen without fixation to the oesophageal wall. The issue of angulation of the stent when used across the oesophago-gastric junction is due to protrusion of the distal part of the stent into the stomach at an angle from posteriorly to anteriorly. Hence, the front wall of the stomach tends to push the stent posteriorly and contributes to the angulation. This angulation decreases the effective lumen of the stent with subsequent limitation to nutritional intake.

The development of gastro-oesophageal reflux following stentin of the lower oesophagus over the GOJ is self-explanatory. The physiological sphincter at the GOJ is rendered non-functional by the stent, which allows gastro-oesophageal reflux freely. Reflux occurs more readily when intra-abdominal pressure is increased or when gravity is eliminated in the supine position. Stenting across the GOJ also increases the risk of aspiration and consequently mortality. Hence, prescribing proton pump inhibitors can control the symptoms of gastro-oesophageal reflux in the majority of patients and may reduce regurgitation and the risk of aspiration.

Over the last few years, stents with anti-reflux valves have been developed and clinically tested but so far the results have not confirmed the effectiveness of these antireflux valves in controlling reflux symptoms or preventing regurgitation. In addition, these stents have been reported to have a higher migration rate and symptoms of post-prandial gas bloating. Due to the additional cost and lack of rigorous efficacy data, the majority of units who use stents with anti-reflux valves restrict their use to patients with tumours at the OGJ and who are expected to survive more than 6 weeks.

Clinical Results

The palliation of dysphagia due to a malignant neoplasm of the oesophagus using stents can be assessed either on the basis of clinical outcome (relief of dysphagia with adequate oral intake of nutrition to meet the individual's requirements) or technical (successful stent insertion across the obstruction without complications). The clinical outcome in terms of restoring a degree of swallowing ability can be assessed with the use of one of the published dysphagia scores (Table **6**). The dysphagia score should decrease by at least one grade in the majority of stented patients. However, it is important to incorporate the development of pain or other complications into the equation. Measuring quality of life is probably the best predictor of clinical success.

Table 6. A recognised dysphagia Scoring system.

Grade	Oral intake
0	Normal diet
1	Semi-solid diet
2	Soft diet
3	Liquids only
4	Complete dysphagia

The overall technical success rate of oesophageal stenting is adequately high at around 96%. Relief of dysphagia (clinical outcome) is around 80%. The remaining 20% includes a small number of patients who are unable to swallow and a much number of patients whose swallowing remains suboptimal. The vast majority of patients can increase nutritional intake to meet the requirement with an improved quality of life (QoL). The majority of patients die within 4-months after stent insertion mainly due to the extent of the disease at the time of diagnosis [20]. Additional palliative treatments, such as chemotherapy or chemoradiotherapy increase the survival of these patients. However, it is noteworthy that the presence of an oesophageal stent can cause problems with radiotherapy dosimetry. A number of reports have suggested an increased incidence of oesophago-tracheal fistulae after radiotherapy in stented patients. There is no good causal evidence to support the claims. In addition, there is no conclusive evidence on the increased risks of oesophageal perforation or haemorrhage following chemoradiotherapy in stented patients. Despite the lack of evidence, most radiotherapists prefer to wait 3-6-week between stenting and commencing chemoradiotherapy.

Complications

The overall rate of technical failure is less than 1% in experienced hands. This includes deployment failure and stent misplacement. Significant complications such as haemorrhage, infection and perforation account for less than 20% and most of these tend to be self-limiting self-limiting. Post-stenting chest pain can occur in up to 20% of patients and is usually associated with flared stent designs. Bleeding is reported in up to 10% of patients and is usually self-limiting. Tumour ingrowth is rare when covered stents are used in comparison to 36% when uncovered stents are used. Perforation is reported in less than 1% and is usually self-limiting with appropriate use of antibiotics, antifungals and fluids and food abstinence. If a perforation is recognised early, it can be managed with the use of a covered stent or co-axial insertion of another overlapping stent (together with antibiotics and fasting). Procedure related mortality is less than 1% [21].

Migration of uncovered stents is infrequent (10%) compared to covered stents (30%). Partial migration can be managed with co-axial insertion of another overlapping stent. Complete migration of the stent can result in obstructive symptoms. In these cases, the stent has to be removed either endoscopically if accessible or surgically. The majority of stents, which migrate, end up in the stomach where they remain silent. Endoscopic retrieval is usually possible but may cause bleeding. Surgery is only indicated if a migrated obstructing stent could not be retrieved endoscopically.

Delayed complications such as tumour ingrowth or overgrowth above or below an existing stent can be treated with repeat coaxial stent placement or by injection of absolute alcohol to the overgrown / ingrown malignant tissue. Other delayed complications, are usually attributable to the stent material including stent fracture and fistulation following oesophageal wall erosion. A fractured stent can be removed endoscopically and fistulation can be managed by the insertion of a covered stent.

Stenting for Malignant Gastric Outlet Obstruction (MGOO)

The syndrome gastric outlet obstruction is characterized by persistent nausea (90%), vomiting (83%), regurgitation (69%) and abdominal pain (66%). A large proportion of patients who have malignant gastric outlet obstruction (MGOO) present with persistent vomiting and are unable to tolerate an adequate food intake, and 40% have no oral intake at all. In Western countries, pancreatic cancer is the most common cause of MGOO, while globally, gastric cancer is the commonest cause. Gastric outlet obstruction can be complete or partial with commensurate symptom severity. MGOO is usually a late symptom of a locally advanced or metastatic neoplasm. The prognosis of these patients is poor with a mean survival of around 3 months after diagnosis, with a poor quality of life. The aim of palliation is to relieve obstructive symptoms in order to enable resumption of oral intake. The available therapeutic options include stent placement (endoscopic/ radiological), surgical bypass by means of a gastrojejunostomy, a percutaneous venting gastrostomy (PEG) serving for gastric decompressing with a simultaneous jejunal feeding tube placement, and pharmacological therapy aiming for improvement in gastric emptying, reduction of secretions, relief of symptoms and comfort [22]. Stenting improves swallowing rapidly with early return to oral intake and shorter hospital stay than surgical gastroenterostomy. In the long term, patients with a stent have more recurrent obstructive episodes and require more medical interventions than surgically treated patients. Therefore, patients with a projected short survival (less than 2 months) would benefit more from stent placement. However, patients expected to survive longer periods should be considered for a palliative gastroenterostomy [23].

Self-expandable metal stents (SEMSs) are used for the endoscopic management of MGOO and are usually covered or partially covered. Patients referred for pyloric stenting should be admitted to hospital 48 hours in advance for gastric lavage using a naso-gastric tube. During this period, intravenous administration of fluids and nutrition is essential.

Technical and Clinical Success of Stenting MGOO

Technical success can be achieved in up to 97% of patients. The factors associated with failure include inability to pass the guide wire across the distal gastric stenosis (1.0%), stent misplacement (0.3%) and failed deployment (0.3%). Procedure-related perforation is rare. The overall rate of a successful clinical outcome is around 85%. In general, partially covered stents have a higher rate of clinical success than uncovered self- stents. After stenting, careful follow-up is necessary, with the possibility of further interventional endoscopic procedures in over a half of the patients stented [24].

Stent Dysfunction

Stent dysfunction is reported to be due to obstruction of the stent by tumour in- or overgrowth (12%) and stent migration (4%). Stent compression and deformation by the tumour mass is a rare phenomenon. Other rare reasons for stent dysfunction include food occlusion, insufficient expansion, and rarely, stent fracture.

Perforation and Bleeding

The overall perforation rate is around 1%. Early perforations are slightly more common than late perforations. Bleeding is reported in 4% of patients and it is self-limiting in the majority of patients. More major bleeding, requiring a haemostatic intervention, occurs in less than 1% of patients.

Stent Patency and Overall Survival

The mean stent patency is around 3 months and the mean overall survival is around 4 months. Patients with gastric cancer tend to survive slightly longer than patients with pancreatic cancer.

SEMS Stenting Procedure

A combined radiological and endoscopic procedure is preferred in most centres [25]. After sedation, per oral endoscopy is carried out. The obstructive pyloric lesion should be assessed and a smooth biliary guide wire (260 Cm) is passed through the instrument channel of the endoscope and guided through the obstructing tumour. The endoscope is withdrawn and a radiological catheter is passed over the guide wire into the duodenum across the obstructing lesion. A water-soluble contrast medium (Gastrograffin) is injected into the catheter and the length of the stricture is measured by fluoroscopy. The flexible guide wire is replaced with a heavy wire through the catheter. The stent mounted on the delivery system is then advanced over the heavy guide wire into position under fluoroscopy and endoscopy. After positioning the stent, it is released from the distal end. A water-soluble contrast medium can be injected through the stent to check position across the obstruction and stent patency using fluoroscopy. Expansion and position of the stent can be confirmed by serial abdominal plain radiography taken at adequate intervals.

Evaluation of Subjective Symptoms after SEMS

The gastric outlet obstruction scoring system (GOOSS) can be used to evaluate obstructive symptoms and compare clinical outcomes (Table **7**).

Table 7. Gastric Outlet Obstruction Scoring System (GOOSS)

Oral Intake	Score
No oral intake	0
Liquids only	1
Soft solids	2
Almost complete or normal diet	3

The ability to take solid diet is indicated by score 2 or 3.

The GOOSS value is assigned on a 4-point scale: 0, no oral intake; 1, liquids only; 2, soft solids only; 3, low residue or full diet. The score could be repeated at several time points before and after the procedure for comparison. The GOOSS score should improve immediately after stent placement.

Future Advances in Oesophageal Stenting

Stents design and performance are in a constant state of improvement. The manufacturing industry has been engaged with the clinical community to meet the clinical demand for stent design and durability. Within this engagement, they have reviewed a variety of clinical reports specifically looking the requirements of a successful clinical outcome. Stent migration has been at the top of the agenda and identified mechanisms to stop this include applying adhesive materials to the outer surface of the stent or technical modifications to both ends of the stent with anchoring mechanisms. In addition, increasing stent flexibility and durability of the covering membrane by using state of the art synthetic membranes. Relatively recently, cytotoxic drug-eluting stents have been designed which may inhibit growth of malignant tissue ingrowth thereby increasing stent patency and durability. These are likely to be on the market shortly.

Biodegradable oesophageal stents (woven polydioxanone) are currently available for use. Polydioxanone is a biodegradable polymer with sufficient flexibility and shape memory ability once it is deployed. Biodegradable stents can remain *in situ* enabling swallowing for up to 6 weeks. After this period, the stents are degraded and swallowing ability deteriorates gradually. This seems ideal for patients with dysphagia receiving neoadjuvant chemo or chemoradiotherapy prior to surgery. However, this period is insufficient for patients with palliative treatment intent without other modalities of treatment. Increasing stent durability is one of the current areas of technical work. Other possible improvements in this stent can incorporate radiopaque markers to facilitate radiographic detection either during insertion, deployment or subsequently. The gradual decrease in radial force and elasticity over time can also limit their functional durability. This could be improved by a variety of means.

CONSENT FOR PUBLICATION

Not applicable.

ACKNOWLEDGEMENT

Declare none.

CONFLICT OF INTEREST

The authors declare no conflict of interest, financial or otherwise.

REFERENCES

[1]   Tsuji K, Yoshida N, Nakanishi H, Takemura K, Yamada S, Doyama H. Recent traction methods for endoscopic submucosal dissection. World J Gastroenterol 2016; 22(26): 5917-26.
[http://dx.doi.org/10.3748/wjg.v22.i26.5917] [PMID: 27468186]

[2]   The Paris endoscopic classification of superficial neoplastic lesions: esophagus, stomach, and colon: November 30 to December 1, 2002. Gastrointest Endosc 2003; 58(6) (Suppl.): S3-S43.
[http://dx.doi.org/10.1016/S0016-5107(03)02159-X] [PMID: 14652541]

[3]   Komeda Y, Bruno M, Koch A. EMR is not inferior to ESD for early Barrett's and EGJ neoplasia: An extensive review on outcome, recurrence and complication rates. Endosc Int Open 2014; 2(2): E58-64.
[http://dx.doi.org/10.1055/s-0034-1365528] [PMID: 26135261]

[4]   Maple JT, Abu Dayyeh BK, Chauhan SS, *et al.* Endoscopic submucosal dissection. Gastrointest Endosc 2015; 81(6): 1311-25.
[http://dx.doi.org/10.1016/j.gie.2014.12.010] [PMID: 25796422]

[5]   Bennett C, Vakil N, Bergman J, *et al.* Consensus statements for management of Barrett's dysplasia and early-stage esophageal adenocarcinoma, based on a Delphi process. Gastroenterology 2012; 143(2): 336-46.
[http://dx.doi.org/10.1053/j.gastro.2012.04.032] [PMID: 22537613]

[6]   Phoa KN, Pouw RE, van Vilsteren FG, *et al.* Remission of Barrett's esophagus with early neoplasia 5 years after radiofrequency ablation with endoscopic resection: a Netherlands cohort study. Gastroenterology 2013; 145(1): 96-104.
[http://dx.doi.org/10.1053/j.gastro.2013.03.046] [PMID: 23542068]

[7]   Phoa KN, van Vilsteren FG, Weusten BL, *et al.* Radiofrequency ablation *vs* endoscopic surveillance for patients with Barrett esophagus and low-grade dysplasia: a randomized clinical trial. JAMA 2014; 311(12): 1209-17.
[http://dx.doi.org/10.1001/jama.2014.2511] [PMID: 24668102]

[8] Orman ES, Li N, Shaheen NJ. Efficacy and durability of radiofrequency ablation for Barrett's Esophagus: systematic review and meta-analysis. Clin Gastroenterol Hepatol 2013; 11(10): 1245-55.
[http://dx.doi.org/10.1016/j.cgh.2013.03.039] [PMID: 23644385]

[9] Blatchford O, Murray WR, Blatchford M. A risk score to predict need for treatment for upper-gastrointestinal haemorrhage. Lancet 2000; 356(9238): 1318-21.
[http://dx.doi.org/10.1016/S0140-6736(00)02816-6] [PMID: 11073021]

[10] Rockall TA, Logan RF, Devlin HB, Northfield TC. Influencing the practice and outcome in acute upper gastrointestinal haemorrhage. Gut 1997; 41(5): 606-11.
[http://dx.doi.org/10.1136/gut.41.5.606] [PMID: 9414965]

[11] Rockall TA, Logan RF, Devlin HB, Northfield TC. Risk assessment after acute upper gastrointestinal haemorrhage. Gut 1996; 38(3): 316-21.
[http://dx.doi.org/10.1136/gut.38.3.316] [PMID: 8675081]

[12] Forrest JA, Finlayson ND, Shearman DJ. Endoscopy in gastrointestinal bleeding. Lancet 1974; 2(7877): 394-7.
[http://dx.doi.org/10.1016/S0140-6736(74)91770-X] [PMID: 4136718]

[13] Changela K, Ona MA, Anand S, Duddempudi S. Self-Expanding Metal Stent (SEMS): an innovative rescue therapy for refractory acute variceal bleeding. Endosc Int Open 2014; 2(4): E244-51.
[http://dx.doi.org/10.1055/s-0034-1377980] [PMID: 26135101]

[14] Aina R, Oliva VL, Therasse E, *et al.* Arterial embolotherapy for upper gastrointestinal hemorrhage: outcome assessment. J Vasc Interv Radiol 2001; 12(2): 195-200.
[http://dx.doi.org/10.1016/S1051-0443(07)61825-9] [PMID: 11265883]

[15] Lu Y, Loffroy R, Lau JY, Barkun A. Multidisciplinary management strategies for acute non-variceal upper gastrointestinal bleeding. Br J Surg 2014; 101(1): e34-50.
[http://dx.doi.org/10.1002/bjs.9351] [PMID: 24277160]

[16] Loffroy R, Rao P, Ota S, De Lin M, Kwak BK, Geschwind JF. Embolization of acute nonvariceal upper gastrointestinal hemorrhage resistant to endoscopic treatment: results and predictors of recurrent bleeding. Cardiovasc Intervent Radiol 2010; 33(6): 1088-100.
[http://dx.doi.org/10.1007/s00270-010-9829-7] [PMID: 20232200]

[17] Glatz T, Marjanovic G, Kulemann B, Hipp J, Theodor Hopt U, Fischer A, *et al.* Management and outcome of esophageal stenting for spontaneous esophageal perforations. Dis Esophagus 2016; (Oct): 28.
[PMID: 27790804]

[18] Griffiths EA, Gregory CJ, Pursnani KG, Ward JB, Stockwell RC. The use of biodegradable (SX-ELLA) oesophageal stents to treat dysphagia due to benign and malignant oesophageal disease. Surg Endosc 2012; 26(8): 2367-75.
[http://dx.doi.org/10.1007/s00464-012-2192-9] [PMID: 22395954]

[19] Diamantis G, Scarpa M, Bocus P, *et al.* Quality of life in patients with esophageal stenting for the palliation of malignant dysphagia. World J Gastroenterol 2011; 17(2): 144-50.
[http://dx.doi.org/10.3748/wjg.v17.i2.144] [PMID: 21245986]

[20] Stewart DJ, Balamurugan R, Everitt NJ, Ravi K. Ten-year experience of esophageal self-expanding metal stent insertion at a single institution. Dis Esophagus 2013; 26(3): 276-81.
[http://dx.doi.org/10.1111/j.1442-2050.2012.01364.x] [PMID: 22676427]

[21] Gray RT, O'Donnell ME, Scott RD, McGuigan JA, Mainie I. Self-expanding metal stent insertion for inoperable esophageal carcinoma in Belfast: an audit of outcomes and literature review. Dis Esophagus 2011; 24(8): 569-74.
[http://dx.doi.org/10.1111/j.1442-2050.2011.01188.x] [PMID: 21418125]

[22] Kiely JM, Dua KS, Graewin SJ, *et al.* Palliative stenting for late malignant gastric outlet obstruction. J Gastrointest Surg 2007; 11(1): 107-13.

[http://dx.doi.org/10.1007/s11605-006-0060-4] [PMID: 17390196]

[23]   Jeurnink SM, Steyerberg EW, Hof Gv, van Eijck CH, Kuipers EJ, Siersema PD. Gastrojejunostomy versus stent placement in patients with malignant gastric outlet obstruction: a comparison in 95 patients. J Surg Oncol 2007; 96(5): 389-96.
       [http://dx.doi.org/10.1002/jso.20828] [PMID: 17474082]

[24]   Fiori E, Lamazza A, Demasi E, Decesare A, Schillaci A, Sterpetti AV. Endoscopic stenting for gastric outlet obstruction in patients with unresectable antro pyloric cancer. Systematic review of the literature and final results of a prospective study. The point of view of a surgical group. Am J Surg 2013; 206(2): 210-7.
       [http://dx.doi.org/10.1016/j.amjsurg.2012.08.018] [PMID: 23735668]

[25]   Lowe AS, Beckett CG, Jowett S, *et al.* Self-expandable metal stent placement for the palliation of malignant gastroduodenal obstruction: experience in a large, single, UK centre. Clin Radiol 2007; 62(8): 738-44.
       [http://dx.doi.org/10.1016/j.crad.2007.01.021] [PMID: 17604761]

CHAPTER 7

Bariatric Anaesthesia

Shaun McLeod[*]

Department of Anaesthesia, Ninewells Hospital and Medical School, Dundee, Scotland, UK

Abstract: Obesity is a complex multi-system disorder, which is increasingly recognized as one of the greatest challenges faced by health care systems throughout the world. Obesity is classified on the basis of both the BMI and the fat distribution. Surgical bariatric procedures can achieve up to 50% weight loss and this is sustained for a longer period of time. The procedures, although not without risk, are relatively safe with low morbidity and mortality rates. A key marker for increased risk of perioperative complications is central obesity. The presence of obstructive sleep apnoea is an independent marker of risk that leads to the doubling of postoperative respiratory and cardiac complications. Obese patients will have a markedly different volume of distribution of drugs as a result of the adipose tissue. To compensate for these changes drug dosing in obese patients is based on a combination of adjusted body weight, total body weight, ideal body weight and lean body mass. Adequate time and preparation is essential to provide safe conditions to anaesthetise obese patients. There are specific considerations for the intra-operative anaesthetic management of obese individuals, which need to be adhered to for the safe conduct and reversal of anaesthesia. Most patients presenting for bariatric surgery can be discharged to a ward environment. However, some patients carry an increased risk and as such may be required to be cared for in a high dependency or an intensive care unit. In addition, a number of patients may require specific measures for safe hospital discharge.

Keywords: Anaesthesia, Anaesthetic management, Analgesia, Bariatric surgery, Monitoring, Obesity hypoventilation syndrome, Obstructive sleep apnoea, Post-operative care, Respiratory function, Risk stratification scores.

ANAESTHESIA IN BARIATRIC SURGERY

Introduction

Obesity is a complex multi-system disorder, which is increasingly recognized as one of the greatest challenges faced by health care systems throughout the world. Obesity is associated with a heavy disease burden that increases both morbidity and mortality. Health and Social Care Center statistics in the United Kingdom

---

[*] **Corresponding author Shaun McLeod:** Department of Anaesthesia, Ninewells Hospital and Medical School, Dundee DD1 9SY, Scotland, UK; Tel/Fax: +44 1382 660111; E-mail: shaun.mcleod@nhs.net

Sami M. Shimi

show that in 2013, 24% of men and 25% of women are classified as obese with a Body Mass Index (BMI) >30. The prevalence of obesity is increasing. It has been predicted that by 2050, 50% of the UK population will be obese. This prevalence is similarly mirrored throughout the Western world with some countries having a higher obesity rate and others less.

Obesity is classified on the basis of both the BMI and the fat distribution. The World Health Organisation classification based on BMI directly and provides a useful tool in stratifying obese patients (Table **1**). Anyone with a BMI >30 is at an increased risk of peri-operative morbidity and mortality but those with a BMI >40 or, a BMI >35 with comorbid disease are at significant risk of peri-operative morbidity and mortality [1].

Table 1. Classification of obesity based on BMI (WHO) [1].

Body Mass Index (kg.m^2)	Classification
<18.5	Underweight
18.5-24.9	Normal
25.0-29.9	Overweight
30.0-34.9	Obese 1
35.0-39.9	Obese 2
>40.0	Obese 3

Fat distribution is classically described as:

- *Android* distribution: involves mainly central fat distribution, which is usually intra-peritoneal and focused on the liver and the omentum.
- *Gynaecoid* distribution: involves mainly peripheral areas such as the arms, legs and buttocks.

Each distribution can occur in both genders but android is more common in men and is associated with increased morbidity and mortality. It is important to note that BMI by itself is a poor predictor of anaesthetic and surgical difficulties but fat distribution is a more accurate predictor of risk.

Obesity, particularly in patients with gynaecoid fat distribution, is associated with several disease processes including:

- Hypertension
- Dyslipidaemia
- Diabetes Mellitus
- Ischaemic Heart disease

- Obstructive Sleep Apnoea
- Obesity Hypoventilation Syndrome
- Liver disease
- Osteoarthritis

A higher BMI with longer duration of obesity are associated with increased prevalence and severity of these disease processes.

It is well recognized that 5-10% weight reduction can improve the health of the obese individual and reduce the incidence of associated diseases. Lifestyle changes and drug therapy are important however they have limited roles, as sustained significant weight reduction is not often achieved. Surgical bariatric procedures can achieve up to 50% weight loss and this is sustained for a longer period of time. The procedures, although not without risk, are relatively safe with low morbidity and mortality rates.

Bariatric services should be provided by an experienced multi-disciplinary team, which includes a Surgeon, Anaesthetist, Physician with interest in endocrinology and/ or obesity, Dietician, Psychologist and a Specialist nurse.

A holistic bariatric service should include advice on diet and lifestyle modifications including increased physical activity for all obese patients. In addition, the Multidisciplinary team should consider a pharmacological approach for obesity and associated or aetiological disorders. In this regard, drug therapy has a very limited role in weight reduction due to lack of long term efficacy and significant side effects. Psychologists play an increasing role in assessing the motivation of obese patients as well as aetiological and emergent emotional factors. Dieticians play a central role in all stages of management. They provide dietary advice as a treatment modality but also in preparation for, and after surgery. Surgeons should be able to offer both restrictive and mal-absorptive surgery. Surgical procedures were traditionally done by open surgery but increasingly surgeons are offering laparoscopic procedures.

Pathophysiology of Obesity

Obesity is a syndrome of physical-related and metabolic-related conditions. The physical changes and comorbidities include degenerative joint disease (DJD), hyperkinetic circulation, increased blood volume, increased renal blood flow, increased intra-abdominal pressure, increased intrathoracic pressure with restrictive pattern, decubital changes, and psychosocial incapacity. The Metabolic Syndrome (Syndrome X) encompasses the cardiovascular, endocrine, and immunologic consequences of obesity. The components of metabolic obesity are linked to energy balance with the major determinant being caloric intake. A rapid eating rate leads to increased production of insulin and pancreatic polypeptides, as well as increased absorptive effects, which, in turn, determine glucotoxicity and lipotoxicity [2].

Atherosclerotic cardiovascular disease and thromboembolic phenomena are commonly seen in obese individuals and may be considered manifestations of the pro-inflammatory condition that is triggered by substrate overload. In addition, obesity encourages resistance to leptin, which cause expression of cytokines with anti-inflammatory and possibly anti-atherogenic properties.

Obese individuals also have a higher incidence of infectious complications, thrombogenesis and a pro-inflammatory state, with behavioural, immune, metabolic, and cardiovascular sequel.

Anti-obesity Surgery

For the anaesthetist, bariatric surgery consists of malabsorptive, restrictive and combined procedures. These have specific benefits and complications profiles. In malabsorptive surgery, the procedure involves bypassing most of the absorptive small bowel and inherently means opening the bowel and an anastomosis. This translates into longer surgery, raises the risk of surgical site infection and the risks of anastomotic leakage in the post-operative period. Restrictive procedures on the other hand, have relatively shorter operating times, less prone to surgical site infection and anastomotic dehiscence. However, they are less popular now and tend to achieve lesser degrees of weight loss. Combined procedures however are still in main practice. The majority of patients are managed laparoscopically. Although this has lessened the impact of surgery on post-operative recovery, this type of surgery has its own risks, complications and limitations. Operating times are generally longer than open surgery, there are more risks to bowel injury and pneumoperitoneum can increase end tidal carbon dioxide and reduce ventilatory volumes. The pros and cons of the exact surgical procedure would have been considered carefully with all members of the multi-disciplinary team before a final decision has been made [3].

A more difficult group of patients to manage are those who have redo surgery due to the occurrence of complications or due to failure of the previous anti-obesity procedure. Naturally, these patients have the additional burden of the complication in addition to obesity. These patients should be optimised before the re-do procedure.

Anaesthetic Considerations

Obesity is a multisystem condition affecting all organ systems. However, there are a number of specific issues regarding the respiratory, cardiovascular and endocrine systems that are important to delineate and make adjustments for, when providing anaesthesia for bariatric surgery. In addition, the volume and distribution of anaesthetic agents necessitates significant adjustments to be effective in obese individuals.

Pre-operative Optimisation

Optimisation of many of the known risk factors must include early implementation of an attitude of healthy lifestyle in the months prior to surgery. This encourages patients to adopt health-promoting behaviors early on, which can be continued postoperatively increasing the success of the operation. Advice regarding regular physical exercise for incremental periods every day will aid cardiac function as well as insulin control. Dietary advice regarding low fat, low salt, and high vegetable diets will decrease atherosclerosis in the long term (although unlikely to make much impact in the short term), as will cessation of all smoking. In many hospitals, patients attend seminars preoperatively that have a strong input from a specialist bariatric dietician, who can advise on pre- and post-operative nutrition. In terms of pre-operative optimisation, the dietician can arrange for nutritional evaluation including selective micronutrient measurements, help patients correct nutritional deficiencies, achieve a significant weight loss including shrinking the liver which is usually enlarged by steatohepatitis.

Anaesthetically, patients should be evaluated for indicators of systemic or pulmonary hypertension, ischaemic heart disease, and heart failure. Despite several studies on predictors for difficult intubation in this group of patients, there is a lack of evidence of predictors and incidence of difficulty of bag–mask ventilation post-induction. As such, a high index of suspicion of a difficult intubation should be maintained. In addition, all patients should be assessed for respiratory, cardiovascular and metabolic risks some of which may prohibit surgery, others require correction and the rest require recognition.

Obstructive Sleep Apnoea (OSA)

There is a greater prevalence of OSA (or sleep disordered breathing) in the obese population with an incidence of up to 77% in patients with BMI >35. A neck circumference of more than 40 Cm in men and 38 Cm in women is a good predictor of OSA. However, it is unrecognized in the majority of cases. The presence of OSA is an independent marker of risk that leads to a doubling of postoperative respiratory and cardiac complications. Its presence should be identified as these complications are reduced if treated pre-operatively with nocturnal Continuous Positive Airway Pressure (CPAP).

OSA can be defined as periods of apnoea occurring during sleep as a result of pharyngeal collapse. An apnoeic episode is defined as 10 seconds or more of total cessation of airflow, despite continuous respiratory effort against a closed airway. These become clinically significant when there are more than 5 per hour or more than 30 per night [4]. It is characterized by pharyngeal collapse occurring during sleep (mostly when patients are sleeping on their back). This may be due to obstruction caused by increased pharyngeal fat deposits resulting in an increase in pharyngeal wall compliance. During sleep this results in a tendency to airway collapse as a result of inspiration, which impedes gas flow.

The consequences of these periods of apnoea are:

- Desensitising central respiratory centres which can result in hypersensitivity to opiates and sedative drugs
- Increasing reliance on hypoxic drive
- Type 2 respiratory failure
- Pulmonary hypertension
- Right heart failure
- Polycythaemia

The goal of management is to keep the airways open and prevent periods of apnoea during sleep. Most patients will have trained to sleep on their side and when they sleep on their back, use different pillow positions to elevate the upper body (above the waist) to reduce airway collapse. Some patients with OSA may have used mandibular advancement or tongue retaining devices. The former is shaped as a mouth guard, which lets the lower jaw, ease forward. The latter, looks like a splint, which holds the tongue in place to keep the airway open. Patients with diagnosed OSA may have been started on Continuous Positive Air Pressure (CPAP) devices. These machines use air at positive pressure delivered through a tight fitting mask to keep the airways open. A minority of patients may have implanted nerve stimulators which monitor breathing patterns and stimulate the nerves, which control the tongue, and laryngeal muscles to move forward and unobstruct air flow.

The management of OSA focuses on detecting its presence and instigating nocturnal Continuous Positive Airway Pressure (CPAP). All obese patients should be screened with the STOP-BANG screening questionnaire (Table **2**) [5]. A score of ≥5 indicates that the patient is at a significant risk of OSA and these patients should proceed to sleep studies prior to surgery.

Table 2. Standard questionnaire to determine the STOP-BANG Score [5].

	Feature	Question / Response
S	Snoring	Do you snore loudly?
T	Tired	Do you often feel tired, fatigued or sleepy during daytime? Do you fall asleep in the daytime?
O	Observed	Has anyone observed you stop breathing, choke or gasping during your sleep?
P	Blood Pressure	Do you have or are treated for high blood pressure?
B	BMI	>35 kg.m^2
A	Age	> 50 years
N	Neck Circumference	>43 cm (males) >41 cm (females)
B	Gender	Male

If significant OSA is present, then nocturnal CPAP should be instigated. However, there may be issues with poor compliance or difficulty in mask fitting. The patient should be re-assessed for symptom improvement after CPAP.

Obesity Hypoventilation Syndrome

This is a condition associated with obesity, which affects control of breathing. It consists of the triad of obesity (BMI > 35), OSA (sleep disordered breathing) and daytime hypercapnia pCO_2 >6 kPa. Obesity results in relative leptin insensitivity and, as leptin has an influence on respiratory drive and carbon dioxide sensitivity, this results in hypoventilation. This effect is accentuated with anaesthetic drugs and other depressant drugs including analgesia and can result in postoperative respiratory depression. Recognition of this condition preoperatively should lead to modification of anaesthetic technique with the avoidance of long acting sedative drugs and minimal use of opiates postoperatively.

Respiratory Function

Basal metabolic rate does not change with obesity but there is an increased oxygen requirement and carbon dioxide production due to the increase in tissue volume from the increased body mass. The ability to deal with this increase in oxygen and ventilation requirements is compromised with the changes that occur to the respiratory system with obesity. Increased adipose tissue in the thorax and abdomen results in reduced chest wall compliance and cephalad displacement of the abdominal contents below the thorax. There is also an increase in pulmonary blood volume.

These changes lead to a reduction to the functional residual capacity (FRC), ventilation-perfusion mismatching and intrapulmonary shunting. This can result in hypoxia at rest and rapid significant oxygen desaturation with apnoea, such as at the induction and emergence from anaesthesia. Airway pressures during controlled ventilation may be higher than would normally be expected with the risk of barotrauma occurring.

Cardiovascular Factors

The cardiovascular system is put under significant strain with obesity as it tries to match the metabolic demand of the increased tissues. This increase in cardiac output results in a number of changes that can be detrimental.

Systemic hypertension is ten times more common in obese patients and can result in left ventricular hypertrophy, diastolic dysfunction and eventually left ventricular failure. In addition, increased workload is placed on the pulmonary circulation resulting in pulmonary hypertension and potentially right heart failure.

Dyslipidaemia is very common and this along with hypertension results in an increased incidence of ischaemic heart disease. This may not be immediately obvious due to a sedentary lifestyle common in this group of patients. Arrhythmias are more common due to ventricular hypertrophy, fatty infiltration of the heart and metabolic upset due to obesity or cardiac drug treatments. Blood volume is increased as a result of changes to the Renin-Angiotensin-System and secondary polycythaemia from chronic hypoxia.

Endocrine Factors

Diabetes Mellitus is much more common in obese patients compared to patients with a normal BMI. Insulin resistance, or type-2 diabetes, is the commonest presentation. The use of insulin as well as oral hypoglycaemic agents is often required for glucose control [6].

Diabetes results in multiple micro- and macro- vascular complications in all organ systems. The longer a patient has diabetes the more complications from the disease they will have. The presence of these should be carefully assessed preoperatively.

Pharmacology of Anaesthetic Agents in Obesity

The adaptation of drug dosages to obese patients is an important consideration, particularly for drugs with a narrow therapeutic index. The main factors that affect the tissue distribution of drugs are body composition, regional blood flow and the affinity of the drug for plasma proteins and/or tissue components. The presence of large amounts of adipose tissue in obese patients causes considerable, and challenging problems with drug dosing for commonly used anaesthetic drugs. Most drug doses are based on 'normal reference' individual's body weight. Using these agents with extrapolations to obese patients' weight would lead to significant overdose that may have serious side effects.

Obese patients have a markedly different volume of distribution of drugs as a result of the adipose tissue. Obese people have larger absolute lean body masses as well as fat masses than non-obese individuals of the same age, gender and height. However, the percentage of fat per kg of total body weight (TBW) is markedly increased, whereas that of lean tissue is reduced. This changes the pharmacokinetics of the drugs resulting in a less predictable effect of the drugs and variations in the duration of their action. Lipophilic drugs will have a larger volume of distribution whereas volume of distribution for polar drugs may be similar. To compensate for these changes drug dosing in obese patients is based on a combination of adjusted body weight, total body weight, ideal body weight and lean body mass (Fig. **1**) [7]. Current recommendations on drug dosing for different anaesthetic agents include a differential on the basis of different weight parameters (Table **3**).

Table 3. Commonly used anaesthetic agents and dosing regimes [8].

Dosing Based On		
Lean Body Weight	**Adjusted Body Weight**	**Total Body Weight**
Propofol (induction)	Propofol (maintenance)	Suxamethonium (max 140kg)
Thiopentone	Antibiotics	
Fentanyl	Low molecular weight heparins	
Rocuronium	Alfentanil	
Atracurium	Neostigmine	
Vecuronium	Sugammadex	
Morphine		
Paracetamol		
Bupivacaine		
Lignocaine		

> **Ideal body weight (IBW)**
>   Kg= height (cm)- 100 for males
>   Kg= height (cm)- 105 for females
> **Lean body mass (LBM)**
>   Male LBM=   1.10 (weight)-128(weight/height)^2
>   Female LBM=   1.07 (weight)- 148 (weight/height)^2
> **Adjusted body weight**
>   ABW= IBW+0.4 (TBW-IBW)

Fig. (1). Example calculation of different weight parameters used in anaesthetic drug dosing for obese patients [7, 8].

Further, cardiac performance and adipose tissue blood flow maybe altered in obesity. There is uncertainty about the binding of drugs to plasma proteins in obese patients. Some data suggest that the activities of hepatic cytochrome P450 isoforms are altered, but no clear overview of drug hepatic metabolism in obesity is currently available. Pharmacokinetic studies provide differing data on renal function in obese patients.

Pharmacokinetic studies in obesity show that the behavior of molecules with weak or moderate lipophilicity (*e.g.* vecuronium) is generally rather predictable, as these drugs are distributed mainly in lean tissues. The dosage of these drugs should be based on the ideal bodyweight (IBW). However, some of these drugs (*e.g.* antibiotics) are partly distributed in adipose tissues, and their dosage is based on IBW plus a percentage of the patient's excess bodyweight.

There is no systematic relationship between the degree of lipophilicity of markedly lipophilic drugs (*e.g.* remifentanil and some β-blockers) and their distribution in obese individuals. The distribution of a drug between fat and lean tissues may influence its pharmacokinetics in obese patients. Thus, the loading dose should be adjusted to the TBW or IBW, according to data from studies carried out in obese individuals. Adjustment of the maintenance dosage depends on the observed modifications in clearance.

In practice, most anaesthetic drugs are titrated to produce the desired effect and this should still be the case in the obese patients. Similarly, for regional anaesthesia, adjustment to the drug dosage, have to be made. Due to excess adipose tissue in the epidural space, drug dosages in both spinal anaesthesia and epidural anaesthesia should be reduced by 25%.

PRE-OPERATIVE PREPARATION

Patients with obesity require a multidisciplinary approach to stratify their risk and to ensure that they are on an appropriate care pathway. The anaesthetist involved in the surgical management of these patients should be an integral part of the multi-disciplinary team. This ensures that patients who require additional time, equipment and preparation to manage their case safely are identified at an early stage. The vast majority of obese patients, are otherwise healthy and carry little additional risk for surgery and anaesthesia. However, there are a significant proportion of patients who carry additional increased risk, which potentially can be optimized. As such it is essential for anaesthetists involved in the pre-operative management of obese patients to screen them and identify those at increased risk in order to manage them appropriately.

A key marker for increased risk of perioperative complications is central obesity. Other markers of increased risk have to be identified and one useful tool is the Obesity Surgery Mortality Risk Stratification score, (Table **4**). This scoring system focuses on the presence of sleep-disordered breathing, metabolic syndrome and risk of veno-thrombo-embolism. It has been validated for bariatric surgical procedures [9].

Table 4. Risk factor scoring recommended for obese patients [9].

Risk Factor	Score
BMI >50 kg.m^2	1
Male	1
Age >45 years	1
Hypertension	1

Risk factor for pulmonary embolism
  Previous venous thromboembolism
  Vena caval filter
  OSA/Sleep disordered breathing
  Pulmonary hypertension
	1

A comprehensive assessment should be carried out routinely on all obese patients prior to any planned surgical procedure to risk stratify them and identify other incidental comorbid diseases, not necessarily arising from obesity. Additional diagnostic tests and appropriate management may be required depending on the findings. Based on this risk stratification, a class risk of predicted mortality can be inferred which can be used primarily for selection of patients [10] but also for consent and to guide surgical decision-making and post-operative management (Table **5**) [11].

Table 5. Obesity Surgical Mortality Risk Stratification score [9].

Score	Risk Class	Mortality Risk
0-1 points	A	0.2-0.3%
2-3 points	B	1.1-1.5%
4-5 points	C	2.4-3.0%

Airway Assessment

Management of the airway is of crucial importance in obese patients as difficulty in maintaining a patent airway can result in significant hypoxia rapidly due to the reduction in the functional residual capacity. Intubation itself may not be difficult but effective mask ventilation can be very difficult.

Up to a 30% of obese patients are reported to have difficult or failed intubation. However, weight itself is a poor predictor of intubation difficulty. Anaesthetic assessment of the airway normally involves a visual assessment of the airway looking at the space from the base of the tongue to the roof of the mouth as described by Mallampati. Obesity together with a Mallampati score ≥ 3, visualisation of only the base of the uvula and the soft palate, and a large neck circumference are associated with difficult laryngoscopy. A neck circumference of 40 cm is associated with a 5% incidence of difficult laryngoscopy and a circumference of >60 cm has a 35% incidence of difficulty in laryngoscopy. It should be noted that the airway size might be smaller than anticipated and so may require smaller endotracheal tubes.

Respiratory System

Anatomical and physical changes to the respiratory system occur in obesity and may cause respiratory impairment or disease. Underlying respiratory disease of significance can be identified by:

- Respiratory wheeze at rest
- Arterial saturation <95% on air
- FVC <3l
- FEV1 <1.5l
- Serum bicarbonate >27 mmol.l^{-1}
- PaCO$_2$ >6.0 kPa

Sleep disordered breathing is associated with significant postoperative risk which can be reduced with appropriate treatment such as nocturnal CPAP. A validated screening tool is STOP-BANG, see table 2, which can identify these patients at risk who can then go forward for sleep studies and treatment if required. It has been suggested a score of ≥5 indicates possible sleep disordered breathing. However even a low STOP-BANG score does not rule out sleep disordered breathing and so evidence of right heart strain should also be explored.

Cardiovascular System

Obese patients should be assessed as any other patients for cardiovascular risk and investigated appropriately as per current guidelines. Central obesity and metabolic syndrome are markers for increased cardiovascular disease and patients with central obesity should be thoroughly screened and investigated for all cardio-vascular risk factors.

It should be noted that there might be difficulty in assessing exercise tolerance due to inability to exercise caused by body habitus. Additionally, there may be difficulty in accessing appropriate equipment to assess exercise tolerance, which can accommodate super obese individuals.

Glucose Control

Type 2 Diabetes is common in obese patients that may be treated with oral hypoglycaemic agents, insulin or both. Blood glucose levels should be stable in the range of 6-10 mmol/l. Long term control can be assessed with HbA1C which should be ≤75 mmol/mol prior to surgery

Nutritional State

Liver shrinking diet and drug therapy used for obesity may cause specific nutritional deficiencies, which should be identified and corrected preoperatively. A nutritional screen carried out before surgery is essential for the diagnosis of these deficiencies. Adequate time should be given to correction of these nutritional deficiencies.

INTRA-OPERATIVE ANESTHETIC MANAGEMENT

Adequate time and preparation is essential to provide safe conditions to anaesthetise obese patients. The operating table should be of adequate size and build to take the required weight without over challenging the movement mechanical gears. Specialized equipment required to position patients and assist manual handling should be available.

Positioning

To minimise moving and handling, which may be hazardous to staff, induction of anaesthesia should be carried out on the operating table in the operating theatre. Ideally the patient should walk into theatre and position themselves on the operating table in such a way that is both dignified and most comfortable to them. This ensures there is minimal movement of the patient and a reduction in risk of damage from traction to nerves or pressure areas with poor patient positioning. An air hover mattress should be in place under the patient as this will aid moving and handling at the end of the surgical procedure.

Patients should be positioned in the supine position for surgery. A ramped head up position is optimal, with the tragus of the ear at the level of the sternum, to provide the best intubation conditions and improved respiratory function during induction of anaesthesia. Arms will be out in a cruciform arrangement and the legs will be split to allow surgical access. As the patient will be placed in the reverse Trendelenberg for the procedure it is crucial that they do not slip down the operating table. Anti- slip sheets are useful to minimise this risk and feet plates should be in place to provide additional protection from slippage. The body and limbs should be securely positioned ensuring that there is no impingement on pressure areas or nerves. Obese patients are at an increased risk of pressure area damage including compartment syndrome of the lower limbs. The split leg position puts the large nerves at risk of stretch through abduction of the limbs and attempts should be made to minimize the angle between the legs as far as possible.

A large oro-gastric or nasogastric tube is usually inserted to ensure that the stomach is deflated and can serve as a guide during surgery. In addition, it can be used to test for anastomotic leaks at the end of the procedure with blue dye injection.

Thrombo-embolism Prophylaxis

The risk of veno-thromboembolism is extremely high in obese patients and anti-thromboembolic stockings and calf compression devices (Sequential compression) should be used in all patients. Chemical prophylaxis is also essential throughout the perioperative period.

Antibiotic Prophylaxis

Obese patients are at increased risk of postoperative infections. These are mainly respiratory tract infection but urine, wound and surgical site infections are not uncommon. These infections are a reflection of the diabetic and respiratory status of these patients and the clean/ contaminated nature of surgery. Antibiotics prophylaxis should be administered prior to the commencement of surgery as per local guidelines. The antimicrobial cover may need to be extended or recommenced depending on the nature of surgery and post-operative course.

Standard Monitoring

This should be applied for all patients undergoing bariatric surgery. It should include ECG, pulse oximetry, carbon dioxide and blood pressure monitoring. Non-invasive blood pressure monitoring is usually adequate if a correctly sized cuff is used, however it may be more appropriate to use invasive blood pressure monitoring for selected patients. For patients who have been deemed to be at a higher risk, additional monitoring is used as appropriate. This includes monitoring of central venous pressure and additional monitoring of cardiac parameters. In these patients post-operative monitoring may be continued in the high dependency or intensive care unit as appropriate until they have recovered sufficiently and the risk is largely obviated.

Venous Access

Venous cannulation should be secured which may be difficult depending on fat distribution. The use of ultrasound can help intravenous cannulation. Occasionally it may not be possible to obtain peripheral venous access and in this situation central venous access is required. While this may be more difficult in obese individuals, it can occasionally be more efficient in administering fluids and pharmaceutical agents both intra-operatively and in the post-operative period.

Pre-oxygenation

This is an essential step in all obese patients since even short periods of apnoea can result in significant hypoxia. Ideally this should be for three minutes or until the end tidal expired oxygen concentration is >85%. There is increasing use of high flow nasal cannula, which can delay time to desaturation during the apnoea time, but this is reserved for the super obese with extremely high BMIs and is usually not required in the majority of cases.

Induction of Anaesthesia

Intravenous induction of anaesthesia is recommended for all patients. It is not recommended to attempt an inhalational technique of induction even for a brief period. A balanced anaesthetic approach is the standard practice using a hypnotic agent, short acting opiate and a rapid acting muscle relaxant. The choice of muscle relaxant is made on personal preference, with some advocating using Suxamethonium and others using the non-depolarising agent Rocuronium as both have rapid predictable onset.

Intubation

Tracheal intubation is required to prevent aspiration and obtain full control of oxygenation and ventilation. If there is a significant risk of aspiration or there is the potential for difficult mask ventilation, then a rapid sequence induction should be performed with or without cricoid pressure depending on the anaesthetists' preference. Otherwise a standard induction is performed with mask ventilation until optimal intubating conditions have been achieved. Occasionally, if there is an anticipated difficulty in securing the airway in the standard manner, it may be necessary to perform an awake fibre optic intubation [12].

The use of laryngeal masks as airway rescue devices has been noted to be less effective than in the non-obese population. Second generation laryngeal masks may be more efficacious. The use of front of neck access to rescue the airway is extremely difficult. As such elective awake fibre optic intubation should be considered in all patients who have anticipated, or known, difficulty with intubation.

Once the trachea has been intubated controlled ventilation is required. No mode of ventilation has been shown to be superior. However, pressure controlled ventilation does give larger tidal volumes for a given pressure compared with volume controlled ventilation thus reducing the incidence of barotrauma. Tidal volumes are ideally between 6-8 mls/kg based on ideal body weight with peak airway pressures <30 cm H_2O [13]. It may not be possible to achieve these values particularly in extreme obesity and if a pneumoperitoneum is present thus higher airway pressures may have to be tolerated. The use of Positive End Expiratory Pressure (PEEP) at 6-8 cm H_2O and recruitment manoeuvres every 30 minutes will improve the FRC thus improving oxygenation.

Maintenance of Anaesthesia

This is achieved by using either short acting volatile anaesthetic agents; Desflurane may be superior to Sevoflurane, or Total Intravenous Anaesthesia (TIVA). The absolute amount of anaesthetic agent delivered could be reduced with the use of depth of anaesthesia monitoring which may reduce postoperative complications as there may be less residual agents causing respiratory compromise.

Neuromuscular blockade should be monitored throughout the procedure. It is now thought that quantitative methods of monitoring the degree of muscular block using acceleromyography are superior to other methods. Deep paralysis is often required to facilitate surgery. Full reversal should be achieved before extubation occurs. The use of Rocuronium is the ideal muscle relaxant in obese patients as it can be completely reversed with Sugamadex- a rapidly acting reversal agent.

Multimodal Analgesia

This should be used to reduce the requirements for opiate analgesia, as these can be associated with postoperative respiratory compromise. Suitable drugs include paracetamol, non-steroidal anti-inflammatory drugs and novel analgesics such as clonidine or ketamine.

Regional anaesthesia in conjunction with general anaesthesia is useful if the surgical procedure is an open one. However due to body habitus these may prove challenging to site. Methods used include epidural anaesthesia, spinal anaesthesia, rectus sheath block, transverse abdominis plane block and wound catheters depending on the incision used. In laparoscopic procedures infiltration of port sites by local anaesthetics is helpful.

Reversal of Anaesthesia

Emergence from anaesthesia can be a very challenging time and is often the time that hypoxia can occur. It is recommended that extubation be performed with the patient sitting upright. This position improves respiratory function and improves the FRC. The patient should be wide-awake and cooperative with a normal respiratory pattern prior to removal of the endotracheal tube.

There is a debate as to whether 100% oxygen should be used during extubation or if a reduction in inspired oxygen concentration, FiO_2 0.7-0.8 O_2, is used instead. The latter is associated with a reduction in postoperative hypoxia as there is a reduction in atelectasis due to the presence of nitrogen splinting [14]. Each patient should be assessed individually when making this decision but if there is any previous difficulty with either securing the airway or bag mask ventilation then 100% O_2 should be used.

POST-ANAESTHETIC MANAGEMENT

All patients should be monitored and cared for in the post-anaesthetic care unit (PACU) immediately postoperatively. They should be nursed sitting up at >45^0 angle. Oxygen should be administered to maintain their oxygen saturation at preoperative values. It may be required to administer CPAP with supplemental oxygen in the immediate postoperative period due to the effects of the anaesthetic agents. High flow nasal cannulas are also useful and may be better tolerated by patients.

Discharge from PACU should occur when-

• Routine discharge criteria are met
• Analgesia is satisfactory for deep breathing and coughing

- Oxygen saturation levels are at preoperative values, with or without supplemental oxygen
- Respiratory rate is normal and there has been no periods of apnoea or hypoventilation for at least one hour

Post-operative Environment

Most patients presenting for bariatric surgery can be discharged to a ward environment. On the ward they should be encouraged to mobilise and sit in a chair at the earliest possible time to reduce respiratory and thromboembolic complications. The use of intravenous infusions, patient controlled intravenous analgesia, urinary catheters and monitoring, hinders mobilisation and should be removed as soon as it is safe to do so.

Some patients presenting for bariatric surgery carry an increased risk and as such may be required to be cared for in a high dependency unit or an intensive care unit. A modified Montefiore Obesity Surgical Score has been suggested to identify patients requiring HDU or ICU care postoperatively (Table **6**) [15].

Table 6. Modified Montefiore Obesity Surgical Score for high level post-operative care. The presence of 4 or more factors merit consideration for higher level of care [15].

• Gastric bypass surgery
• Male gender
• BMI ≥ 50kg m^{-2}
• Age ≥ 50 yr. old
• Confirmed OSA
• Significant surgical or medical comorbidities
• Previous abdominal surgery

If the patient normally uses nocturnal CPAP then they should continue to do so whilst on the ward. It is advisable that they bring in their own unit and use it, as they would do at home.

Particular attention should be paid to blood glucose levels as these may fluctuate in the immediate postoperative period and modification may be required to hypoglycaemic agents. Different units have strict protocols on the frequency of glucose monitoring and these should be adhered to. However, individual patients may require additional monitoring depending on the fragility of their diabetes control and on their glucose levels.

Supplementary Oxygen

It is essential to use continuous pulse oximetry to monitor oxygen saturation at least in the first 24 hours after surgery. After this period, oximetry can be intermittent and depend on the individual patient. Supplementary oxygen should be continued until oxygen saturations are sustained at baseline on air. This is usually achieved 24-48 hours after surgery but can be as long as one week for a minority of patients. If parental opiates are required, then supplemental oxygen should continue. Patients with obstructive sleep apnoea who use A CPAP device can have additional oxygen connected to the CPAP device when it is in use. Otherwise, supplementary oxygen can be delivered by a ventimask or nasal cannulae depending on the oxygen requirement and the comfort of the individual patient.

Post-operative Analgesia

Apart from the abhorrent discomfort that post-operative pain can cause, pain impacts on cardiovascular and respiratory parameters and can be detrimental to the post-operative course. Analgesia in the early post-operative period can be provided with oral opiates. However, a multimodal approach is preferred especially if the procedure has been laparoscopic. If the surgical procedure is opened, then intravenous opiate analgesia or a regional technique will be required and the patient should be cared for in a suitable environment as they will require additional monitoring. After the acute phase, patients will continue to experience discomfort and an analgesia step down approach protocol should be adopted. By the time of hospital discharge, most patients should be comfortable using oral simple analgesia.

Shoulder tip pain can be a frequent complaint. After laparoscopy, this is not uncommon and reflects stretching of the diaphragm caused by pneumoperitoneum at the time of surgery. This type of referred pain can last up to two weeks after surgery. This usually responds to simple analgesia in most patients. In other patients, shoulder tip pain may represent diaphragmatic irritation from tube drains or inflammation caused by infection. Withdrawal of tube drains by a few centimetres may help some patients. In others, 3 dimensional scans may be indicated to investigate the cause of the irritation.

Thrombo-embolism Prophylaxis

Intra-operatively, immediately post operatively and for the first 24-hours, sequential compression stockings should be applied ensuring that the machine is operational to achieve sequential compression of the calf muscles. Thrombo-embolic deterrent stockings should be used until discharge from hospital.

Chemical anti-thrombotic prophylaxis such as low-molecular weight heparins should be administered to reduce the risk of deep venous thrombosis. Mobility should be encouraged as early as possible. This may necessitate removal or securing intravenous lines, drains and catheters if present. Short assisted walks should be encouraged from the first post-operative day with increasing the walking distance on subsequent days. After discharge from hospital, all patients should be encouraged to be mobile. Some patients may benefit from continuing to wear thrombo-embolic deterrent stockings particularly during sleep. Others may require an extended period of chemical antithrombotic prophylaxis while at home. The discharging physician should make an objective assessment of each patient's motivation and stamina to remain mobile. Patients should be advised to avoid prolonged car journeys and to pre-plan stop breaks if such journeys are undertaken.

Mobilisation

There is sufficient evidence in the literature to support early post-operative mobilisation after any abdominal surgery but specifically after upper abdominal surgery. Early mobilisation reduces the incidence of post-operative pulmonary complications by increasing lung volumes and increasing inspiratory muscle strength. It also reduces anxiety and the period required for return to physical activity and contributes to early discharge from hospital. This is best achieved when the culture of the recovery environment staff is familiar and engaged with the principles of early mobilisation and recovery. A structured programme of early mobilisation and physical therapy should start on the first post-operative day and continued until discharge. Goal directed mobilisation establishes the mobility aspirations set for each individual based on their pre-operative mobility profile. The programme is incremental subject to patient's tolerance, stamina and the onset of complications. The programme can start with the first session in or around the patient's bed and progress to venturing incremental distances away from the bed. The programme should be discussed with patients before surgery and patients are encouraged to follow the daily mobility programme. Prior to mobilisation, intravenous catheters and drains should be secured to prevent accidental withdrawal. Obstacles in the mobility path should be removed or minimised. Resting stations should be installed at various distances. Additional members of staff should be on standby for patients encountering difficulties during mobilisation particularly postural hypotension or tachypnoea. When difficulties arise, patients should be encouraged to attempt a repeat of the exercise at a later time rather than abandon it.

Fluids and Diet Reintroduction

In general, the surgeon who carried out the operation should direct the timing of fluid and diet reintroduction. This is due to the fact that the surgical procedure carried out may be different depending on the anatomy of the individual patient. In addition, the surgical findings during the procedure may indicate a less than ideal environment for anastomotic healing, which would suggest a delay fluid and diet reintroduction. Notwithstanding any surgical issues, a protocol of fluid reintroduction should commence once the patient is sufficiently awake and able to sit upright post-operatively. Clear fluids include water, tea, diluted juice, jelly and clear soup. This should be followed by a liquid diet for the first post-operative week including milk, thicker soup and yoghurt. A pureed diet can be started in the second postoperative week and includes cooked and blended vegetables, and meats with mashed potatoes and cereals. A soft diet can be commenced after 2 weeks. This diet includes foods, which can be mashed easily on the plate or cut with a fork. By 4 weeks, a healthy normal diet could be commenced. Nausea can be an issue in up to 50% of patients particularly in the early stages after surgery and this should be managed by pharmacotherapy. It is not however unusual for patients to be sated by a small volume. Blood sugar monitoring is essential for all patients but particularly in diabetic patients.

In a small number of patients, the surgeon may be anxious about anastomotic healing. In these patients, different surgeons adopt different protocols. Some prefer to carry out a water-soluble contrast study to examine the anastomoses at a certain period post surgery (from day 1 to day 3). During this period, they recommend abstinence from oral intake. Others suffice with abstinence from oral intake for a period after surgery (from 1 to 5 days) but do not test the anastomoses with a water-soluble contrast study for all patients. Instead, they focus on the vital parameters for each patient and adopt selective contrast studies on the basis of untoward signs or symptoms.

Hospital Discharge

The majority of patients should be planned for discharge home by the third post-operative day. Ideally, all drains should be removed prior to discharge. However, some patients can be discharged with drains after appropriate advice on drain care together with community support. Discharge planning should include preparation of discharge care advice including wound care, medication, transport and a diet plan. All patients should be seen by a specialist dietician prior to discharge for advice on progressing their diet after discharge. This includes some sample menus and advice on portion sizes and eating habits. In addition, most centres tend to hand out a post-discharge protocol giving important information on the recovery process and contact numbers for additional help and support. This protocol should itemise important information and remedies for common difficulties after bariatric surgery including constipation, hair loss and dumping syndrome. In addition, the protocols should give helpful advice on alcohol intake; vitamin and mineral supplementation and long term follow up. All patients should be given an appointment with the community practitioner for wound(s) toilet and removing wound sutures. After hospital discharge, patients will need at least one review appointment with the surgical team. In addition, the patient will need an early appointment with the dietetic team and possibly the diabetic team. Vulnerable patient may also need an appointment with the specialist psychologist.

CONSENT FOR PUBLICATION

Not applicable.

ACKNOWLEDGEMENT

Declare none.

CONFLICT OF INTEREST

The author declares no conflict of interest, financial or otherwise.

REFERENCES

[1]   Aronne LJ. Classification of obesity and assessment of obesity-related health risks. Obes Res 2002; 10 (Suppl. 2): 105S-15S.
        [http://dx.doi.org/10.1038/oby.2002.203] [PMID: 12490659]

[2]   Redinger RN. The pathophysiology of obesity and its clinical manifestations. Gastroenterol Hepatol (N Y) 2007; 3(11): 856-63.
        [PMID: 21960798]

[3]   Waitman JA, Aronne LJ. Obesity surgery: pros and cons. J Endocrinol Invest 2002; 25(10): 925-8.
        [http://dx.doi.org/10.1007/BF03344059] [PMID: 12508958]

[4]   Benumof JL. Obstructive sleep apnea in the adult obese patient: implications for airway management. J Clin Anesth 2001; 13(2): 144-56.
        [http://dx.doi.org/10.1016/S0952-8180(01)00232-X] [PMID: 11331179]

[5]   Chung F, Yegneswaran B, Liao P, *et al.* STOP questionnaire: a tool to screen patients for obstructive sleep apnea. Anesthesiology 2008; 108(5): 812-21.
        [http://dx.doi.org/10.1097/ALN.0b013e31816d83e4] [PMID: 18431116]

[6]   Propst M, Colvin C, Griffin RL, *et al.* Diabetes and prediabetes are significantly higher in morbidly obese children compared with obese children. Endocr Pract 2015; 21(9): 1046-53.
        [http://dx.doi.org/10.4158/EP14414.OR] [PMID: 26121438]

[7]   Ingrande J, Lemmens HJ. Dose adjustment of anaesthetics in the morbidly obese. Br J Anaesth 2010; 105 (Suppl. 1): i16-23.
        [http://dx.doi.org/10.1093/bja/aeq312] [PMID: 21148651]

[8]   Nightingale CE, Margarson MP, Shearer E, *et al.* Members of the Working Party; Association of Anaesthetists of Great Britain; Ireland Society for Obesity and Bariatric Anaesthesia. Peri-operative

management of the obese surgical patient 2015: Association of Anaesthetists of Great Britain and Ireland Society for Obesity and Bariatric Anaesthesia. Anaesthesia 2015; 70(7): 859-76.
[http://dx.doi.org/10.1111/anae.13101] [PMID: 25950621]

[9]   DeMaria EJ, Murr M, Byrne TK, *et al.* Validation of the obesity surgery mortality risk score in a multicenter study proves it stratifies mortality risk in patients undergoing gastric bypass for morbid obesity. Ann Surg 2007; 246(4): 578-82.
[http://dx.doi.org/10.1097/SLA.0b013e318157206e] [PMID: 17893494]

[10]   Orłowski M, Janik MR, Paśnik K, Jędrzejewski E. Usefulness of the obesity surgery mortality risk score (OR-MRS) in choosing the laparoscopic bariatric procedure. Wideochir Inne Tech Malo Inwazyjne 2015; 10(2): 233-6.
[http://dx.doi.org/10.5114/wiitm.2015.52390] [PMID: 26240623]

[11]   Thomas H, Agrawal S. Systematic review of obesity surgery mortality risk score--preoperative risk stratification in bariatric surgery. Obes Surg 2012; 22(7): 1135-40.
[http://dx.doi.org/10.1007/s11695-012-0663-7] [PMID: 22535443]

[12]   Brodsky J B, Lemmens H J, Brock-Utne J G, Vierra M, Saidman L J. Morbid obesity and tracheal intubation 2002.
[http://dx.doi.org/10.1097/00000539-200203000-00047]

[13]   Futier E, Constantin JM, Paugam-Burtz C, *et al.* A trial of intraoperative low-tidal-volume ventilation in abdominal surgery. N Engl J Med 2013; 369(5): 428-37.
[http://dx.doi.org/10.1056/NEJMoa1301082] [PMID: 23902482]

[14]   Benoit Z, Wicky S, Fischer J F, Frascarolo P, Chapuis C, Spahn D R, *et al.* The effect of increased FIO(2) before tracheal extubation on postoperative atelectasis 2002.

[15]   Levi D, Goodman ER, Patel M, Savransky Y. Critical care of the obese and bariatric surgical patient. Crit Care Clin 2003; 19(1): 11-32.
[http://dx.doi.org/10.1016/S0749-0704(02)00060-X] [PMID: 12688575]

CHAPTER 8

Bariatric and Metabolic Surgery

Jamie Young[*]

Department of Surgery, Borders General Hospital, Melrose, Roxburghshire, Scotland, UK

Abstract: Obesity is a complex condition, one with serious social and psychological dimensions, that affects virtually all age and socioeconomic groups. It is a consequence of abundance, convenience and underlying biology. Preventing obesity requires changes in the environment and organisational behaviour, as well as changes in groups, family and individual behaviour. Treatment strategies vary in different centres and treatment sectors. Non-surgical management consists of diet, exercise, psychology and pharmacology. Non-surgical management can achieve weight loss. Anti-obesity drugs may be effective as adjunctive therapy to diet and physical activity in those subjects who struggle to lose weight despite following an appropriate weight loss programme. The problem with non-surgical treatment is of long-term sustainability. Bariatric surgery is the only management, which has long-term sustainability of weight loss and reversal of comorbidities. However, it is not applicable to all obese patients. Both restrictive and malabsorptive procedures have a relatively high success rate in weight loss and improvement of blood sugar control. However, these procedures have many pitfalls and complications. Experienced bariatric surgeons in high-volume centres have achieved minimal morbidity and mortality after weight loss surgery. Patient selection and preparation is key to success. Special anaesthetic considerations and modifications must be adhered to. The choice of procedure for any individual patient is a complex process and depends on many factors. Follow-up after bariatric surgery must be rigorous to monitor and correct micronutrient deficiency and provide psychological support to patients who have had to change their life style albeit to a healthier existence.

Keywords: Audit of outcomes, Bariatric surgery, Complications, Diabetes, Diet, Exercise, Medical management, Obesity, Psychology, Re-do bariatric surgery.

GLOBAL OBESITY

Obesity became recognised as an aesthetic issue in the late 19th century and was recognised as a health problem in the 20th century. Jaw wiring was the earliest attempt to alleviate obesity on the basis of the assumption that enforced reduction in food intake would result in sustained weight loss. This procedure proved

[*] **Corresponding author Jamie Young:** Department of Surgery, Borders General Hospital, Melrose, Roxburghshire, TD6 9BS, Scotland, UK; Tel/Fax: +44 1382 660111; E-mail: jamie.young@nhs.net

unsuccessful because it allowed patients to consume high-calorie liquids, which eventually resulted in weight regain. The procedure also caused additional health problems. Jaw wiring was therefore discontinued. Surgeons reported that patients who lost a portion of their small intestine lost weight despite increased caloric intake. These observations sparked the beginning of bariatric surgery, as we know it today. The earliest surgical procedures were predominantly malabsorptive. Although they were successful in achieving weight loss, they also resulted in significant nutritional complications due to malabsorption of essential vitamins and minerals. This has led to a surge of predominantly restrictive procedures, with varying degrees of success, in achieving sustainable weight loss. Multiple procedures related complications were also reported. The last decade has seen the emergence of new and mixed malabsorptive and restrictive procedures practiced by specialist bariatric surgeons in working with multidisciplinary teams catering for the complex needs, pre-assessment and follow up of these patients. Bariatric surgery has gained recognition as the only method of achieving sustainable weight loss. Initially, bariatric surgery was the generic term used to describe weight loss surgery. However, there was growing recognition that obesity is a metabolic disorder and metabolic surgery has gained acceptance as the term best used to describe this type of surgery.

Background

Obesity is one of today's most blatantly visible public health problems. An escalating global epidemic of overweight and obesity – "globesity" – is taking over many parts of the world. If immediate action is not taken, millions will suffer from an array of serious health disorders.

Obesity is a complex condition, one with serious social and psychological dimensions, that affects virtually all age and socioeconomic groups and threatens to overwhelm both developed and developing countries. In 1995, there were an estimated 200 million obese adults worldwide and another 18 million under-five children classified as overweight. As of 2000, the number of obese adults has increased to over 300 million. Contrary to conventional wisdom, the obesity epidemic is not restricted to industrialized societies. It is estimated that over 115 million people suffer from obesity-related problems in developing countries.

In general, although men may have higher rates of being overweight, women have higher rates of obesity. For both, obesity poses a major risk for serious diet-related diseases, including diabetes mellitus, cardiovascular disease, hypertension and stroke, and certain forms of cancer. Its health consequences range from increased risk of premature death to serious chronic conditions that reduce the overall quality of life.

Aetiology and Epidemiology

Obesity is a consequence of abundance, convenience and underlying biology. There are multiple causes of obesity, and the aetiology is not well known. Obesity is at least in part attributable to overconsumption of calorie-dense foods and physical inactivity. Other factors such as personality traits, depression, side effects of pharmaceuticals, food addiction, or genetic predisposition may also contribute. Obesity may result from a combination of dysfunction of brain circuits and neuroendocrine hormones related to pathological overeating, physical inactivity and other pathophysiological conditions. In simple terms obesity is caused by a positive imbalance between calories consumed and calories expended. In practice, the problem is far more complex. The energy imbalance is determined by a complex multifaceted system of causes where no single influence dominates. The foresight report suggested several predominant interactive themes in the development of obesity. At the heart of the issue of excess weight lies a homeostatic *biological system* with an underlying propensity to accumulate energy and conserve it. Obesity is linked to broad social developments and shifts in values, such as changes in food production, motorised transport and work/home lifestyle patterns. The technological revolution of the 20th century has left in its wake an *'obesogenic environment'* that serves to expose the biological vulnerability of human beings. The *life course component* is also at play. Obesity takes time to develop and excess weight takes time to be lost. The risks of becoming obese may also start at an early stage. Growth patterns in the first few weeks and months of life affect the risk of later obesity and chronic disease. There is also a *generational dimension* with the most significant predictor of childhood obesity being parental obesity. In addition, vulnerability in physiological factors, eating habits, decreased activity levels and psychosocial influences all contribute in some form or other to the development of obesity.

Definition of Obesity

Overweight and obesity are the nutrition-related disorders, which are caused by the accumulation of extra body fat to such an extent that health and well-being may be adversely affected. Body mass index (BMI) is universally used as a measure for overweight and obesity. BMI = weight (kg) divided by height (m^2) (Table **1**).

In children and adolescents age 2 to 18 years, BMI is used in reference to body weight percentile reference tables. It is recommended that a percentile scale based on the child's sex and age be used. In this population, overweight is defined as a BMI in the 85th to 94th percentile, and obesity is a BMI at or above the 95th percentile. To a large extent this definition applies also to adults. Although BMI is useful on a population scale, it has limitations on an individual level, where more specific means of body composition complex measurement may be more useful and accurate. This is not routinely done nor indeed required in every case. BMI defines general obesity but does not account for body fat distribution. Abdominal obesity (central obesity), as assessed by waist circumference (WC), is more strongly associated with the risk of type 2 diabetes, hypertension, dyslipidaemia, cardiovascular disease, cancer, and all-cause mortality than general obesity. Abdominal obesity is defined as waist circumference of ≥90 cm for men and ≥80 cm for women. However, waist measurements are not routinely taken, and are subject to a measurement error due to difficulties in accurately and reproducibly identifying the waist. Specialised clinics rely on markers and schematic diagrams for repeat measurements.

Table 1. BMI based classification of individuals (Adapted from various sources). Morbidities pertain to hypertension, cardiovascular disease and diabetes. The super obese category is a sub-class of the grossly obese class.

BMI	Classification	Risk of Co-morbidities	
		For Waist circumference	
		Men ≤102Cm Women ≤ 88Cm	Men > 102Cm Women > 88Cm
< 18.5	Underweight		
18.5 – 24.9	Normal Range		
≥ 25.0	Overweight		
25.0 – 29.9	Pre-obese	Increased	High
30 – 34.9	Obese (Class I)	High	Very high
35 – 39.9	Morbidly obese (Class II)	Very High	Very high
≥ 40.0	Grossly obese (Class III)	Extremely high	Extremely high
≥ 50	Super obese	Extremely high	Extremely high

Consequences of Obesity

There is good evidence that obesity causes a wide range of health related problems. For the circulatory system there is an increased risk of coronary heart disease. Obesity also increases the risk of hypertension which is a risk for coronary heart disease, stroke and renal disease. There are also increased rates of deep venous thrombosis (DVT) and thrombo-embolic disease. The effect on the respiratory system includes asthma and obstructive sleep apnoea. It also causes non-alcoholic fatty liver disease (NAFLD), gallstones, hernias and gastro-oesophageal reflux disease. In women it raises the risk of stress incontinence, menstrual abnormalities, polycystic ovarian syndrome and sub-fertility. In men it causes erectile dysfunction. The excess weight puts strain on joints and increases the risk of back pain and arthritis particularly in the knees. Obesity raises the risk of several cancers especially colon, breast and endometrial cancer. Obesity is also linked to low mood, poor self-esteem, depression and reduced libido. Metabolically, obesity is attributable for the development of type-2 diabetes and dyslipidaemia. Being obese increased the risk of pregnancy and birth complications.

The burden of obesity is significant, and is estimated to be responsible for 58% of all Type 2 Diabetes, 21% of all heart disease, 10% of all non-smoking related cancers and hundreds of thousands of premature deaths per year around the globe. There is sufficient evidence to incriminate obesity in a variety of cancers.

Apart from the personal and social costs such as morbidity, mortality, discrimination and social exclusion, there are significant health and social care costs associated with the treatment of obesity and its consequences, as well as costs to the wider economy arising from chronic ill health. The costs of obesity are very likely to grow significantly in the next few decades.

Prevention of Obesity

The distinction between prevention and treatment is important. Once gained, weight is very difficult to lose. Preventing obesity requires changes in the environment and organisational behaviour, as well as changes in groups, family and individual behaviour. Interventions based on improved nutrition and increased physical activity can be effective for individuals. Shifting the *population* distribution of obesity will require interventions that target elements of the 'obesogenic' environment (including both the activity- and food-related environment) as well. Changes in transport infrastructure and urban design can be difficult and costly. However, they are more likely to affect multiple pathways within the obesity system in a sustainable way. Early life interventions such as breast-feeding, healthy weaning practices and appropriate maternal nutrition have all been linked to reduced obesity later in life. New drugs that can help regulate appetite control and energy intake are being developed that do not have the side effects and limited efficacy of current treatments. However, alone this is not a long-term sustainable solution. Devices to monitor and provide feedback on energy intake and energy expenditure, along with biomarkers of health, such as blood pressure, and blood glucose in real time are evolving. However, people may not act on this information. Altering the composition and manufacture of food products could help address obesity by seeking to control the release of macronutrients, by reducing energy- dense ingredients and by structuring food to slow the rate at which the stomach empties. However, the acceptability of such foods is uncertain. Once the interventions begin to influence behaviour, it is essential that behavioural change be maintained.

In practice, a strategy to tackle obesity needs a comprehensive portfolio of interventions with in-built sustainability targeting a broad set of variables and different levels within the obesity system.

Management of Obesity

Even modest weight loss (by 5–10% of initial weight) reduces the risk of developing type 2 diabetes, improves blood pressure and reduces total cholesterol. However, many people find it very difficult to maintain weight loss and there is often a gradual regain.

Treatment strategies vary in different centres and treatment sectors. However, a population-based strategy is based on a four-tiered model (Fig. **1**) working from a community based, self-care approach towards a more specialist based service [1]. In general, patients progress through the system in a step-wise manner:

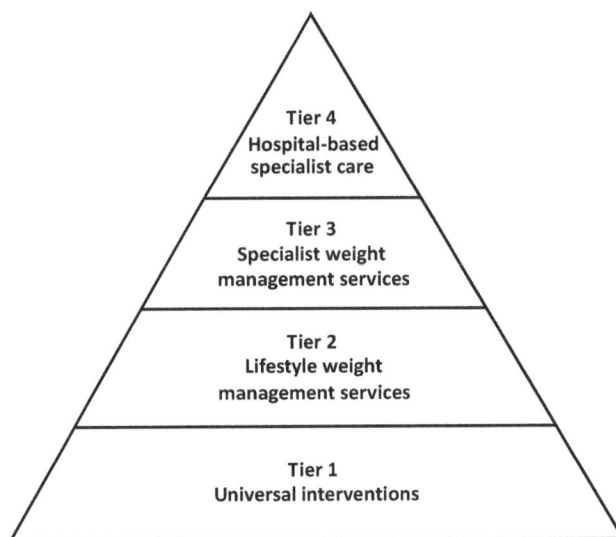

Fig. (1). Population based strategy for the management of obesity [1].

Tier 1 is universal and can be applied to the whole population both for management and as a prevention activity. The measures involve self-care dietary modifications and healthy eating with life-style changes with an aim of reducing calorie intake and increasing physical activity. This is often achieved by indirect contact using telephony advice or printed self-help leaflets. Lifestyle interventions of dietary restriction and increased physical activity can be successful as primary treatments. However, maintaining weight loss is often difficult. Sustained changes in diet and physical activity can lead to modest but sustained reductions in body weight, of approximately 5%, over many years. In reality, many people do not achieve sustained changes in either diet or physical activity.

Tier 2 involves the use of formal lifestyle weight management programs to reduce energy intake with increase in physical activity by changing behaviour. The programs are usually provided by public, private or voluntary sectors. The programs focus on changing behaviour to adopt a healthy life style, which entails calorie reduction and increased physical activity. Referral is often from a health practitioner but many programs will accept self-referrals. Enrolled people will usually be assigned an advisor who will provide support through an agreed program for a limited period (12 weeks) initially. In practice, people tend to drop in and out of these programs at will.

Tier 3 involves referral by a community medical practitioner (GP) or other secondary care practitioner *e.g.* cardiologist, orthopaedic surgeons or diabetologist to the local multidisciplinary team. This team will then progress and prioritise referral to the specialist weight management services. Referral criteria can vary but most patients need to have engaged with tier 1 and 2 and have a BMI of 40+ or a BMI 35 with co morbidities.

Tier 4 involves the use of anti-obesity drugs, supervised very low calorie diets and metabolic surgery.

Multidisciplinary Team

The multidisciplinary team consists of weight loss dieticians, metabolic (endocrine) physicians, specialist bariatric surgeons and psychologists. Ideally an anaesthetist with special interest in bariatric anaesthesia and a radiologist with an interest in gastrointestinal radiology can also be part of the team along with a nurse specialist.

After referral and discussion at the MDT, patients are seen at an introductory (group session) meeting. After a detailed explanation of the program, patients are invited to "opt in". This is followed by individual initial consultations to obtain a detailed history both medical and dietetic with major psychological issues identified in this consultation. The aim of the program is to influence sustained behavioural change and to demonstrate improvement. There is emphasis that the change needs to be gradual, sustained and has to be measurable *e.g.* pre-set weight loss of 5-10% over 6 months. The role of tier 3 service practitioners in those patients progressing to tier 4 has not been shown to improve outcomes but does help to identify patients who may not benefit from non- reversible surgery.

The program is based on a tailored approach for each individual patient. A good attendance record, ability to address change, psychological readiness and improvement in diet, all point towards a positive outcome after potential surgery. A sensitive goal directed approach should be adopted with all patients. There is good evidence that multi-component interventions are more likely to be effective than single component interventions *e.g.* diet alone outcomes vs diet and exercise. Patients with particular endocrine problems must be identified at an early stage and their endocrine problems managed appropriately by specialist physicians.

NON-SURGICAL MANAGEMENT

Dietary Management

Lifestyle interventions of dietary restriction and increased physical activity can be successful as primary treatments. For the majority of obese patients, a sustained positive calories balance led to the weight gain. It is essential to tackle this component sensitively. An initial one to one dietetic counselling session is essential to probe drivers and lifestyle, agree objectives and ensure engagement. The diet modification should aim for a healthy, nutritious eating plan, which fits into the patient's lifestyle. This often involves utilising a structured regular eating plan of improved quality foods focused on fresh food with low fat content. Advice on portion size and menu planning is integral. A discussion on eating out including fast foods should account for their calorific content. The calorific value of alcohol intake should also be accounted. For many patients, a simple reduction of 600 Kilocalories per day is all that is required. For others major lifestyle changes are required to address the significant dietary imbalances. Regular meetings focused on support and positive feedback with charting of achievements including weight loss should follow the initial counselling session.

Very Low Calorie Diets

There have been promising insights into using very low calorie diets using diets of between 600 and 1000Kcal per day under expert supervision as part of Tier 4 program in a research setting using either a combination of meal replacement sachets and vegetables or as a nasogastric infusion. In the short term they showed many of the benefits of weight loss surgery such as reversal of diabetes but in the long-term weight regain was observed when normal food was reintroduced. These diets are sold commercially and in enthusiasts, achieve significant (more than 5%) weight loss. However, the diets tend to have a bland taste and tolerance can be short lasting. Consequently, sustainability of weight loss is rarely achieved. However, these diets tend to produce early weight loss and may be used initially in a longitudinal program.

Exercise

Exercise improves overall health and helps with weight loss. The exercise component of the program is based on making small manageable changes to the patient's lifestyle by incorporating exercise and physical activity into daily routine. There should be emphasis on being realistic with small gradual incremental changes. The patient's medical history and current exercise ability should be taken into account. An otherwise fit and well young person with a BMI of 40 will have very different exercise ability in comparison with an older diabetic person with a BMI of 50 or more.

Psychology

Psychological input is important in anti-obesity programs. However, there has been variable uptake of psychological assessment and behavioural modification therapies in different programs. Food is consumed for pleasure and to satiate a craving. For many people, the daily routine is structured around meal times and food breaks. Others use food (or alcohol) to complement other social activities. Others still use food to help with stress and negative emotions. In contrast, obese individuals can be locked into psychological negativity with self-esteem, body image and societal acceptability issues. Many people view obesity as a physical issue and are not readily able or willing to discuss the impact of psychology or behavioural modification. For all these reasons, it is important to introduce psychological assessment and interventions sensitively and gradually. During psychology sessions, patients should have the opportunity to explore their relationship with food and the triggers around emotional eating. Some patients will have an eating disorder. They need help to learn new coping strategies and goal setting. Patients find it far easier to adopt dietary change and become more active once they have addressed the psychological issues that have underpinned their weight gain in the first place. Whether every patient or only selected patients need to see a psychologist remains controversial.

Pharmacology

Anti-obesity drugs may be effective as adjunctive therapy to diet and physical activity in those subjects who struggle to lose weight despite following an appropriate weight loss programme, most particularly those individuals who face or have developed medical complications as a result of their obesity. There is short-term evidence, which confirm that anti-obesity drugs induce weight loss in the region of 5-10% in the majority of patients during the first six months of treatment, and this is generally maintained while the drug is taken.

Over the years many drugs have been used for weight loss but all the amphetamine type drugs have now been withdrawn. Some drugs taken for other reasons may help weight loss but this is not their primary aim *e.g.* metformin, topiramate.

There are currently two classes of anti-obesity drugs: lipase inhibitors that work within the bowel to restrict fat absorption and centrally acting drugs that suppress appetite. Orlistat, is an example of the first group. This drug is licenced throughout the world. It works by ensuring that patients reduce fatty foods in their diet to avoid diarrhoea. It is licenced for use at a BMI of 28+ with co-morbidities or BMI 30 without. Treatment is initiated as a trial for 3 months and only continued if a 5% weight loss is demonstrated. Type 2 diabetics tend to achieve less than 5% weight loss and this goal may need to be modified in this group. In practice, the effectiveness of Orlistat is modest with patients losing 2-3 kg per year more than diet and exercise alone. The GI side effects include steatorrhoea and flatulence. Rarely, faecal leakage or incontinence can be reported due to unabsorbed fats reaching the large intestine. The results of therapy tend to be good in patients who are able to modify their diet and reduce fat content. They tend to tolerate the drug. Due to the side effects, treatment compliance tends to be low in those who do not modify their diet. Examples of the second group of drugs are Sibutramine and Rimonabant. These agents suppress appetite by making people feel full. This property is particularly helpful for obese patients because it deters overeating and encourages compliance with a sensible eating plan. The effectiveness of these drugs tends to be in the short term with significant weight loss in the first 6 months. The weight loss subsequently plateaus. However, patients tend to regain weight if the drugs are stopped. This group of drugs is not licenced throughout the world.

Outcomes of Non-Surgical Treatment

The problem with medical treatment is of long-term sustainability. Many patients will discuss the cycle of successful weight loss followed by weight gain (often more than they lost). This weight cycle reflects a combination of patients slipping back to old dietary and sedentary habits and losing the drive to change but also that the body adapts to the calorie deficit. There is a need to identify individuals most likely to benefit from specific treatment of their obesity. BMI is a useful measure for population surveillance but it has limited sensitivity at an individual level. Instead, it needs to be combined with information on the distribution of body fat, as well as other risk factors including family history, to make better risk assessments.

SURGICAL MANAGEMENT

Bariatric surgery is the only management, which has long-term sustainability of weight loss and reversal of comorbidities. However, it is not applicable to all obese patients. Bariatric surgery is an option for patients' subject to certain criteria. All non-surgical measures should have been attempted but have not resulted in meaningful weight loss. The patient has to be sufficiently fit to withstand anaesthesia and surgery. In addition, the patient has to be committed to long-term follow up. However, different surgical providers, have their own variations on the common theme. Most providers agree to enlist patients with BMI 35 kg/m^2 with comorbidities such as diabetes, sleep apnoea, osteoarthritis, hypertension, asthma or BMI 40 kg/m^2 without comorbidities for surgery. There is growing evidence that South-eastern Asians need a lower threshold and in select groups with new onset type 2 diabetes a lower threshold (BMI 30) may be appropriate. Smoking is seen as a relative contraindication, as the risks of smoking generally outweigh those of obesity. Others however see the risks as additive and therefore would consider surgery in smokers but the per-operative risks of complications in smokers are higher and more difficult to treat. In general, surgical interventions are the options of choice in patients with a BMI of greater than 50. Lifestyle or drug interventions are unlikely to be successful in this group of patients.

The risks of anti-obesity surgery, whether done laparoscopically or open should not be underestimated. Surgery has a powerful effect on cumulative mortality from all causes as seen in the Swedish obesity study. However, more recent data is less convincing. Discussions with patients on the merits of surgery should include the potential benefits, perioperative mortality, complication, associated risks and longer term implications. To date, there is no perfect weight loss surgical procedure, which would be suitable for all patients. Every surgical procedure has potential benefits and disadvantages. It is important that any specialist anti-obesity surgeon is able to offer more than procedure and can tailor the selected operation for the individual needs and circumstances of the patient.

Pathophysiology of Anti-Obesity Surgery

Originally anti-obesity surgery was broadly classified into restrictive and malabsorptive procedures. More recently, this concept has been challenged. Gastric banding restricts the ingested volume and is described as restrictive. By contrast, a biliopancreatic diversion procedure does not restrict the intake volume but reduce the absorption channel to only a meter in length. Hence, this procedure is termed malabsorptive.

Roux-en Y gastric bypass (RYGB) is the most frequently performed bariatric procedure, providing significant and sustained weight loss at long-term follow-up. However, the mechanisms of action in RYGB that result in weight loss are not well understood. A significant proportion of the resulting reduction in caloric intake is unaccounted for by the restrictive and malabsorptive mechanisms and is thought to be mediated by neuroendocrine function. RYGB is thought to cause substantial and simultaneous changes in gut peptides, brain activation, the desire to eat, and taste preferences. Some authors have assigned these changes to the 'foregut theory' whereby exclusion of the proximal intestine from food suppresses anti-incretin hormones. This leads to changes in blood sugar control and may be part of the explanation for improvement in blood glucose control (by stimulating insulin secretion and suppressing glucagon secretion) [2]. The alternative 'hindgut theory' suggests that the rapid delivery of nutrients to the distal small bowel stimulates release of hormones such as glucagon like peptide 1 (GLP1). The exaggerated secretion of satiety hormones such GLP-1 and peptide YY3-36 (PYY) from the distal small bowel have provided new insight into the physiological changes that occur after surgery which may be regarded as beneficial. However, the overall physiological changes, which occur after gastric bypass are unlikely to be due to a single hormone or indeed a single mechanism.

The physiological changes after anti-obesity surgery are probably a combination of multiple hormone effects in combination with complex-gut brain signalling which is poorly understood. The initial weight loss probably augments and modifies the effects with multiple mechanisms opting in and out in the post-surgery course. After surgery, patients display diverse changes, which can be beneficial such as improvement in blood sugar control, hypertension and hypercholesterolemia but also detrimental such as hypertriglyceridaemia and hyperuricaemia [3].

Outcomes after anti-obesity surgery are recorded in either percentage weight loss (total), percentage of initial excess weight or resolution of comorbidities. As a general rule the technically more difficult procedures, those which expose a greater risk with a greater potential long-term problems confer better improvement in potential weight loss and comorbidities. Bilio-pancreatic diversion (BPD) confers better improvement than Roux-en-Y gastric bypass (RYGB) then sleeve gastrectomy and gastric banding in that order. Over the years there has been a trend for using gastric bands in patients in whom a low risk procedure is required. Likewise, a sleeve gastrectomy was advocated for "volume eaters" and a gastric bypass for "sweet eaters". Other surgeons would advocate that a sleeve gastrectomy would be the primary option for the super morbidly obese due to the technical difficulties of other procedures in this group of patients. Blood sugar control measure using HbA1c in diabetics is best achieved by BPD followed by RYGB [4].

Bariatric Surgery and Pregnancy

Women are often advised to avoid pregnancy for the first twelve to eighteen months following surgery. The evidence base for this recommendation is limited, but it helps to ensure that the patient has reached a stable weight and facilitates appropriate planning of pregnancy and associated care [5].

Women who become pregnant after obesity surgery should take 5 mg folic acid until the 12th week of pregnancy (Compared to 400 mcg/day in normal healthy women) as there may be an increased risk of neural tube defects in born babies. As part of preconception care, women are advised to avoid vitamin and mineral preparations, which contain vitamin A in the retinol form in the first trimester of pregnancy as this may increase the teratogenicity risk. However, avoidance of supplements containing vitamin A may place women more at risk of low vitamin A levels especially if they have had a distal bypass or BPD/DS. Supplements containing vitamin A in the beta-carotene and not retinol form should be used.

Women who become pregnant following bariatric surgery should undergo nutritional screening every trimester. This should include ferritin, folate, vitamin B12, calcium and fat-soluble vitamins. Pregnant patients, especially those who have had distal bypass or BPD/DS procedures, may be at risk of low vitamin A levels and possibly vitamins E and K. Vitamin A levels (and possibly vitamin E and K levels) should be monitored during pregnancy. A more frequent review with the specialist bariatric dietician is advisable.

Preoperative Assessment

All patients who will potentially have bariatric surgery require a comprehensive assessment and a number of interventions to stratify their risks with a view to modifying the risk factors [6]. The vast majority of obese patients are relatively healthy and of a similar peri-operative risk to patients of a normal weight. Patients with central obesity and metabolic syndrome are however high risk. In addition to general considerations particular attention should focus on the risk of sleep disordered breathing and thromboembolism.

Although several risk stratification scores have been proposed, the obesity surgery mortality risk stratification score (OSMRS) is the most useful guide. The OSMRS was the first scoring system for risk assessment and stratification in bariatric surgery and is the only system validated independently by multiple centres throughout the world. The OSMRS assigns 1 point to each of the following five preoperative variables: age ≥ 45 years, male gender, body mass index (BMI) ≥ 50

kg/m2, hypertension and known risk factors for pulmonary embolism or 'PE risk' (previous thromboembolism, presence of inferior vena cava filter placement, a history of right heart failure or pulmonary hypertension and obesity hypoventilation syndrome). Patients with score 0 to 1 are classified as class 'A' (lowest) risk group, score 2 to 3 as class 'B' (intermediate) risk group and score 4 to 5 as class 'C' (high) risk group.

In order to assess for obstructive sleep apnea the STOP-BANG score is used and a score of 5 or more is significant in indicating obstructed sleep apnoea. These are loud Snoring, Tired during the day, Observed choking/gasping or stopping breathing, high blood Pressure (with or without treatment), BMI of 35+, Age 50+, Neck with collar size 17 men, 16 women and male Gender [7].

Patients with sleep apnoea should be asked to bring their continuous positive airways pressure (CPAP) devices to hospital with them for all hospital episodes particularly if they have surgery. Many of the obese patients have gastro-oesophageal reflux disease and preoperative treatment with proton pump inhibitors and antacids may reduce the risk of harmful aspiration particularly in the peri-operative period.

Pre-operative psychological assessment is controversial. Some centres recommend a psychological assessment for all patients before bariatric surgery. Others request a psychological assessment on a more selective basis after the first surgical assessment and a questionnaire psychological screen. This is claimed to be more cost effective. There is no hard and fast rule as to which patients will require psychological support after surgery and hence the selective approach is probably more cost effective. However, most units provide psychologists support after the procedure. With regards to using the psychological assessment for selection of patients for surgery, this is also controversial.

Some centres enrol patients in a dietetic programme to lose 10 – 20% of excess body weight as a demonstration of commitment towards the principle of weight loss, but also to help make the surgical procedure easier particularly by shrinking the liver.

Anaesthetic Considerations

Although regional anaesthesia is preferable, this is rarely possible for bariatric surgery. The use maximum tolerable doses of local anaesthetic agents complements post-operative analgesia regimens and reduce the risk of narcolepsy particularly in the presence of obstructed sleep apnoea.

Easily reversible drugs with fast onset and washout are the agents of choice for anti-obesity surgery. Anaesthetists must be prepared to recognise and plan for potential airway problems. Rescue techniques such as supra-glottic airway devices and emergency cricothyroidotomy have an increased failure rate and adverse events in obese patients.

The use of the ramped up position (tragus of ear at the same level as the sternum) during induction and reversal of anaesthesia improves lung mechanics and assists with intubation. This can be achieved by adjusting the head of the trolley position, by using additional pillows or with one a number of specially designed devices marketed specifically for the purpose (Fig. **2**).

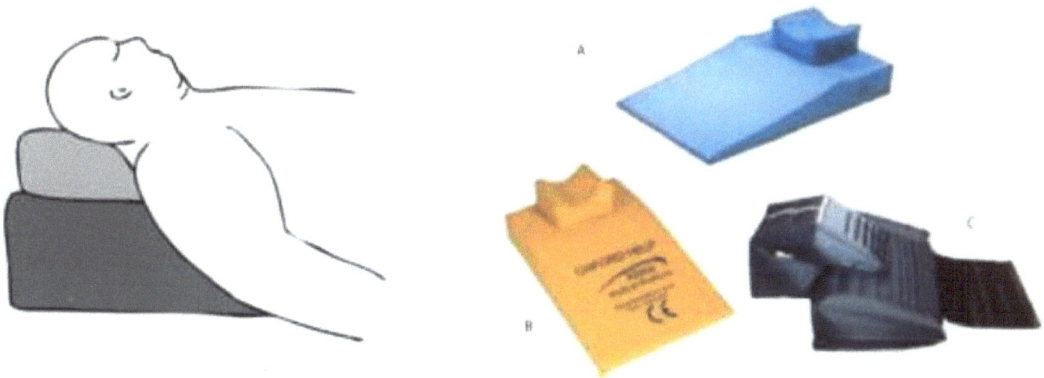

Fig. (2). (*left*) The ramped up position during induction and reversal of anaesthesia using custom made operating theatre standard foam support pillows (*right*).

There is limited information on the effect of obesity on the pharmacology of drugs used in anaesthesia. Much of the excess weight is adipose tissue, which has a relatively poor blood supply. Lipophilic drugs will have a larger volume of drug distribution than hydrophilic drugs. As a general guide, drug dosages should be calculated on the basis of lean or adjusted body weight. However, in practice, most drugs should be titrated (within the tolerance of the guide) according to effect. Drug dose calculations based on body weight can result in accidental awareness under anaesthesia due to abnormal distribution of drugs. To overcome this problem, monitoring of anaesthesia should be used routinely particularly with target controlled infusion (TCI) techniques and neuromuscular blockers.

Obesity is regarded as a prothrombotic state and thrombotic events are high. Pulmonary embolism is one of the major causes of mortality after surgery. The increased risk status remains elevated for up to 4 weeks after surgery. Multimodal anti-thrombotic prophylaxis is essential and includes avoidance of stasis, early mobilization, thromboembolic deterrent stockings (TEDS), Chemoprophylaxis (*e.g.* Clexane 40 mg, Fragmin 5000 iu with larger doses in larger patients) and sequential calf compression systems during surgery (Fig. **3**).

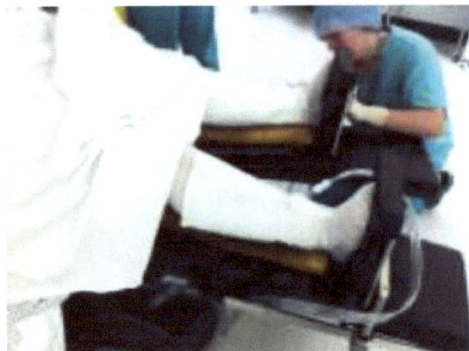

Fig. (3). The sequential calf compression system can be used intra-operatively and 48-hours post-operatively for thrombo-prophylaxis.

Gastric bypass surgery can cause a dramatically rapid neuro-humeral response reducing insulin requirements post-surgery. Adequate monitoring, anticipation, recognition and rapid correction are all very important.

An extubation plan must be in place in accordance with the Difficult Airway Society extubation guidelines. A nerve stimulator should guide reversal of neuromuscular blockade. Anaesthetists usually ensure that patients have regained airway reflexes and are breathing with an adequate tidal volume before tracheal extubation. Extubation is usually performed with the patient awake and in the sitting position. In those patients with confirmed obstructed sleep apnoea (OSA), the insertion of a nasopharyngeal airway before waking helps mitigate partial airway obstruction, which may be encountered during emergence from anaesthesia.

Post-operative Care

In the immediate post-operative recovery period, patients should have full monitoring of vital signs. Throughout recovery, patients are nursed in the sitting or 45-degree head up position. Patient with OSA who normally uses CPAP at home should have this commenced either in the recovery room or on the ward. Before discharge from the recovery room, all obese patients should be observed whilst unstimulated for signs of hypoventilation, (apnoea or hyperpnoea with associated oxygen desaturation). This warrants an extended period of monitoring in the recovery room. On-going hypoventilation will necessitate anaesthetic reassessment to establish the need for further respiratory support and/ or level-2 care.

For the vast majority of elective patients, a return to the ward environment with an enhanced recovery protocol is advocated. This protocol implies patient return from theatre without restricting equipment (IV lines, catheters, drains) wherever possible with early mobilization encouraged. Pulse oximetry should be continued until baseline oxygen saturations are maintained without supplemental oxygen and parental opioids are no longer needed.

Operative Considerations

The average BMI of patients operated on in the UK for weight loss surgery in 2015 was 49.8 kg/m^2 and the vast majority of procedures were carried out laparoscopically. In experienced high-volume centres, the operative setup should be geared towards the laparoscopic approach, with its acclaimed benefits in this patient group. However open conversion instruments should always be readily available for rapid conversion should the need arise.

Surgery should be carried out in a high volume unit with experienced personnel. These units should have adequate facilities and recognition for education, training and accreditation. The recommended learning curve is thought to include 50 cases with mixed banding and stapling procedures. The imaging setup should consist of a modern high-definition (HD) laparoscopic stack and dual screens with a 30 degrees high quality optical telescope. Whilst specialist long instruments and ports are generally not needed they should always be available if required. The operating table should have the facility to function in the head up position and must be able to withstand 250 kg weight load as a minimum. Footplates should be available as they help to stop a patient sliding off the table in the head up (anti-Trendelenberg) position. A "seatbelt" type strap can also help as an adequate restraint. The ideal position for surgery for most patients is the split leg, head up position with a degree of hip flexion, the so-called "deck chair position". The majority of bariatric surgeons prefer to operate with the surgeon standing between the split legs for all or significant portions of the operation. Some surgeons exchange positions with the assistant or scrub nurse during relevant parts of the operation. The assistant (positioned on the side of the patient) must be able to use the camera in one hand and retract with the other. The scrub nurse is usually positioned on the other side of the patient opposite the assistant. The assistant and scrub nurse should have direct, unobstructed view to the screen throughout these long and complex operations (Fig. **4**). Supplementary instruments required in cases of conversion to open surgery must include deep, mechanical, self-retaining retractors and long instruments similar to those used in conventional open surgery.

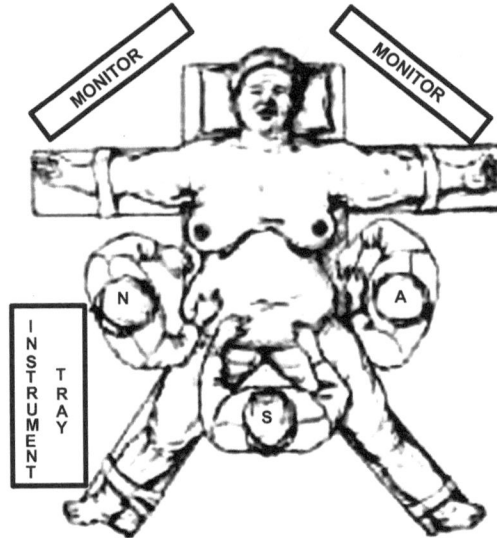

Fig. (4). Standard positioning of patient and surgical team for bariatric surgery (S: Surgeon, A: Assistant, N: Scrub Nurse).

All operating theatre personnel should have completed an instruction course in manual handling and transfer of patients. A "Hovermat®" system is popular for transferring patients onto and off the operating table. Due to the head up operating position, a step for the anaesthetist to stand on is usually necessary.

Most surgeons use standard ports, which are used in conventional laparoscopic surgery *e.g.* fundoplication. Some surgeons use specialized long ports designed for obese patients.

Port positions and sizes can be variable and depend on the surgeon's experience and training (Fig. **5**). The 5 mm liver retractor is usually positioned sub-xiphisternum and the other ports are usually positioned along the circumference of a semi-circle in the sub-sternal triangle. The camera port is usually positioned supra-umbilically. The other ports need to be of a sufficient size to accommodate the optical telescope, stapler and or band. Most surgeons use 12 mm ports with the exception of the left hand side assistants retract port, which can be 5 mm. The patient position is almost always head-up although some surgeons reduce the head up angle when working in the infra-colic compartment.

Entry to the abdomen is dependent on the individual surgeon but an open cut down is rarely appropriate in this group. The use of a Verres needle in Palmers point is common and as many standard ports allow a camera directed entry this has become common place

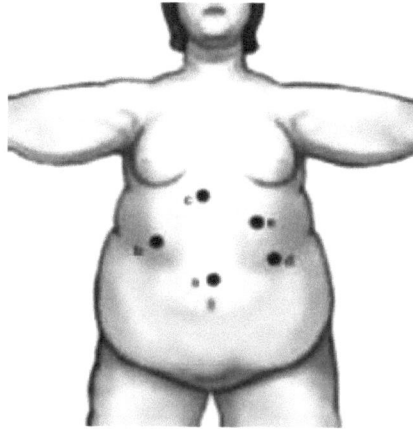

Fig. (5). Port positions for bariatric surgery. The camera could be introduced via ports a or b. Port c is for the liver retractor. Ports d and e are for dissection and retraction respectively.

Follow Up after Bariatric Surgery

Follow up after anti-obesity surgery falls into two broad categories. The first category includes early follow-up to detect and deal with post-operative complications and delayed emergencies. The unit performing surgery must be available to give advice to patients and to other health professionals should patients present to their local general medical facility. On discharge, patients should receive instructions on how to make urgent contact with the bariatric surgical unit. Although complication after discharge are uncommon, delayed presentation of leaks or internal hernias can be potentially life threatening.

The second category of follow-up is continuous clinical follow up to provide appropriate dietary and nutritional assessment and to offer support and guidance in the short and long term on weight loss, appropriate goals and maintenance. It is also important to monitor nutrients and micronutrients and to signpost to patient support groups. Many commissioned services and specialized centres provide this follow up for 2 years before handing it over to the patient's general medical practitioner (GP) for an annual review.

Nutritional deficiencies are common after some types of surgery [8]. Full guidance is available from specialist surgical and nutritional associations. Patients who have had a gastric balloon or band will need a once daily multivitamin tablet. As balloons only remain in-situ for 6 months, long-term follow up is unnecessary. In the short term, weight, blood glucose, urea, haemoglobin, electrolytes and liver enzymes measurements should be monitored routinely. Gastric band patients should have these checked annually along with lipids if this has been abnormal. Sleeve gastrectomy is a common procedure and patients require close monitoring for the first year including measurement of urea, electrolytes, liver enzymes, haemoglobin, Ferritin, folate, Calcium, Vitamin D and Parathyroid hormone at 3, 6, and 12 months before annual testing. Lipids and glucose monitoring is appropriate but micronutrients assessments are not recommended unless clinically indicated. It is suggested that sleeve gastrectomy patients should be taking lifelong multivitamins, minerals, B12 (hydroxyl cobalamine) injections every 3 months starting 6 months after surgery, iron and calcium tablets. Patients who have had gastric bypass procedures need the same monitoring as sleeve gastrectomy patients but with the addition of annual zinc and copper measurements. After duodenal switch/ BPD, patients should have the same follow up and monitoring as gastric bypass patients with the addition of routine monitoring of vitamin A. Monitoring of vitamins E (neuropathy or anaemia), K (bleeding disorders) and selenium (anaemia, heart failure, chronic diarrhoea, and fatigue) are indicated by symptoms.

A number of studies have shown an increased suicide risk reported in patients after bariatric surgery [9]. There is a great need to identify persons at risk pre-operatively and provide post-operative psychological monitoring and support for these individuals. Most bariatric surgical units provide an urgent support line for patients in despair. Suicide advice cards with contact numbers of key trained personnel are issued to all patients after bariatric surgery in some centres [10].

Audit / Outcomes

Despite tremendous recent progress, bariatric surgery remains in its infancy and there is a lot of room for improvement. Bariatric surgery has rapidly gained acceptance by the public, primary care physicians, and surgeons. The resulting exponential growth of bariatric surgery has increased scrutiny by governmental bodies and the media regarding the safety of bariatric surgery. To date, the outcome of bariatric surgery has been derived from large, single-institution series reflecting practice of bariatric surgery by enthusiasts at a few experienced centers. Although the beneficial effects of bariatric surgery have been documented, the perioperative death rates of up to 2% is concerning [11]. Long-term audit data suggest that weight loss after bariatric surgery is sustainable [12], Type 2 diabetes [13] and other comorbidities are decreased [14] and overall mortality is decreased [15].

The results of audit outcomes should inform the basis of informed consent for the procedures in general and for the centre's outcomes. It is important that all staff involved with bariatric surgery facilitate quality control in the interest of patients. This engagement and facilitation should be at both the local and national level. This could be by formal audit studies of selected important parameters or by adding data to a recognised registry. Key indicators include morbidity, mortality, co-morbidity improvement, BMI/ weight loss, re-operation, satisfaction and quality of life. Additional measures should include long-term sustainability of weight loss, effect on overall mortality. Co-morbidity improvement should be general but also include improvement in specific diseases such as type 2 diabetes, high blood pressure, dyslipidaemia, sleep apnoea and functional status.

SURGICAL PROCEDURES

Choice of Procedure

There is no perfect weight loss operation. Each operation has advantages and disadvantages. It is important that surgeons have a repertoire of more than one procedure to offer their patients. Patients with co-morbidities such as diabetes would benefit more from a bypass or BPD. Super obese patients with a high BMI (> 50) are better served with a staged procedure such as an intra-gastric balloon or sleeve gastrectomy followed by a duodenal switch. A sleeve gastrectomy should be avoided in patients with a hiatus hernia or past history of gastro-oesophageal reflux. The type of procedure should be determined during the MDT discussion based on all the available information. Additional information may be required to reach a decision such as the need for preoperative endoscopy. A laparoscopic approach has the established benefits of reduction in morbidity, mortality and hospital stay, should always be preferred to open surgery whenever possible. Current evidence suggests that unless the patient has pre-existing gallstone symptoms then cholecystectomy is unnecessary at the primary procedure.

Intra-Gastric Balloon

Gastric balloons create an artificial bezoar filling the stomach and restricting excess food intake (Fig. **6**). The balloon results initially in nausea but more importantly it increases satiety. Patients can lose 10-20% of excess weight in the 6-month period they are inserted for. They are indicated as part of a staged procedure for the super obese. Alternatively, they are indicated in patients who need to lose weight due to co-morbidities and are unable to withstand formal weight loss surgery. The balloons are licensed for 6 months' maximal use. However, they can be replaced after 6 months but the benefits become limited. Some patients tolerate a balloon remarkably well (80%) and others don't. Those who do not tolerate the balloon complain bitterly of nausea despite a cocktail of anti-nausea medicines. In these patients, the balloon is usually removed before leaving hospital. Balloons have a role in improving the operative risks of the super morbidly obese and may have a role together with psychology input in trying to break the food craving cycle.

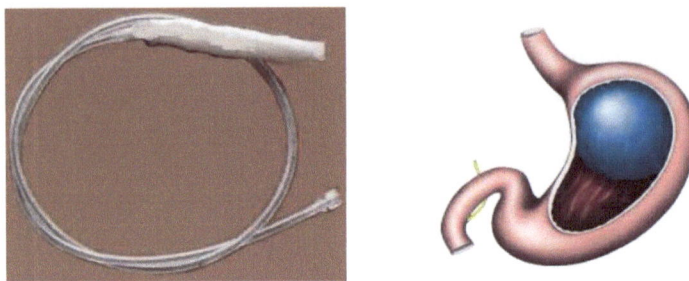

Fig. (6). The intra-gastric balloon oro-gastric introducer (*left*) and a schematic diagram of the intra-gastric balloon in situ (*right*).

Insertion is performed under conscious sedation. An experienced interventional endoscopist can safely complete the procedure. The endoscopist should pay particular attention to the diaphragmatic hiatus looking for evidence of gastro-oesophageal reflux or a hiatus hernia. Active peptic ulceration in the stomach is a contra-indication. The balloon is supplied preloaded into a small oro-gastric introducer. The tube is placed in the stomach and the sheath withdrawn to deploy the balloon into the stomach. The position of the balloon is confirmed by reinsertion of the endoscope. Under endoscopic vision 500-700 mls of methylene blue dyed saline is inserted into the access port. Some endoscopists use air / saline mix to aid positioning in the gastric fundus. Once the balloon is inflated a sharp tug removes the delivery device and the balloon valve seals. Patients are advised to stick to liquids for 24-hours progressing to a semi liquid diet initially along with anti-emetics. Removal of the balloon involves endoscopic needle aspiration of the contents followed by grasping the deflated balloon and pulling it up the oesophagus (Fig. **7**). The removal procedure can also be done under conscious sedation.

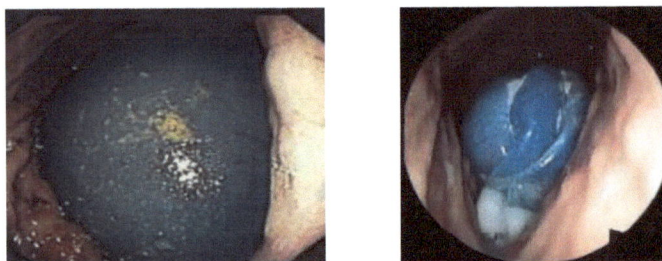

Fig. (7). The intra-gastric balloon in situ. (*left*) the balloon is fully inflated. (*right*) the balloon is partially inflated.

The benefits of the balloon include that it can be done under conscious sedation, works instantly and is easily removable. Disadvantages include the temporary nature, intolerance, reflux, ulceration and spontaneous rupture. The latter manifests with the patients passing green urine due to the methylene blue dye being absorbed in the small bowel and excreted in urine. Patients should be advised to report this manifestation urgently and the balloon must be removed early before it exists the stomach into the intestine where it can cause obstruction. Damage to the oesophagus has been reported during insertion and removal.

Vertical Banded Gastroplasty

Vertical Banded Gastroplasty (VBG) is a primarily restrictive anti-obesity procedure, which was popular 30 years ago but is seldom performed now. It suited the open era of surgery but staple line disruption was common. The aim of the procedure was to produce a small gastric pouch with an exit stoma of controlled size. The procedure can be done laparoscopically. The ports and theatre equipment setup is similar to standard laparoscopic upper GI procedures. The Angle of his is mobilized. The lesser sac is then entered to form the small pouch. A 32 Fr. bougie is placed across the oesophago-gastric junction. The anvil of a 33 circular stapler is inserted into the abdomen and placed into the lesser sac with the spike puncturing posterior and anterior walls of the stomach. The circular staple gun is inserted into the abdomen, attached to the anvil (after removal of the spike) and fired. This creates a circular defect in the walls of the stomach adjacent to the intraluminal bougie. A linear stapler is inserted through this circular defect cephalad towards the angle of his and fired. Some surgeons divide this staple line. A 1.5 cm wide Goretex band is placed around the lower portion of the pouch and held with at least 3 non-absorbable sutures (Fig. **8**). The advantages of this procedure are that it is relatively easy to perform and is reversible. Many surgeons regard the procedure technically difficult especially in positioning the anvil laparoscopically. Other procedures achieve similar or better results. Staple line problems were common especially if not divided. As a result, this procedure is largely abandoned.

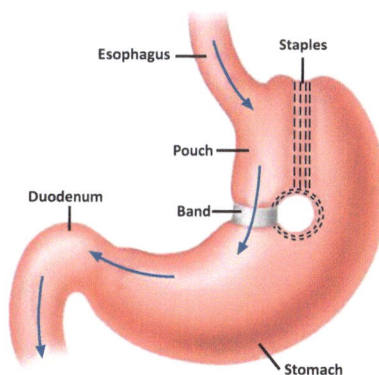

Fig. (8). Schematic diagram of the vertical banded gastroplasty.

Duodeno-Jejunal Bypass Sleeve

The Duodenal–jejunal bypass sleeve (DJBS, EndoBarrier Gastrointestinal Liner; GI Dynamics Inc., Lexington, Massachusetts, USA) is an endoscopically and fluoroscopically inserted implant. It consists of an impermeable flouro-polymer sleeve that is reversibly fixated to the duodenal bulb and extends 80 cm into the small bowel, usually terminating in the proximal jejunum (Fig. **9**). It allows transit of chyme from the stomach through to the jejunum without contact with the duodenal or jejunal mucosa. By not allowing mixing with pancreatic exocrine secretions and bile in the jejunum, it mimics a duodenal-jejunal bypass and encourages weight loss through malabsorption.

The insertion procedure is done with the patient under general anaesthesia or sedation, using image guidance. The sleeve is positioned and deployed endoscopically. Using a delivery catheter, a capsule containing a single-use impermeable DJBS is positioned in the duodenal bulb just distal to the pylorus and is secured there using an integral spring metal anchor. The sleeve is advanced distally into the jejunum with the aid of a tension wire, which is part of the introducer device. It extends down the small intestine and forms a barrier between food and the intestinal wall. The sleeve is regarded as malabsorptive.

After the procedure, patients are placed on a diet that typically involves progression from fluids to semi-solid foods, before returning to solid foods.

After a maximum of a year, the sleeve is removed under sedation, using endoscopy and image guidance. The anchor incorporates a drawstring mechanism that enables it to be collapsed and partly withdrawn into a plastic hood fitted to the endoscope. The entire device is then withdrawn.

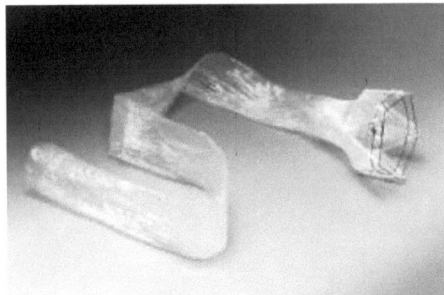

Fig. (9). The duodeno-jejunal bypass Sleeve (DJBS).

The advantages of this device are that it can be inserted as a day case procedure without scars and is reversible with a lifetime of 12 months. Mean weight loss is 10 kg (10% excess weight) and 50-75% of patients showed improvements in diabetic control during treatment. Side effects are common with nausea (77%) and cramps (30%) reported by the majority of patients. The symptoms generally settled within a week with medication [16]. A small number of patients have needed explantation of the device. Serious risks include device migration, failure to deploy or and liver abscesses. Some patients have had serious bleeding due to the duodenal bulb anchoring spikes injuring the mucosa either during insertion or after removal.

Gastric Bands

The Adjustable Gastric Band involves placing a plastic ring with an inflatable insert around the upper portion of the stomach, creating a small stomach pouch above the band with food emptying slowly through the band constricted section of the stomach. In theory a small amount of food will fill the pouch above the band to satisfy hunger, and produce the feeling of satiety promoting less food consumption. The feeling of fullness depends on food retention in the pouch above the band and this is controlled by the diameter of the band-constricted stomach. This diameter is adjustable by filling the band with sterile saline, which is injected through a port placed subcutaneously. Reducing the size of the opening is done gradually over time with repeated adjustments or "fills". The gastric band is purely restrictive. The technique for gastric band placement has been modified over the years to try and reduce complications by using the pars flaccid route and by stitching the band in situ.

The procedure is done under general anaesthesia. The laparoscopic ports are inserted in standard positions. A larger port (12 or 15 mm) on the left of the patient is used to allow intra-abdominal insertion of the band. The procedure commences with mobilization of the angle of His. The pars flaccida is incised and the right diaphragmatic crus is identified. A blunt dissector *e.g.* "Goldfinger™" device is inserted behind the stomach, anterior to the right diaphragmatic crus to form a retro-gastric tunnel exiting at the angle of His. Some surgeons use a calibrating device to assist with pouch formation. If a hiatus hernia is encountered the crura should be repaired with non-absorbable sutures. Once the "Goldfinger™" is in place the prepared band is inserted into the abdomen and attached to the "Goldfinger™". By withdrawing the "Goldfinger™", the band is passed behind the stomach. The band is then locked in front of the stomach. Three gastro-gastric sutures are placed to secure the band in position (Fig. **10**).

The fill tubing attached to the band is the exited from the abdomen and tunnelled to a suitable position immediately above the muscle layer. The port is attached to the tubing and secured to the rectus muscle with non-absorbable sutures or using the inbuilt locking mechanism present on some systems. Wounds are then closed.

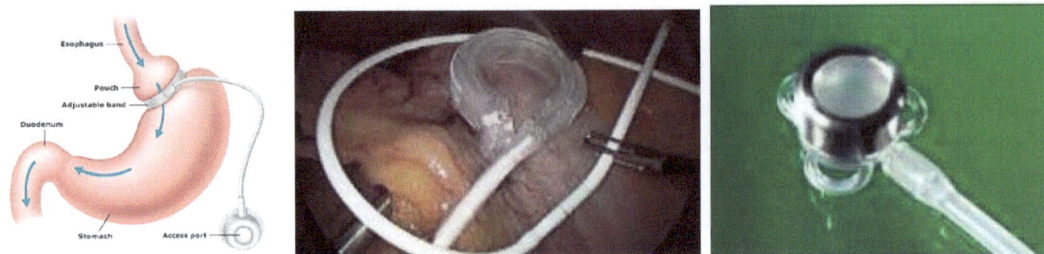

Fig. (10). (*left*) Schematic diagram of the adjustable gastric band system. (*centre*) The band introduced into the abdomen for placement. (*right*) The filling port is implanted subcutaneously and connected to the band.

The advantages of the gastric band are that it can result in loss of approximately 40 – 50 per cent of excess weight, requires a short hospital stay (often less than 24 hours, with day cases in some centres), involves no division of the stomach or rerouting of the intestines and is reversible and adjustable [17]. It has the lowest rate of early postoperative complications and mortality among the approved bariatric procedures. The procedure is very popular amongst private care physicians. Additionally, it has the lowest risk for vitamin/ mineral deficiencies. The disadvantages are that weight loss is slow and less than other procedures with the highest failure rate despite s strict adherence to the postoperative diet and to postoperative follow-up visits. It can take a period of time to adjust the band correctly to "the sweet spot". It entails a foreign device to remain in the body and can result in band infection, slippage or erosion (Fig. **11**) into the stomach in a small percentage of patients. Mechanical problems can arise with the band, tube or port.

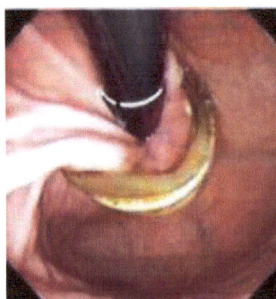

Fig. (11). Endoscopic review of an intra-gastric erosion of band. The band can be removed endoscopically.

All of these problems have led to the highest rate of reoperation. Irreversible oesophageal dilation has been reported in patients who persistently overeat. Although the bands remain popular and have received a large amount of media coverage, they are beginning to be abandoned by the surgical community. However, they continue to have a place in the surgical armamentarium to combat obesity. It will be a matter of time to determine whether they will still occupy a prominent place in that surgical armamentarium. Technical advances in the design and placement of the bands is focussed on negating some of the surgical complications and these steps may encourage their continued use and popularity.

Sleeve Gastric Resection

This procedure permanently removes 80% of the stomach volume. It was originally described as the first stage before a bilio-pancreatic diversion (BPD) but resulted in many patients losing a sufficient amount of weight that the second stage procedure was deemed unnecessary. The stomach remnant holds a considerably smaller volume than the normal stomach and helps to significantly reduce the amount of food (and thus calories) that can be consumed. It results in secretion of hunger induced GI hormones including Ghrelin and this effect improves hunger, satiety, and blood sugar control. Sleeve gastric resection is primarily regarded as a restrictive procedure [18].

The technique involves mobilization of the greater curve of the stomach using an energy device such as Harmonic scalpel or 'Ligasure™' and separating the stomach from the omentum. The gastric remnant from the pylorus to the gastro-oesophageal junction is calibrated around a bougie. The remnant size varies between surgeons (32 Fr to 50 Fr) but almost all surgeons use a bougie to calibrate the remnant gastric tube to their preferred size. The stomach is then stapled starting distally aiming towards the bougie on the initial firing and then parallel to the bougie to complete the resection of the greater curve of the stomach (Fig. **12**). Care is taken not to staple the bougie. The bariatric surgical community remains divided about the use of staple line reinforcement. The divided stomach is then removed. Some surgeons perform a leak test using injected methylene blue dye intraluminally.

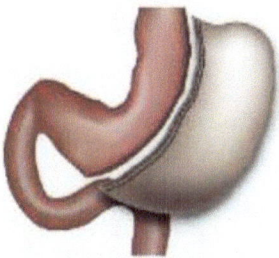

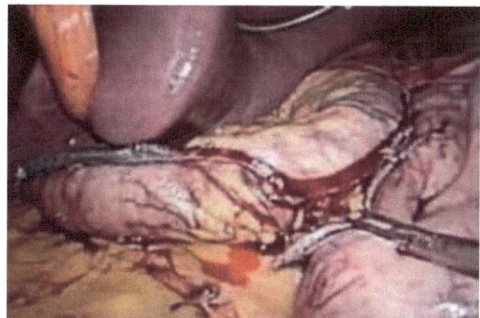

Fig. (12). (left) Schematic diagram of sleeve gastric resection. (right) intra-operative view of sleeve gastric resection.

Studies have suggested that the results of sleeve gastric resection are nearly as good as gastric bypass surgery with excess weight loss of around 50%. There are no foreign bodies or rerouting of intestines (endoscopy and ERCP can be performed when necessary). The disadvantages of this procedure are that it is permanent and that the sleeve can progressively increase in size. Post-operative bleeding or leaks are uncommon but can be serious. Leaks tend to be near the oesophagogastric junction and are difficult to heal due to the high pressure of the intact pylorus. Chronic leaks can turn into entero-cutaneous fistulae (Fig. **13**). These leaks should be treated in an identical fashion to leaks after other surgeries with drainage, antibiotics and alternative nutrition until they heal. Rarely conversion to a low-pressure gastric bypass is necessary. This procedure has the potential of incurring vitamin and mineral deficiencies.

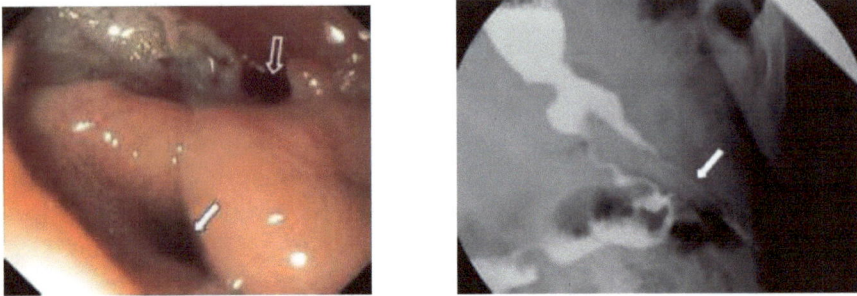

Fig. (13). Radiological and endoscopic view of a sleeve fistula.

Roux-en-Y Gastric Bypass

The Roux-En-Y Gastric bypass (RYGB) is considered the gold standard anti-obesity procedure and involves two components. The first component entails creation of a small gastric pouch. Secondarily, the small bowel is used to bypass the duodenum and a metre of proximal jejunum. This results in a small stomach pouch promoting reduced calorie consumption (restrictive), some degree of malabsorption due to the duodeno-jejunal by pass and gut hormone changes which contribute to satiety and blood sugar control.

A number of different techniques have been described to perform RYGB but all involve making a small gastric pouch, identifying the proximal jejunum and dividing it. The rerouted small bowel (in front or behind the colon) is approximated to the stomach remnant (gastroenterostomy) and the distal jejunum is approximated to the small bowel as an end to side entero-enterostomy. The small bowel can be rerouted in front or behind the colon to form the gastroenterostomy. The retrocolic approach requires a shorter segment of small bowel but requires additional dissection in the transverse mesocolon and the potential for bleeding.

The procedure is carried out under general anaesthesia and a single dose of antibiotics is given for prophylaxis. Pneumoperitoneum is achieved before inserting ports and a liver retractor. A laparoscopic survey excludes gross adhesions, which may affect the mobility of the small bowel. The angle of His is dissected free and a 60 ml gastric pouch (long and thin) is created from the lesser curvature of the stomach. A calibrated bougie and a stapling device are used to create the gastric pouch. A 45 mm transverse staple line used to divide the stomach and the pouch completed using a bougie for guidance, stapling cephalad lateral to the OGJ. This staple line is checked for haemostasis and additional clips applied if necessary. In the antecolic approach, the transverse colon is carefully reflected and the omentum split if appropriate. The DJ flexure is positively identified and the jejunum walked distally using atraumatic graspers to approximately 60 cm. The jejunum is divided using the linear stapler and the distal small bowel is brought over the colon and anastomosed to the gastric pouch. The gastroenterostomy can be fashioned using linear staplers or a circular stapler. An end-to-side or side-to-side entero-enterostomy is fashioned a further 150 cm down the small bowel using liner staplers (Fig. **14**). A blue methylene blue dye leak test is performed. Hernia defects are closed either with staples or non-absorbable sutures and haemostasis is checked and secured.

In the retrocolic approach, the DJ flexure is identified and a defect is made in the transverse mesocolon. The proximal jejunum is then measured and divided with the jejuno-jejunal anastomosis performed first. The distal divided end is passed through the window in the transverse colon mesentry and retrieved above the colon and anastomosed to the stomach pouch.

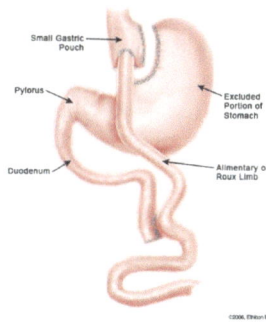

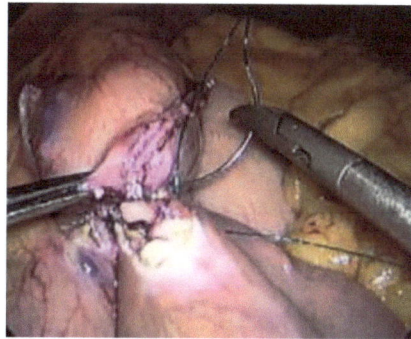

Fig. (14). (left) Schematic diagram of Roux-en-Y gastric bypass procedure. Intra-operative view of the gastric-pouch enterostomy.

The main advantage of the RYGB is that it reliably produces significant long-term weight loss (60 to 80 per cent of excess weight) [19]. The disadvantages are that it is more technically demanding. The per-operative risks include bleeding, leaks, incorrect rerouting (Roux-en-O), internal hernias resulting in bowel obstruction, marginal ulceration (Fig. **15**) and can lead to long-term vitamin/mineral deficiencies particularly deficits in vitamin B12, iron, calcium, and folate unless life-long vitamin/mineral supplementation is taken. It is important that these patients comply with long-term follow-up to recognize and identify the nutritional deficiencies. Dumping syndrome affects many patients after RYGB as the lack of pylorus means food can rapidly be transported into the small bowel. Early dumping happens 10 to 30 minutes after a meal whereas late dumping occurs 1 to 3 hours after food. Early dumping occurs when foods especially carbohydrates are "dumped" quickly into the intestine. The small bowel senses the hyperosmolar contents and the body react by shifting fluids into the small bowel causing nausea, vomiting, cramps, diarrhoea, flushing, dizziness, an urge to lie down and a rapid heart rate. Late dumping occurs in response to the carbohydrates absorbed from the small bowel. An exaggerated insulin response to counteract the hyperglycaemia ensues. Since the carbohydrates have rapidly left the small bowel, the patient is left in a hypoglycaemic state. The symptoms of late dumping include sweating, dizziness, weakness, hunger, fatigue, weakness and a rapid heart rate. To avoid dumping a dietary modification is necessary avoiding high carbohydrate meals and fluids during meals. The unpleasant symptoms of dumping can reinforce the required dietary changes with gastric bypass surgery. Patients should be advised to eat smaller more frequent meals based on complex carbohydrates like whole grains rather than simple carbohydrates like bread or sweets. They should avoid liquids with their meals, which aid gastric emptying. Glucose response tests and radioactive gastric emptying studies may be used to aid diagnosis. If this dietary modification fails treatment is limited to somatostatins and in rare cases revision surgery.

Internal hernias can cause life-threatening complications at any point after gastric bypass surgery. They can block the intestine depending on which part is obstructed. Although patients will experience pain and nausea, they may not vomit due to the reformed anatomy. Clinical suspicion and confirmation with contrast enhanced three-dimensional scanning (CT) or laparoscopy will usually reveal the diagnosis and site of obstruction. Weight loss may make the risk of obstruction higher due to loss of occupying fat protecting the potential hernia spaces. There are three potential sites for internal hernias. The first is at the defect in the transverse mesocolon through which the Roux limb passes if it is placed in the retrocolic position. The second is at the mesenteric defect at the entero-enterostomy (jejuno-jejunostomy) and thirdly behind the Roux limb mesentery placed in a retrocolic or antecolic position (Petersen type hernia) [19]. Closure of these potential hernia defects at the time as surgery should avoid this untoward complication.

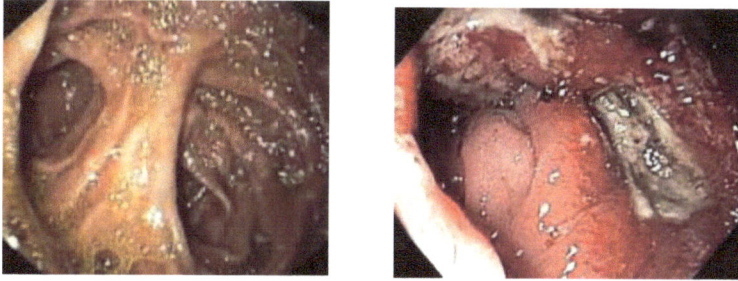

Fig. (15). (*left*) Normal view at gastro-jejunal anastomosis after RYGB. (*right*) Non healing marginal ulcer after gastric bypass.

Due to the depth of the subcutaneous fat layer, port site fascia is rarely closed. Port site hernias can occur at any stage and are often not clinically palpable. A high index of suspicion and appropriate imaging will usually reveal the diagnosis and the site of herniation (Fig. **16**).

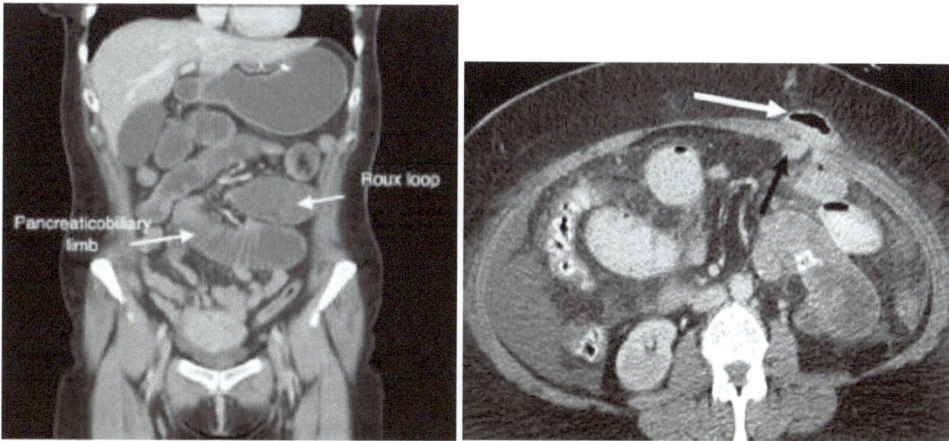

Fig. (16). (*left*) Obstruction due to internal hernia in common limb after RYGB. (*right*) Port site hernia.

Loop Gastric Bypass

Over the past few years the "mini gastric bypass" or single anastomosis gastric bypass has gained popularity. The procedure is partly restrictive due to the size of the gastric pouch and partly malabsorptive as food preferentially travels down the pro-peristaltic distal small bowel.

The technique involves mobilizing the angle of His, entering the lesser sac through the lesser omentum at the level of the crow's foot. A long thin gastric pouch is created over a 36Fr bougie using linear staplers in similar fashion to a bypass/ sleeve (Fig. **17**). Once the gastric pouch is completed, the omentum is retracted from the left to the right to allow positive identification of the DJ flexure. The proximal small bowel is measured to 200 cm and a gastric pouch-enterostomy is created at this measured point along the small bowel. Some surgeons add an anti-reflux procedure at the end. The operation time is usually shorter than RYGB.

The use of a single anastomosis reduces the potential of leaks by 50% and also removes one of the hernia defects. Long-term data are still awaited but this procedure appears to be at least as effective in terms of weight loss as RYGB and weight loss may be quicker. Many of the other risks are similar to RYGB but as digestive enzymes and bile are not diverted away from the stomach after mini gastric bypass this can lead to bile reflux gastritis which can cause pain that is difficult to treat. Bile reflux gastritis may also theoretically increase the risk of cancer in the stomach pouch or oesophagus.

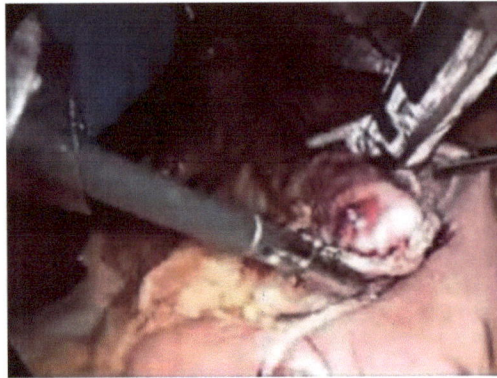

Fig. (17). Intra-operative view of the completed gastric pouch.

Bilio-Pancreatic Bypass with Duodenal Switch (BPD/DS)

The BPD/DS is a procedure with two components. Firstly, removing a portion of the stomach akin to the sleeve gastrectomy creates a tubular stomach pouch and secondly a large portion of the small intestine is bypassed. The procedure is partly restrictive due to the size of the gastric pouch and partly malabsorptive as food is diverted from the proximal small bowel.

This procedure is not very popular among bariatric surgical community but it produces the most profound weight loss and best control of diabetes. The stomach size is reduced and hence calorie intake is reduced. In addition, the food stream bypasses three-quarters of the small intestine. The bile and pancreatic enzymes necessary for the breakdown and absorption of protein and fat only mix with the food stream in the last portion of the small intestine. Gut hormonal changes are similar to those after RYGB.

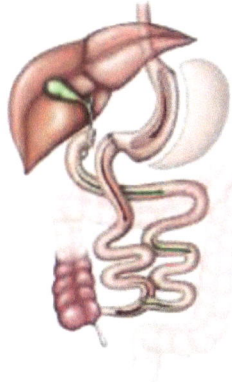

Fig. (18). Schematic diagram depicting the bilio-pancreatic bypass with duodenal switch procedure.

The key steps to the operation include mobilization of the greater curve of the stomach using an energy device, creation of a long, thin gastric pouch over a bougie as in a sleeve gastrectomy and small intestinal bypass. The procedure is partly restrictive and partly malabsorptive.

After creation of the gastric pouch, the duodenum is carefully dissected avoiding bleeding and preserving the gastroepiploic vessels. The duodenum is then transected using a linear stapler. For the diversion, measurements are taken from the caecum (rather than DJ flexure) with 100 cm (common channel) marked and the ileum divided at 250 cm. The entero-enterostomy is performed at the 100 cm mark in the same manner as in RYGB. The proximal end of ileum is passed antecolic and anastomosed with proximal duodenum using either sutures or staples (Fig. **18**). The omentum may need to be divided to foreshorten the route. All hernia defects are closed and a blue methylene blue dye leak test is performed at the end of the procedure.

The BPD/DS results in greater loss of excess weight (60 – 70%) than RYGB, LSG, or LAGB at 5 year follow up and this procedure is the most effective in obviating diabetes [20]. The procedure allows patients to eventually eat near normal meals. Fat absorption is reduced by 70%. The disadvantages of BPD/DS are greater operative risks than other surgical techniques with a higher morbidity and mortality. The procedure is more complex and consists of different parts and the operating time is considerably longer. The risks of bleeding, anastomotic leak, bowel injury, internal hernia and DVT/PE are all higher. Due to the significant malabsorptive component the procedure, there is a greater potential to cause protein deficiencies and long-term deficiencies in a number of vitamin and minerals, *e.g.* iron, calcium, zinc and fat-soluble vitamins such as vitamin A and D. Patients who have had a BPD/DS must comply with long-term follow-up visits and strict adherence to dietary and vitamin supplementation to avoid serious complications from protein and certain vitamin deficiencies.

Novel Procedures

A number of novel procedures have been described which result in weight loss. They remain experimental at this stage. These include gastric plication where instead of excising the greater curvature of the stomach (as in a sleeve gastrectomy) it is plicated using sutures so that it cannot function anatomically [21]. Gastric pacing has also been used in an attempt to reduce hunger. More recently, embolisation of the fundus region of the stomach using conventional radiological techniques usually used for bleeding in order to reduce ghrelin secretion has been attempted [22].

Re-do bariatric surgery

Re-do bariatric surgery is indicated to deal with complications of the primary operation, incorrect primary surgery and regain of weight. All patients should have a similar primary work up including history, examination, dietetic assessment, upper GI endoscopy, barium swallow /meal and follow through and often a CT scan. Patients should then be discussed at the MDT. The options are variable and depend on the primary surgery, the presentation, patient commitment, comorbidities and funding arrangements.

For acute presentations, treatment to deal with complications such as eroded or slipped bands are urgent before the onset of malnutrition (Fig. **19**). Similarly, fistulae or non-healing marginal ulcers should be dealt with along with intolerable acid or bile reflux after a sleeve. Marginal ulcers can be difficult to heal but are more prevalent in smokers, when permanent suture material has been used along with gastric irritants. If they remain persistent despite reversal of aggravating factors and prolonged antacid treatment, then resection and redo of the anastomosis may be necessary.

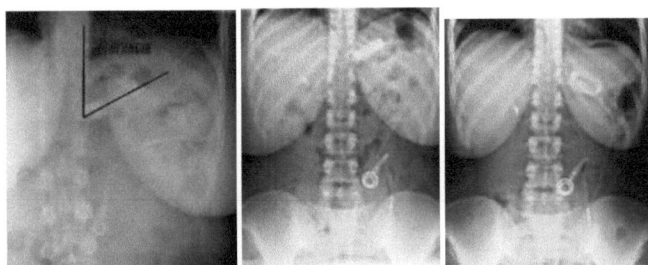

Fig. (19). (*left*) Gastric band in normal position with no lumen visible (O sign) and a phi angle (4-58 degrees from vertical spinal column). (*middle*) Normal position of gastric band. (*right*) Slipped gastric band.

In patients with inadequate weight loss or indeed regain after primary surgery, the situation is more complex and the decision for revision surgery should be made after thoroughly balancing the risks and benefits. All patients will expect some weight regain after 18 months. It is important to reassess dietary intake and give patients appropriate advice. The majority of patients who have had a functioning procedure and regained weight would benefit from dietetic and psychological input. It is equally important to ensure the absence of technical complications, which contribute to weight regain. If revision surgery is contemplated, referral to a specialist centre may be appropriate as "re-sleeving", adjustment of limb lengths and banded bypasses are possible options. Experts in high volume centres best do these procedures since the potential for untoward complications in redo surgery is immense.

CONSENT FOR PUBLICATION

Not applicable.

ACKNOWLEDGEMENT

Declare none.

CONFLICT OF INTEREST

The author declares no conflict of interest, financial or otherwise.

REFERENCES

[1]   Barth JH. How should we deliver obesity services? British Journal of Obesity 2015; 1: 123-67.

[2]   Lim EL, Hollingsworth KG, Aribisala BS, Chen MJ, Mathers JC, Taylor R. Reversal of type 2 diabetes: normalisation of beta cell function in association with decreased pancreas and liver triacylglycerol. Diabetologia 2011; 54(10): 2506-14.
[http://dx.doi.org/10.1007/s00125-011-2204-7] [PMID: 21656330]

[3]   Buchwald H. Introduction and current status of bariatric procedures. Surg Obes Relat Dis 2008; 4(3) (Suppl.): S1-6.
[http://dx.doi.org/10.1016/j.soard.2008.04.001] [PMID: 18501310]

[4]   Mingrone G, Panunzi S, De Gaetano A, *et al.* Bariatric surgery versus conventional medical therapy for type 2 diabetes. N Engl J Med 2012; 366(17): 1577-85.
[http://dx.doi.org/10.1056/NEJMoa1200111] [PMID: 22449317]

[5]   Beard JH, Bell RL, Duffy AJ. Reproductive considerations and pregnancy after bariatric surgery: current evidence and recommendations. Obes Surg 2008; 18(8): 1023-7.
[http://dx.doi.org/10.1007/s11695-007-9389-3] [PMID: 18392904]

[6]   Mahawar KK, Parmar C, Carr WR, *et al.* Preoperative interventions for patients being considered for bariatric surgery: separating the fact from fiction. Obes Surg 2015; 25(8): 1527-33.
[http://dx.doi.org/10.1007/s11695-015-1738-z] [PMID: 25994780]

[7]   Nightingale CE, Margarson MP, Shearer E, *et al.* Members of the Working Party; Association of Anaesthetists of Great Britain; Ireland Society for Obesity and Bariatric Anaesthesia. Peri-operative management of the obese surgical patient 2015: Association of Anaesthetists of Great Britain and

Ireland Society for Obesity and Bariatric Anaesthesia. Anaesthesia 2015; 70(7): 859-76.
[http://dx.doi.org/10.1111/anae.13101] [PMID: 25950621]

[8]   Xanthakos S A. Nutritional deficiencies in obesity and after bariatric surgery 2009.
[http://dx.doi.org/10.1016/j.pcl.2009.07.002]

[9]   Peterhänsel C, Petroff D, Klinitzke G, Kersting A, Wagner B. Risk of completed suicide after bariatric surgery: a systematic review. Obes Rev 2013; 14(5): 369-82.
[http://dx.doi.org/10.1111/obr.12014] [PMID: 23297762]

[10]   Wise J. Suicide screening should be given to patients who have bariatric surgery, study recommends. BMJ 2015; 351: h5367.
[http://dx.doi.org/10.1136/bmj.h5367] [PMID: 26450999]

[11]   Nguyen NT, Silver M, Robinson M, *et al.* Result of a national audit of bariatric surgery performed at academic centers: a 2004 University HealthSystem Consortium Benchmarking Project. Arch Surg 2006; 141(5): 445-9.
[http://dx.doi.org/10.1001/archsurg.141.5.445] [PMID: 16702515]

[12]   Wise J. Weight loss is sustained over four years after bariatric surgery, study finds. BMJ 2015; 351: h6917.
[http://dx.doi.org/10.1136/bmj.h6917] [PMID: 26705346]

[13]   Sjöström L, Lindroos AK, Peltonen M, *et al.* Swedish Obese Subjects Study Scientific Group. Lifestyle, diabetes, and cardiovascular risk factors 10 years after bariatric surgery. N Engl J Med 2004; 351(26): 2683-93.
[http://dx.doi.org/10.1056/NEJMoa035622] [PMID: 15616203]

[14]   Wise J. Bariatric surgery is linked to more diabetes remission than lifestyle intervention alone, study finds. BMJ 2015; 351: h3603.
[http://dx.doi.org/10.1136/bmj.h3603] [PMID: 26138811]

[15]   Sjöström L, Narbro K, Sjöström CD, *et al.* Swedish Obese Subjects Study. Effects of bariatric surgery on mortality in Swedish obese subjects. N Engl J Med 2007; 357(8): 741-52.
[http://dx.doi.org/10.1056/NEJMoa066254] [PMID: 17715408]

[16]   Patel SR, Mason J, Hakim N. The duodenal-jejunal bypass sleeve (endobarrier gastrointestinal liner) for weight loss and treatment of type II diabetes. Indian J Surg 2012; 74(4): 275-7.
[http://dx.doi.org/10.1007/s12262-012-0721-3] [PMID: 23904712]

[17]   O'Brien PE, Dixon JB, Laurie C, *et al.* Treatment of mild to moderate obesity with laparoscopic adjustable gastric banding or an intensive medical program: a randomized trial. Ann Intern Med 2006; 144(9): 625-33.

[18]   Rosenthal RJ, Diaz AA, Arvidsson D, *et al.* International Sleeve Gastrectomy Expert Panel. International Sleeve Gastrectomy Expert Panel Consensus Statement: best practice guidelines based on experience of >12,000 cases. Surg Obes Relat Dis 2012; 8(1): 8-19.
[http://dx.doi.org/10.1016/j.soard.2011.10.019] [PMID: 22248433]

[19]   Abdeen G, le Roux CW. Mechanism underlying the weight loss and complications of roux-en-y gastric bypass. review. Obes Surg 2016; 26(2): 410-21.
[http://dx.doi.org/10.1007/s11695-015-1945-7] [PMID: 26530712]

[20]   Dumon K R, Murayama K M. Bariatric surgery outcomes. Clin North Am 2011; 91: 1313-38.

[21]   Brethauer SA, Harris JL, Kroh M, Schauer PR. Laparoscopic gastric plication for treatment of severe obesity. Surg Obes Relat Dis 2011; 7(1): 15-22.
[http://dx.doi.org/10.1016/j.soard.2010.09.023] [PMID: 21144804]

[22]   Weiss CR, Gunn AJ, Kim CY, Paxton BE, Kraitchman DL, Arepally A. Bariatric embolization of the gastric arteries for the treatment of obesity. J Vasc Interv Radiol 2015; 26(5): 613-24.
[http://dx.doi.org/10.1016/j.jvir.2015.01.017] [PMID: 25777177]

SUBJECT INDEX

A

Abdominal aorta 166
Abdominal obesity 286
Abdominal pain 11, 13, 20, 57, 83, 85, 181, 254
Abdominal surgery 50, 277, 279
Abdominal wall, anterior 54, 155, 156
Ablative techniques 225
Acid secretion 17, 19, 23, 24
Acute gastric dilation (AGD) 49, 50, 51
Acute gastritis 5, 8, 12
Adenocarcinomas 9, 93, 94, 95, 98, 99, 100, 106, 107, 108, 109, 114, 115, 131, 133, 140, 142, 152, 153, 164, 186, 187, 195, 196, 197, 198, 199, 201, 202, 203, 205, 216, 220, 224
  gastric 9, 140, 142, 164, 186, 187, 197, 199, 201, 205
  junctional 201, 202, 205
  true 108, 152
Adjuvant chemotherapy (AC) 98, 99, 110, 149, 195, 196, 197, 199, 200, 201
Adjuvant therapy 183, 192, 195, 200
Admission risk marker 41, 42
Advanced disease 68, 69, 93, 102, 131, 132, 134, 174, 180, 202, 244
Advanced gastric cancer (AGC) 145, 146, 147, 149, 154, 163, 169, 174, 175, 180, 204
Advanced lesions 113, 114
Advanced oesophageal 201, 202, 204
AJCC staging manual 108, 109, 152, 153
American joint committee on cancer (AJCC) 105, 106, 107, 152, 164, 167
Amoxicillin 22, 23, 24
Anaemia 3, 12, 13, 45, 69, 95, 142, 145, 146, 181, 186, 302
  iron deficiency 45, 145, 146
Anaesthesia, general 34, 73, 74, 77, 245, 276, 306, 307, 311

Anaesthetic agents 264, 267, 268, 275, 276
Anaesthetic drugs 266, 268, 269
Anaesthetists 26, 109, 128, 262, 263, 269, 270, 275, 289, 297, 298, 300
Analgesia 180, 223, 260, 266, 276, 278
Anastomosis 15, 35, 38, 39, 51, 115, 116, 117, 118, 119, 121, 126, 127, 172, 173, 185, 186, 219, 244, 263, 280, 316
  oesophago-gastric 119, 185, 186
Ankaferd blood stopper (ABS) 234, 235
Anticipated complications 15, 27, 29, 39, 172, 178, 179
Anti-obesity surgery 263, 293, 294, 297, 301
Anti-reflux valves 211, 243, 248, 251, 252
Aperistalsis 64, 69, 70, 71
Apnoea 265, 267, 274, 277, 298
Approach, retrocolic 14, 177, 310, 311
Argon plasma coagulation (APC) 175, 219, 220, 221, 225, 230, 237, 238
Atrophic gastritis 1, 6, 7, 8, 12, 44, 144, 186
  chronic 8, 12, 186
Autoimmune gastritis 5, 9, 10, 186
Azygos vein 116, 118, 119, 120, 128, 129

B

Balloon 33, 73, 179, 221, 222, 224, 245, 301, 303, 304, 305
  intra-gastric 303, 304
Balloon catheter 222, 223
Band ligation 233, 237, 240
Bariatric surgeons 283, 299
Bariatric surgery 260, 263, 264, 274, 277, 281, 283, 284, 293, 295, 296, 300, 301, 302
Barrett's oesophagus 93, 94, 96, 146, 220
Benign gastric tumours 140
Benign tumours 30, 93, 96, 141
Bilio-pancreatic diversion (BPD) 294, 302, 303, 309
Biodegradable oesophageal stents 256
Biodegradable stents 248, 256